POCKET MEDICINE

Second Edition

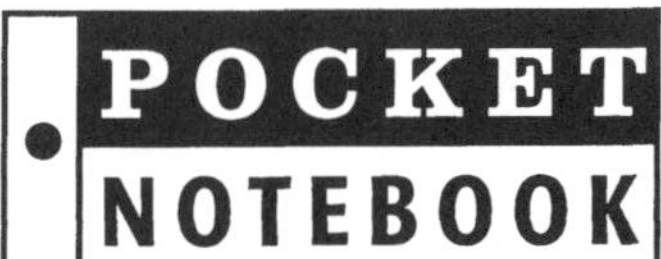

POCKET MEDICINE

Second Edition

Edited by

Marc S. Sabatine, M.D., M.P.H.

The Massachusetts General Hospital Handbook of Internal Medicine

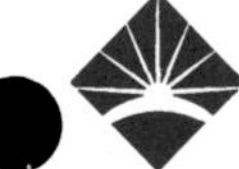

LIPPINCOTT WILLIAMS & WILKINS
A **Wolters Kluwer** Company
Philadelphia • Baltimore • New York • London
Buenos Aires • Hong Kong • Sydney • Tokyo

Acquisitions Editor: Danette Somers
Developmental Editor: Erin McMullan
Production Editor: Jeff Somers
Manufacturing Manager: Ben Rivera
Printer: Victor Graphics

530 Walnut Street
Philadelphia, PA 19106-3780 USA
LWW.com

Printed in the USA

Library of Congress Cataloging-in-Publication Data
ISBN: 0-7817-4447-4
ISBN: 978-0-7817-4447-8

Care has been taken to confirm the accuracy of the information presented and to describe generally accepted practices. However, the author and publisher are not responsible for errors or omissions or for any consequences from application of the information in this book and make no warranty, expressed or implied, with respect to the currency, completeness, or accuracy of the contents of the publication. Application of this information in a particular situation remains the professional responsibility of the practitioner.

The author and publisher have exerted every effort to ensure that drug selection and dosage set forth in this text are in accordance with current recommendations and practice at the time of publication. However, in view of ongoing research, changes in government regulations, and the constant flow of information relating to drug therapy and drug reactions, the reader is urged to check the package insert for each drug for any change in indications and dosage and for added warnings and precautions. This is particularly important when the recommended agent is a new or infrequently employed drug.

Some drugs and medical devices presented in this publication have Food and Drug Administration (FDA) clearance for limited use in restricted research settings. It is the responsibility of the health care provider to ascertain the FDA status of each drug or device planned for use in their clinical practice.

10 9 8 7 6

Contents

Contributing Authors

Karen V. Atkinson, MD
Chief of Rheumatology, Atlanta Veterans Affairs Medical Center
Assistant Professor of Medicine, Emory University

Ednan K. Bajwa, MD
Internal Medicine Resident, Massachusetts General Hospital

Ishir Bhan, MD
Internal Medicine Resident, Massachusetts General Hospital

F. Richard Bringhurst, MD
Physician, Endocrine Unit and Senior Vice President for Medical Services, Massachusetts General Hospital
Associate Professor of Medicine, Harvard Medical School

Annabel A. Chen, MD
Internal Medicine Resident, Massachusetts General Hospital

Salvatore A. Cilmi, MD
Infectious Diseases Fellow, Massachusetts General Hospital

Karen H. Costenbader, MD
Assistant Physician, Division of Rheumatology, Allergy and Immunology, Massachusetts General Hospital
Instructor in Medicine, Harvard Medical School

Benjamin T. Davis, MD
Infectious Diseases Unit, Massachusetts General Hospital
Instructor in Medicine, Harvard Medical School

Daniel J. DeAngelo, MD, PhD
Attending Physician, Department of Medical Oncology
Dana-Farber Cancer Institute & Brigham and Women's Hospital
Instructor in Medicine, Harvard Medical School

David G. Forcione, MD
Gastroenterology Fellow, Massachusetts General Hospital

Lawrence S. Friedman, MD
Chair, Department of Medicine, Newton-Wellesley Hospital
Assistant Chief of Medicine, Massachusetts General Hospital
Professor of Medicine, Harvard Medical School

Levi A. Garraway, MD, PhD
Hematology-Oncology Fellow, Dana-Farber/Partners Oncology Program

David M. Greer, MD
Director, Neurology Evaluation Center, Massachusetts General Hospital
Instructor in Medicine, Harvard Medical School

Alyssa K. Johnsen, MD, PhD
Internal Medicine Resident, Massachusetts General Hospital

Anne G. Kasmar, MD
Internal Medicine Resident, Massachusetts General Hospital

Sekar Kathiresan, MD
Cardiology Fellow, Massachusetts General Hospital

Atul Malhotra, MD
Assistant Physician, Pulmonary and Critical Care Unit,
Massachusetts General Hospital and Brigham and Women's Hospital
Assistant Professor of Medicine, Harvard Medical School

Majd Mouded, MD
Pulmonary and Critical Care Fellow, Massachusetts General Hospital

Juan C. Pallais, MD, MPH
Endocrinology Fellow, Massachusetts General Hospital

Sahil A. Parikh, MD
Internal Medicine Resident, Massachusetts General Hospital

Ina P. Rhee, MD, PhD
Internal Medicine Resident, Massachusetts General Hospital

Andrew S. Ross, MD
Internal Medicine Resident, Massachusetts General Hospital

Marc S. Sabatine, MD, MPH
Associate Physician, Cardiovascular Division, Brigham and Women's Hospital
Affiliate Physician, Cardiology Division, Massachusetts General Hospital
Instructor in Medicine, Harvard Medical School

Michael V. Seiden, MD, PhD
Associate Physician, Hematology-Oncology Unit,
Massachusetts General Hospital
Assistant Professor of Medicine, Harvard Medical School

Karen V. Smirnakis, MD, PhD
Renal Fellow, Massachusetts General Hospital

David M. Systrom, MD
Associate Physician, Pulmonary and Critical Care Unit,
Massachusetts General Hospital
Program Director, Training Program in Pulmonary & Critical Care Medicine
Assistant Professor of Medicine, Harvard Medical School

Deborah J. Wexler, MD, MSc
Internal Medicine Resident, Massachusetts General Hospital

Myles S. Wolf, MD, MMSc
Assistant Physician, Renal Unit, Massachusetts General Hospital
Instructor in Medicine, Harvard Medical School

Foreword to the 1st edition

It is with the greatest enthusiasm that I introduce *Pocket Medicine*. In an era of information glut, it will logically be asked, "Why another manual for medical house officers?" Yet, despite enormous information readily available in any number of textbooks, or at the push of a key on a computer, it is often that the harried house officer is less helped by the description of differential diagnosis and therapies than one would wish.

Pocket Medicine is the joint venture between house staff and faculty expert in a number of medical specialties. This collaboration is designed to provide a rapid but thoughtful initial approach to medical problems seen by house officers with great frequency. Questions that frequently come from faculty to the house staff on rounds, many hours after the initial interaction between patient and doctor, have been anticipated and important pathways for arriving at diagnoses and initiating therapies are presented. This approach will facilitate the evidence-based medicine discussion that will follow the work-up of the patient. This well-conceived handbook should enhance the ability of every medical house officer to properly evaluate a patient in a timely fashion and to be stimulated to think of the evidence supporting the diagnosis and the likely outcome of therapeutic intervention. *Pocket Medicine* will prove to be a worthy addition to medical education and to the care of our patients.

Dennis A. Ausiello, MD
Physician-in-Chief, Massachusetts General Hospital
Jackson Professor of Clinical Medicine, Harvard Medical School

Preface

Written by residents, fellows, and attendings, the mandate for *Pocket Medicine* was to provide, in a concise a manner as possible, the information a house officer needs to know to approach and manage the most common inpatient medical problems.

The tremendous response to the first edition suggests we were able to help fill an important need for clinicians. With this second edition come several major improvements, including a thorough updating of every topic, incorporation of references to the most recent reviews and important studies published through the start of 2004, the addition of a Neurology section, and the use of a larger and cleaner typeface. We welcome any suggestions for further improvement.

Obviously, medicine is far too vast a field to ever summarize in a textbook of any size. Whole textbooks have been devoted to many of the topics discussed herein. *Pocket Medicine* is meant only as a starting point to guide one during the initial phases of diagnosis and management until one has time to consult more definitive resources. Although the recommendations herein are as evidence-based as possible, medicine is both a science and an art. As always, sound clinical judgment must be applied to every scenario.

I am grateful for the support of the house officers, fellows, and attendings at the Massachusetts General Hospital, who simultaneously served as friends, colleagues, and teachers. In particular, my time there as Chief Resident was the best job I have ever had. It was a privilege to work with such a knowledgeable, dedicated, and compassionate group of physicians. I am grateful to several outstanding mentors, including Hasan Bazari, Denny Ausiello, Larry Friedman, Lloyd Axelrod, Nesli Basgoz, Mort Swartz, Eric Isselbacher, Bill Dec, Mike Fifer, Peter Yurchak, and Roman DeSanctis. Special thanks to my parents for their perpetual encouragement and love and, of course, to my wife, Jennifer Tseng, who, despite being a surgeon, is my closest advisor, my best friend, and the love of my life.

I hope that you find *Pocket Medicine* useful throughout the arduous but incredibly rewarding journey of medical residency.

Marc S. Sabatine, MD, MPH

• ELECTROCARDIOGRAPHY •

Approach *(a systematic approach is vital)*
- **Rate** and **rhythm**
- **Intervals** (? BBB) and **axis** (? LAD or RAD)
- **Chamber enlargement** (? LAE and/or RAE, ? LVH and/or RVH)
- **QRST changes** (? Q waves, poor R wave progression, ST Δ, or T wave inversions)

	Left Axis Deviation (LAD)	Right Axis Deviation (RAD)
Definition	axis > -30°	axis > +90°
Determination	S > R in lead II	S > R in lead I
Etiologies	left anterior hemiblock LBBB LVH inferior MI elevated diaphragm	RVH left posterior hemiblock (LPHB) lateral MI COPD (usually not > +110°)

Hemiblocks (axis deviation w/o another cause and with QRS <120 msec)	
Left anterior hemiblock (LAHB)	**Left posterior hemiblock (LPHB)**
LAD (often > -60°) + qR in I & rS in III	RAD (often > +110°) + rS in I & qR in III

Left Bundle Branch Block (LBBB)	Right Bundle Branch Block (RBBB)
1. QRS ≥120 msec 2. Broad, slurred, monophasic R wave in I, V_5, & V_6 (± S wave if cardiomegaly) 3. Absence of Q in I, V_5, and V_6 4. Displacement of ST and T wave opposite to major deflection of QRS 5. ± PRWP, LAD, Q's in inferior leads	1. QRS ≥120 msec 2. rsR' pattern in right precordial leads 3. Wide S wave in I, V_5, and V_6

Prolonged QT interval (*JAMA* 2003;289:2120; *NEJM* 2004;350:1013)
- QT measured from beginning of QRS complex to end of T wave
- No consensus on what is absolutely prolonged, but generally, normal QT <500 msec
- QT varies with HR, correct with Bazett formula: $QTc = \frac{QT}{\sqrt{RR}}$ (normal QTc ≤440 msec)
- Etiologies
  - CAD, cardiomyopathy
  - Severe bradycardia or high-grade AV block
  - **Anti-arrhythmics**: class IA, class IC, and class III
  - **Psychotropic drugs**: phenothiazines, tricyclic antidepressants
  - **Other drugs**: nonsedating antihistamines, macrolides, antifungal azoles
  - **Electrolyte disturbances**: hypocalcemia, ? hypokalemia, ? hypomagnesemia
  - Autonomic nervous system dysfunction: intracranial bleed (usually with deep TWI), stroke, radical neck dissection, carotid endarterectomy
  - Miscellaneous: hypothyroidism, hypothermia
  - Congenital (Long QT Syndrome, LQTS): K and Na channelopathies; often w/ abnl Tw; depending on subtype, can be triggered by exercise, auditory stimuli, stress

	Left Atrial Enlargement (LAE)	Right Atrial Enlargement (RAE)
ECG P wave Criteria	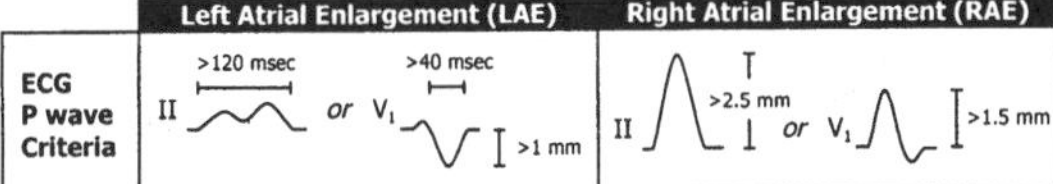	

Left ventricular hypertrophy (LVH)
- Etiologies: HTN, AS/AI, HCMP, coarctation of aorta
- Criteria
  - Romhilt-Estes point-score system (see below): 4 points = probable, 5 points = definite
  - Sokolow-Lyon: S in V_1 + R in V_5 or V_6 ≥35 mm
  - Cornell: R in aVL + S in V_3 >24 mm in men or >20 mm in women
  - Other: R in aVL ≥11 mm (or, if LAD, ≥13 mm *and* S in III ≥15 mm)

Romhilt-Estes LVH Point-Score System	
Criterion	**Points**
Amplitude (any of the following): largest R or S in limb leads ≥20 mm *or* S in V_1 or V_2 ≥30 mm *or* R in V_5 or V_6 ≥30 mm	3
ST-T Δs (displacement opposite to major deflection of QRS complex)	
without digoxin	3
with digoxin	1
Left atrial enlargement	3
Left axis deviation (≥ -30°)	2
QRS duration ≥90 msec	1
Intrinsicoid deflection in V_5 or V_6 ≥50 msec	1

Right ventricular hypertrophy (RVH)
- Etiologies: cor pulmonale, congenital (tetralogy, TGA, PS, ASD, VSD), MS, TR
- Criteria (all tend to be insensitive, but highly specific, except in COPD)
  - R/S ratio in V_1 >1 or R in V_1 ≥7 mm
  - drop in R/S ratio across precordium
  - RAD ≥ +110°

COPD
- P waves: vertical axis (≥ +80°) → ⊖ P wave in V_1, V_2, aVL and isoelectric in I; RAE
- RVH (if cor pulmonale) → S wave in V_6, R/S ratio in V_6 <1, and $S_1S_2S_3$ pattern
- Downward displacement of the heart: low voltage in precordial leads only; PRWP

Low Voltage
- Amplitude of QRS voltage (R+S) <5 mm in all limb leads & <10 mm in all precordial leads
- Etiologies: COPD (precordial leads only), pericardial effusion, myxedema, obesity, pleural effusion, restrictive or infiltrative cardiomyopathy, diffuse CAD

Pathologic Q waves
- Definition: ≥40 msec or >25% height of the R wave in that complex
- Small (septal) q waves in I, aVL, V_5 & V_6 are normal as can be isolated Qw in III, aVR, V_1

Poor R wave progression (PRWP) (*Archives* 1982;142:1145)
- Definition: loss of anterior forces without frank Q waves; R wave in V_3 ≤3 mm
- Etiologies
  - old anteroseptal MI (usually R wave in V_3 ≤1.5 mm, ± persistent ST ↑ or TWI in V_2 & V_3)
  - cardiomyopathy
  - LVH (delayed RWP with prominent left precordial voltage)
  - RVH/COPD (small R wave and prominent S wave in lead I)
  - LBBB
  - clockwise rotation of the heart
  - lead misplacement

ST elevation (STE, *NEJM* 2003;349:2128)
- **Acute MI** (upward convexity ± TWI) or prior MI with persistent STE
- **Coronary spasm** (Prinzmetal's angina)
- **Pericarditis** (diffuse, upward concavity STE; associated with PR ↓; Tw usually upright while ST segments elevated); myocarditis; cardiac contusion
- **Normal early repolarization**: most often seen in leads V_2-V_5 and in young adults
  J point ↑ 1-4 mm; notch in downstroke of R wave; upward concavity of ST; large Tw; ratio of ST elevation / T wave amplitude <25%; pattern may disappear with exercise
- Repolarization abnormality in association with LBBB or LVH (usually only in leads V_1-V_2)

ST depression
- **Myocardial ischemia** (± T wave abnormalities)
- Digitalis *effect* (*not* a sign of *intoxication*; in fact, poorly correlated with dig levels)
- Hypokalemia (± U wave)
- Repolarization abnormality in association with LBBB or LVH (usually in leads V_5, V_6, I, aVL)

T wave inversion (TWI)
- Myocardial ischemia or infarct; pericarditis; cardiomyopathy
- Repolarization abnormality in association with LBBB or LVH
- Post-tachycardia or post-pacing
- Electrolyte, P_aO_2, P_aCO_2, pH, or core temperature disturbances
- Intracranial bleed (usually with ↑ QT)
- Normal variant in leads in which QRS complex predominantly ⊖

• CHEST PAIN •

Cardiac Causes		
Disorder	**Typical characteristics**	**Other S/S; Dx studies**
Angina	substernal pressure → neck, jaw, arm duration <30 min ± dyspnea, diaphoresis, N/V aggravated by exertion relief by nitroglycerin or rest however, relief by nitroglycerin in ED not reliable indicator of angina (*Annals* 2003;139:979)	ECG Δs (ST ↓/↑, and/or TWI)
MI	same as angina but ↑ intensity duration >30 min	ECG Δs (ST ↑/↓, and/or TWI) ⊕ troponin or CK-MB
Pericarditis	sharp pain radiating to trapezius aggravated by respiration relieved by sitting forward	± pericardial friction rub ECG Δs (diffuse concave ST ↑) ± pericardial effusion
Aortic dissection	sudden onset tearing, knife-like pain anterior or posterior mid-scapular	asymmetric BP/pulses; new AI widened mediastinum on CXR false lumen on imaging

Pulmonary Causes		
Disorder	**Typical characteristics**	**Diagnostic studies**
Pneumonia	pleuritic dyspnea, fever, cough, sputum	fever, tachypnea, crackles infiltrate on CXR
Pleuritis	sharp, pleuritic	± pleural friction rub
Pneumothorax	unilateral, sharp, pleuritic sudden onset	unilateral hyperresonance, ↓ BS, PTX on CXR
PE	pleuritic sudden onset	tachypnea, tachycardia, hypoxemia ⊕ V/Q scan or angiogram
Pulmonary HTN	dyspnea, exertional pressure	hypoxemia, loud P_2, right-sided S_3 & S_4

GI Causes		
Disorder	**Typical characteristics**	**Diagnostic studies**
Esophageal reflux	substernal burning acid taste in mouth; water brash aggravated by meals, recumbency relieved by antacids	esophageal pH probe Bernstein acid perfusion test EGD
Esophageal spasm	intense substernal pain aggravated by swallowing relieved by nitroglycerin or CCB	upper GI series manometry
Mallory-Weiss tear	precipitated by vomiting	EGD
Peptic ulcer disease	epigastric pain relieved by antacids ± hematemesis, melena	EGD ± *H. pylori* test
Biliary disease	RUQ pain, nausea/vomiting aggravated by fatty foods	RUQ U/S LFTs
Pancreatitis	epigastric/back discomfort	↑ amylase and lipase, abdominal CT

Musculoskeletal and Miscellaneous Causes		
Disorder	**Typical characteristics**	**Diagnostic studies**
Costochondritis	localized sharp or dull pain	tenderness to palpation
Cervical spine disease/OA	precipitated by motion, lasts sec to hrs	X-rays
Herpes zoster	intense unilateral pain	dermatomal rash & sensory findings
Anxiety	"tightness"	

• NON-INVASIVE EVALUATION OF CAD •

Pretest Likelihood of CAD						
Sx	Nonanginal ≤ 1 of 3 sx		Atypical = 2 of 3 sx		Typical = 3 of 3 sx	
Age	**Men**	**Women**	**Men**	**Women**	**Men**	**Women**
30-39	5%	1%	22%	4%	70%	26%
40-49	14%	3%	46%	13%	87%	55%
50-59	22%	8%	59%	32%	92%	80%
60-69	28%	19%	67%	54%	94%	91%

sx: (1) substernal chest pain, (2) provoked by exertion, (3) relieved by rest or NTG (*NEJM* 1979;300:1350)

Exercise tolerance test ("Stress test")

- **Indications**: dx CAD, evaluate Pts w/ known CAD & Δ in clinical status, risk stratify Pts s/p ACS, localize ischemia (radionuclide imaging required)
- **Contraindications**:
  - **Absolute**: AMI w/in 48 hrs, high risk UA, acute PE, severe AS, uncontrolled CHF, uncontrolled arrhythmias, myopericarditis, acute aortic dissection
  - **Relative**: left main coronary stenosis, moderate valvular stenosis, severe hypertension, HCMP, high-degree AVB, severe electrolyte abnormalities, inability to exercise
- **Exercise options**: standard or modified Bruce protocol, submaximal, or sx-limited
- **Pharmacologic options** (Pts unable to exercise)
  - coronary vasodilators (will reveal coronary stenoses, but will *not* tell you if Pt *ischemic*): dipyridamole or adenosine (may precipitate bradycardia and bronchospasm)
  - chronotropes/inotropes (~physiologic): dobutamine (may precipitate tachyarrhythmias)
- **Imaging options** (Pts with uninterpretable ECG, pharm tests, or localization of ischemia)
  - uninterpretable ECG: paced, LBBB, resting ST↓ >1mm, dig., LVH (=sens., ↓ spec.), WPW
  - **radionuclides** (thallium-201 or ^{99m}Tc-sestaMIBI) or **echocardiography**

Test	Sens.	Spec.	Comments
ETT	~60	~80	Sens. ~90% for 3VD, but <50% for 1VD
ETT-Thal or MIBI	80-90	70-90	↑ sens./spec. but ↑ cost; localize ischemia
Adenosine/dobuta MIBI	80-90	70-90	Side effects of agents as above
Exercise/dobuta ECHO	80-90	~80	Localize ischemia, assess EF; operator-dep.

(*JACC* 2002;40:1531, *Circ* 2002;106:1883, *Am Heart J* 1995;130:373, *JAMA* 1998;280:913)

Test results

- **HR** (must achieve ≥85% of maximal predicted HR for *exercise* test to be diagnostic), **BP** response, and peak **double product** (HR x BP)
- **Max exercise capacity** achieved (METS or mins)
- Occurrence of **symptoms** (at what level of exertion and similarity to presenting sx)
- **ECG changes**: *downsloping* or *horizontal* ST ↓ predictive of CAD; ST ↑ highly predictive
- **Imaging**: radionuclide defects or echocardiographic wall motion abnormalities (reversible = ischemia; fixed = infarct)

Duke Treadmill Score and Prognosis						
= exercise time (min) – (5 × max ST deviation in any lead) – (4 × angina index) where angina index is 0 if none; 1 if non-limiting; 2 if angina was reason for stopping						
		Inpatients			**Outpatients**	
Category	**Score**	**% of**	**1-yr CV mort.**	**4-yr surv.**	**% of**	**4-yr surv.**
Low	≥ 5	34%	< 1%	98%	62%	99%
Mod	-10 to +4	57%	2-3%	92%	34%	95%
High	≤ -11	9%	≥ 5%	71%	4%	79%

(*Annals* 1987;106:793 and *NEJM* 1991;325:849)

High-risk test results (PPV ~50% for LM or 3VD, ∴ consider coronary angiography)

- ECG: ST ↓ ≥2 mm *or* ≥1 mm in stage 1 *or* in ≥5 leads *or* ≥5 min in recovery; ST ↑; VT
- Physiologic: ↓ BP, exercise capacity <6 METS, angina pectoris during exercise
- Radionuclide: ischemia in multiple territories, reversible cavity dilation, ↑ lung uptake
- High risk treadmill score (see above)

Myocardial viability

- Goal: ID stunned or hibernating myocardium that could regain fxn after revascularization
- Options: **rest-redistribution thallium** (~90% sens., ~55% spec.), **dobutamine stress echo** (~70% sens., ~85% spec.); **PET** (~90% sens., ~70% spec.), **MRI** (inversely proportional to degree of hyperenhancement; *NEJM* 2000;343:1445)

• ACUTE CORONARY SYNDROMES •

Definition

- Any constellation of clinical symptoms compatible with acute myocardial ischemia thought secondary to acute plaque rupture and coronary artery thrombosis
- Includes: **unstable angina** (UA), **non-ST-elevation MI** (NSTEMI), and **ST-elevation MI** (STEMI)

Etiologies

- **Atherosclerosis → plaque rupture → coronary artery thrombosis**
- Other causes of myocardial ischemia/infarction
  coronary artery spasm: Prinzmetal's variant, cocaine-induced
  embolism to coronary artery: endocarditis, prosthetic valve, mural thrombus, myxoma
  aortic dissection extending into coronary artery (usually RCA → IMI)
  vasculitis: Kawasaki's syndrome, Takayasu's disease, polyarteritis nodosa, Churg-Strauss
  myocarditis (myocardial necrosis, although not caused by CAD)

Clinical manifestations

- **Angina**: typically retrosternal pressure/pain/tightness ± radiation to neck, jaw, or arms; precip. by exertion, relieved by rest or NTG; in ACS, new-onset, crescendo, or at rest
- Associated symptoms: dyspnea, diaphoresis, N/V, palpitations, or lightheadedness
- ~23% of MIs are initially unrecognized b/c silent or atypical sx (*AJC* 1973;32:1)

Physical exam

- Signs of ischemia: S_4, new MR murmur 2° papillary muscle dysfunction, paradoxical S_2
- Signs of heart failure: ↑ JVP, crackles in lung fields, ⊕ S_3
- Signs of other areas of atherosclerotic disease: carotid or femoral bruits, ↓ distal pulses

Diagnostic studies

- **ECG**: ST deviation and/or TWI; ✓ at presentation, with any Δ in symptoms, and at 24 hrs (always compare to baseline ECG if available)
- **Cardiac biomarkers**: serial testing at presentation, 8 hrs, and 16 hrs
  troponin (I or T): most sens. & spec. biomarker; rise & fall in appropriate clinical setting is gold standard for dx MI
    detectable 4-6 hrs after injury, peaks 24 hrs, elevated for 48 hrs in NSTEMI and up to 7-10 d in STEMI
    "false ⊕" (non-ACS myonecrosis): myocarditis, toxic CMP, severe CHF, PE or severe respiratory distress (RV microinfarctions), cardiac trauma, sepsis, SAH
    renal failure: ? false ⊕ (↓ clearance, skeletal myopathy) *vs.* true microinfarctions (pressure & volume overload or subclinical ACS);
    in Pts w/ ACS & ↓ CrCl, ↑ Tn → poor prognosis (*NEJM* 2002;346;2047)
  CK-MB: less sens. & spec. (skel. muscle, tongue, diaphragm, intestine, uterus, prostate)
- Echocardiogram: new wall motion abnormality (but very operator & reader dependent)
- Myocardial perfusion: inject sestaMIBI during sx; image later to see if reversible defect

Spectrum of Acute Coronary Syndromes			
Coronary thrombosis	Subtotal		Total
History	angina that is new-onset, crescendo, or at rest usually <30 mins		angina at rest usually ≥30 mins
ECG	± ST depression and/or TWI		ST elevations
Biomarkers	⊖	⊕	⊕ ⊕
Dx	UA	NSTEMI	STEMI

Pre-discharge checklist for ACS patients (*Circ* 2001;104:1577)

- **Risk stratification**: stress test if anatomy undefined; echo to assess EF
- **Lifestyle modification**: low chol. (<200 mg/d) & low fat (<7% saturated) diet; exercise (≥30 mins 3-4× per wk); smoking cessation; weight loss (BMI goal 18.5-24.9 kg/m^2)
- **Medical Rx**: ASA; clopidogrel; β-blockers; ACEI; statin (high-intensity lipid-lowering with, e.g., atorvastatin 80 mg, PROVE-IT TIMI 22, *NEJM* 2004); nitrates (if sx; SL NTG prn for all)
- **Risk factor management**: BP <130/85 mm Hg; LDL <100 mg/dl; HbA1c <7%

UA/NSTEMI

Definition

- **UA**: acute myocardial ischemia without evidence of myocardial necrosis
  angina that is new-onset, crescendo, or at rest
  as may or may not see ECG Δs and as biomarkers ⊖ by def'n, *UA remains a clinical dx*
- **NSTEMI**: acute myocardial ischemia w/ evidence of myocardial necrosis (⊕ Tn or CK-MB)

Prinzmetal's (variant) angina

- Coronary spasm → transient STE usually w/o MI (*but* MI, AVB, VT can occur)
- Pts usually young, smokers, ± other vasospastic disorders (e.g., migraines, Raynaud's)
- Tends to occur in morning; precipitated by hyperventilation or cold, *not* exertion
- Angiography → nonobstructive CAD, focal spasm w/ hypervent., methylergonovine, ACh
- Treatment: high-dose CCB, nitrates (+ SL NTG PRN), ? α-blockers; d/c smoking

UA/NSTEMI Risk Stratification and Triage

Factors	High risk (≥1 of the following)	Intermediate risk (≥1 of the following)	Low risk (± any of following)
History	Accelerating tempo of sx in preceding 48 hrs	Prior MI, PAD, CVD, CABG, prior ASA use	
Pain	Ongoing rest angina >20 min	>20 min rest angina, now resolved, *or* <20 min rest angina relieved w/ NTG	New onset or crescendo angina w/o prolonged rest pain
Clinical	Pulmonary edema, rales, S_3 New or worsening MR Hypotension Age >75 yrs	Age >70 yrs	
ECG	ST Δ ≥0.05 mV	TWI >0.2 mV Q waves	Normal or unΔ'd during episode of chest discomfort
Markers	⊕ troponin	slightly ⊕ troponin	⊖ troponin
Triage	CCU or SDU	SDU or floor + telem	Outpt eval w/in 72 hr

(SDU = step-down unit = intermediate level care telemetry unit. Adapted from ACC/AHA 2002 Guideline Update for UA/NSTEMI.)

TIMI Risk Score for UA/NSTEMI

Calculation of Risk Score		Application of Risk Score	
Characteristic	**Point**	**Score**	**D/MI/UR by 14 d**
Historical		0-1	5%
Age ≥65 yrs	1	2	8%
≥3 Risk factors for CAD	1	3	13%
Known CAD (stenosis ≥50%)	1	4	20%
ASA use in past 7 days	1	5	26%
Presentation		6-7	41%
Severe angina (≥2 episodes w/in 24 hrs)	1	Higher risk Pts (TRS ≥3) derive ↑ benefit from LMWH, GP IIb/IIIa inhibitors, and early angiography (*JACC* 2003;41:89S)	
ST deviation ≥0.5 mm	1		
⊕ cardiac marker	1		
RISK SCORE = Total points	**(0-7)**		

(UR = urgent revascularization; *JAMA* 2000;284:825)

Anti-Ischemic Treatment in UA/NSTEMI

Agent	Comment
Nitrates (SL, PO, topical, or IV)	↓ anginal sx, no ↓ in mortality
β-blockers metoprolol 5 mg IV q 5 min × 3 then 25 mg PO q 6 hrs titrate to HR 55-60	13% ↓ in progression to MI (*JAMA* 1988;260:2259). *Contraindicated* if HR <60, SBP <100, moderate or severe CHF, 2°/3° AVB, severe bronchospasm.
Calcium channel blockers (non-dihydropyridines)	Consider in Pts who cannot tolerate β-blockers due to bronchospasm.
Morphine	Consider if persistent sx or CHF.
Oxygen	Use if necessary to keep S_aO_2 >90%.

(Adapted from ACC/AHA 2002 Guideline Update for UA/NSTEMI)

Antithrombotic Treatment in UA/NSTEMI	
Agent	**Comment**
Aspirin 162-325 mg PO (1st dose crushed/chewed) then 75-162 mg PO qd	50-70% ↓ in death or MI (*NEJM* 1988;319:1105; RISC, *Lancet* 1990;336:827)
Clopidogrel 300 mg PO x 1 → 75 mg PO qd	Give if conservative strategy or if PCI planned. 20% ↓ in D/MI/stroke (CURE, *NEJM* 2001;345:494). Not studied w/ upstream GP IIb/IIIa.
UFH 60-75 U/kg IVB (max 5000 U) 12-15 U/kg/hr (max 1000 U/hr) titrate to aPTT 50-70 sec	Give if hx c/w ACS, ECG Δs, or ⊕ marker. 24% ↓ in death/MI (*JAMA* 1996;276:811)
LWMH enoxaparin 1 mg/kg SC bid ± initial 30 mg IVB dalteparin 120 IU/kg SC bid	Consider instead of UFH. Enoxaparin preferred to UFH. 20% ↓ in death/MI/UR (ESSENCE, *NEJM* 1997;337:447; TIMI-11B, *Circ* 1999;100:1593).
GP IIb/IIIa inhibitors abciximab: 0.25 mg/kg IVB → 0.125 µg/kg/min × 18-24 hrs eptifibatide: 180 µg/kg IVB → 2 µg/kg/min × 72 hrs tirofiban: 0.4 µg/kg/min × 30 min → 0.1 µg/kg/min × 48-108 hrs	Give in Pts in whom PCI is planned. 50% ↓ in death/MI (CAPTURE, *Lancet* 1997;349:1429; ESPRIT, *Lancet* 2000;356:2037). Consider upstream eptifibatide or tirofiban in high-risk Pts (⊕ Tn, TRS ≥4) or refractory sx. 10-20% ↓ in death/MI (PURSUIT, *NEJM* 1998;339:436; PRISM-PLUS *NEJM* 1998;338:1488).

(UR = urgent revascularization. Adapted from ACC/AHA 2002 Guideline Update for UA/NSTEMI.)

Angiography

- **Conservative approach**: medical therapy with predischarge stress test; angiography only if recurrent ischemia or ⊕ submaximal ETT or a markedly ⊕ full-level ETT
- **Early invasive approach**: angiography w/in 24-48 hrs
  ~25% ↓ in death/MI (with stents & upstream GP IIb/IIIa inhibitors; FRISC-II, *Lancet* 1999;354:708; TACTICS-TIMI 18, *NEJM* 2001;344:1879; RITA-3, *Lancet* 2002;360:743)
  indicated if high-risk: recur. ischemia, ⊕ Tn, STΔ, TRS ≥3, CHF, ↓ EF, recent PCI, CABG
  angiography w/in 6 hrs superior to "cooling-off" for 3-5 d (ISAR-COOL, *JAMA* 2003;290:1593)

Fig. 1-1. Approach to UA/NSTEMI

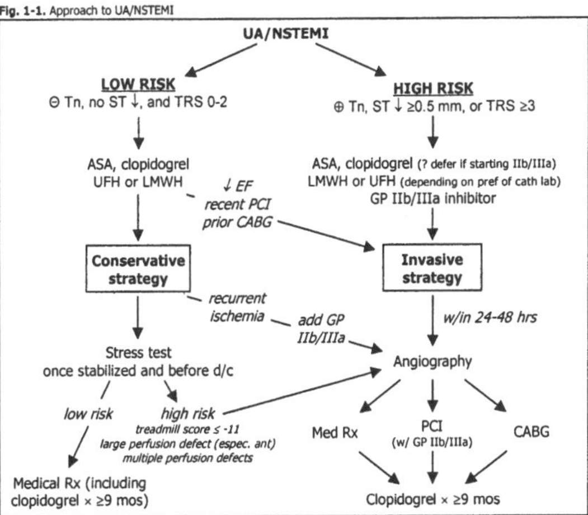

STEMI

Primary PCI

- Should be performed **within 90 mins** by skilled operator at experienced center
- Superior to lysis: 27% ↓ death, 65% ↓ reMI, 54% ↓ stroke, 95% ↓ ICH (*Lancet* 2003;361:13)
- Especially consider if cardiogenic shock, CHF, anterior MI, sx for >3 hrs
- *Transfer* to center for 1° PCI may also be superior to lysis (DANAMI-2, *NEJM* 2003;349:733) *but* was low use of rescue PCI *and* door-to-balloon <120 mins (avg in U.S. ~200 mins)
- Do not let decision regarding *method* of reperfusion delay *time* to reperfusion

Fibrinolysis	
Door-to-needle time should be ≤30 mins	
Indications	**Contraindications**
Sx c/w MI × ≥30 min and <12 hrs *and either* STE ≥1 mm in ≥2 contiguous leads *or* LBBB not known to be old	***Absolute*** • Any prior ICH • Non-hemorrhagic stroke or closed head trauma within 3 (? 6) mos • Intracranial neoplasm, aneurysm, AVM • Active internal bleeding • Suspected aortic dissection
Age limitation: Pts >75 have less of *relative* ↓ in mort., but b/c very high mort. in this group, have more of *absolute* ↓ in mort. ∴ lysis in >75 reasonable, but ↑ risk of ICH. *Time limitation:* earlier lytic is started, greater the benefit. Benefit after 12 hrs less clear but lysis should be considered in Pts presenting 12-24 hrs after onset of pain and still with STE.	***Relative*** • SBP >180 on presentation • INR >2 or known bleeding diathesis • Trauma or major surgery w/in 2-4 wks • Prolonged CPR (>10 min) • Recent internal bleed (w/in 2-4 wks) • Noncompressible vascular punctures • Prior SK exposure (if considering SK) • Pregnancy
~20% ↓ in mortality in anterior MI or LBBB; ~10% ↓ in mortality in inferior MI ~1% risk of ICH (high-risk groups include elderly, women, low wt) Pre-hospital lysis: further 17% ↓ in mortality (*JAMA* 2000;283:2686)	

Thrombolytic	Dose
Reteplase (RPA)	10 U IV over 2 mins, repeat in 30 min × 1
Tenecteplase (TNK)	Single IV bolus over 5 secs <60 kg → 30 mg 60-69 kg → 35 mg 70-79 kg → 40 mg 80-89 kg → 45 mg ≥90 kg → 50 mg
Alteplase (TPA)	15 mg IV bolus, then 0.75 mg/kg (max 50 mg) over 30 min, then 0.5 mg/kg (max 35 mg) over 60 min
Streptokinase (SK)	1.5 MU IV over 30-60 min

Antithrombotic Treatment in STEMI	
Agent	**Comment**
Aspirin 162-325 mg PO (crushed/chewed)	23% ↓ in death; 49% ↓ in death (ISIS-2, *Lancet* ii;349:1988)
UFH 60 U/kg IVB (max 4000 U) 12 U/kg/hr (max 1000 U/hr)	No demonstrated mortality benefit ↑ patency with fibrin-specific lytics titrate to aPTT 50-70 sec
LWMH enoxaparin 30 mg IV × 1 then 1 mg/kg SC bid	*Consider instead of UFH in lysis, age ≤75, Cr <2.0* 25% ↓ death/MI/recurrent ischemia (ASSENT-3, Lancet 2001;358:605)
GP IIb/IIIa inhibitors abciximab: 0.25 mg/kg IVB 0.125 µg/kg/min × 18-24 hrs ? eptifibatide: 180 µg/kg IVB 2 µg/kg/min infusion 2nd 180 µg/kg IVB 10 mins later	*1° PCI: start as early as possible* 60% ↓ D/MI/urg TVR (ADMIRAL, NEJM 2001;344:1895) *Lysis: no indication* ½ dose lytic + GP IIb/IIIa → ↓ reMI, ∅ Δ mort., (GUSTO V, *Lancet* 2001;357:1905 & ASSENT-3, *Lancet* 2001;358:605)

(Adapted from ACC/AHA 1999 Guideline Update for STEMI)

Adjunctive Therapy	
Drug	**Comment**
β-blockers metoprolol 5 mg IV q 5 min × 3 then 25 mg PO q 6 hrs titrate to HR 55-60	15% ↓ in vascular mortality (ISIS-1, *Lancet* 1986;2:57) *Contraindicated* if HR <60, SBP <100, moderate or severe CHF, 2°/3° AVB, severe bronchospasm
Nitrates SL or IV	35% ↓ mortality in pre-lytic era (*Lancet* 1988;1:1088) ? ~5% ↓ mortality w/ oral nitrates (GISSI-3, *Lancet* 1994;343:1115 & ISIS-4, *Lancet* 1995;345:669) *Contraindicated* in hypovolemia, RV infarcts, sildenafil
Oxygen	Use if necessary to keep S_aO_2 >90%.
Morphine	Relieves pain, ↓ anxiety, venodilation → ↓ preload
ACE inhibitors captopril 6.25 mg tid or lisinopril 5 mg qd, then titrate up as tolerated	~10% ↓ mortality at 4-6 wks (GISSI-3, *Lancet* 1994;343:1115; ISIS-4, *Lancet* 1995;345:669) Greatest benefit in ant. MI, EF<40%, or prior MI *Contraindicated* in severe hypotension or renal failure
ARBs	Appear ≈ ACEI (VALIANT, *NEJM* 2003;349:20)
Insulin	Consider insulin infusion in 1st 48 hrs to normalize glc

(Adapted from ACC/AHA 1999 Guideline Update for STEMI)

IMI Complications (*Circ* 1990;81:401; *Annals* 1995;123:509)

- **Heart block** (~20%)
  - 2° AVB in 7%, 3° AVB in 12%; 40% on present., 20% w/in 24 hrs, 40% w/in 24-72 hrs
  - ½ of those who develop high-grade AVB do so gradually, ½ abruptly
  - Rx: atropine, epi, isoproterenol, aminophylline (100 mg/min × 2.5 mins), temp wire
- **Precordial ST** ↓ (15-30%)
  - anterior ischemia *vs.* true posterior MI *vs.* reciprocal Δs
- **RV infarct** (30-50%, but only ½ of those clinically significant)
  - hypotension; ↑ JVP, ⊕ Kussmaul's; 1 mm STE in V_4R; RA/PCWP ≥0.8
  - Rx: optimize preload (RA goal 10-14, *BHJ* 1990;63:98); ↑ contractility (dobutamine); maintain AV synchrony; reperfusion (*NEJM* 1998;338:933); mechanical support (IABP or RVAD); pulmonary vasodilators (e.g., NO)

Mechanical Complications Post-MI		
Complication	**Clinical features**	**Treatment**
Cardiogenic shock	<5% incid.; <48 hrs post-MI	PA catheter, inotropes, pressors, IABP, revasc.
Free wall rupture	<6% incid.; 2-3 d post-MI Transient ↓ BP & HR (epicardial tear) → tamponade or sudden death (PEA)	Volume resuscitation, inotropes, surgery, ? pericardiocentesis
VSD	2-4% incid.; <5 d post-MI 90% → new harsh murmur ± thrill	Inotropes, IABP, diuretics, vasodilators, surgery
Papillary muscle rupture	1% incid.; <5 d post-MI 50% → new murmur, rarely a thrill	Vasodilators, diuretics, IABP, surgery

Arrhythmias Post-MI	
Arrhythmia	**Treatment**
Atrial fibrillation (10-16% incid.)	Cardioversion if hemodynamically unstable or ischemic. β-blocker and/or digoxin, ± amiodarone and heparin.
VT/VF Early monomorphic (<48 hrs post-MI) does *not* carry bad prognosis	Antiarrhythmics and cardioversion/defibrillation per ACLS. Lidocaine or amiodarone × 6-24 hrs, then reassess. ↑ β-blocker as tolerated, replete K & Mg, r/o ischemia ? ICD if VT/VF >3 d post-MI & not due to reversible ischemia
Sinus bradycardia	If symptomatic → atropine; if sx *and* refractory → pacing
Asystole	Atropine and epinephrine → pacing
1° AVB	None
2° AVB type I	If symptomatic → atropine; if sx *and* refractory → pacing
2° AVB type II or 3°	Pacing
Bifascicular block	= LBBB *or* RBBB + either LAHB or LPHB. Consider pacing.
Alternating BBB or trifascicular block	= LBBB alternating with RBBB *or* bifascicular + 1° AVB Pacing

(When pacing is indicated, **transcutaneous pacing** should be attempted first as a bridge to transvenous pacing. When using transcutaneous pacing as a "backup" in standby mode you must ensure that the pacer electrically captures *and* generates a pulse as skeletal muscle activity can mimic ventricular depolarization on the monitor. **Transvenous pacing** is best accomplished under fluoroscopic guidance.)

Other Post-MI Complications		
Complication	**Clinical features**	**Treatment**
LV thrombus	20-40% incid. Risk factors: large antero-apical MI	Anticoagulate × 3-6 mos
Ventricular aneurysm	Noncontractile outpouching of LV; 8-15% incid. Persistent STE do *not* always imply aneurysm.	Surgery if recurrent CHF, thromboemboli, arrhythmia
Ventricular pseudoaneurysm	Rupture → sealed by thrombus and pericardium	Surgery
Pericarditis	10-20% incid.; 1-4 d post-MI ⊕ pericardial rub; ECG Δs rare	High-dose aspirin, NSAIDs Minimize anticoagulation
Dressler's syndrome	<4% incid.; 2-10 wks post-MI Fever, pericarditis, pleuritis.	High-dose aspirin, NSAIDs

Prognosis

- In general, 30-day mortality in RCTs is 6.0-7.5% (~5% for IMIs; ~8% for AMIs)

Killip Class		
Class	**Definition**	**Mort.**
I	no CHF	6%
II	⊕ S_3 and/or basilar rales	17%
III	pulmonary edema	30-40%
IV	cardiogenic shock	60-80%

(*Am J Cardiol* 1967;20:457)

Forrester Class Mortality			
		PCWP (mm Hg)	
		<18	>18
CI	>2.2	3%	9%
	<2.2	23%	51%

(*NEJM* 1976;295:1356)

TIMI Risk Score for STEMI			
Calculation of Risk Score		**Application of Risk Score**	
Characteristic	**Points**	**Score**	**Mortality (%)**
Historical		0	0.8
Age ≥65-74 / ≥75 yrs	2/3	1	1.6
DM or HTN or angina	1	2	2.2
Exam		3	4.4
SBP <100 mm Hg	3	4	7.3
HR >100 bpm	2	5	12.4
Killip class II-IV	2	6	16.1
Weight <67 kg	1	7	23.4
Presentation		8	26.8
Anterior STE or LBBB	1	>8	35.9
Time to Rx >4 hrs	1		
RISK SCORE = Total points	**(0-14)**		

(*Circ* 2000;102:2031)

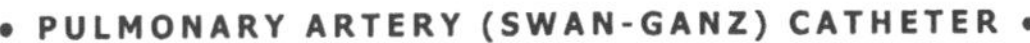

• PULMONARY ARTERY (SWAN-GANZ) CATHETER •

Theoretical considerations

- Frank-Starling principle: SV is dependent in part on LV end-diastolic volume (LVEDV)
- ∴ optimize CO (= SV × HR) and minimize pulmonary edema by manipulating LVEDV
- Balloon at tip of catheter inflated → floats into "wedge" position. Column of blood extends from tip of catheter, through PA, capillaries & veins, to a point just proximal to LA. Under conditions of no flow, PCWP ≈ LA pressure ≈ LVEDP, which is proportional to LVEDV.
- Situations in which these basic assumptions fail:
  1) Catheter tip not in West lung zone 3 (PCWP = alveolar pressure ≠ LA pressure)
  2) PCWP > LA pressure (e.g., mediastinal fibrosis, pulmonary veno-occlusive disease)
  3) Mean LA pressure > LVEDP (e.g., MR, MS)
  4) Altered LVEDP-LVEDV relationship (i.e., abnormal compliance, ∴ normal LVEDP may not be optimal in that Pt)

Indications (*JACC* 1998;32:840)

- **Diagnosis**
  - Ddx of shock
  - Ddx of pulmonary edema
  - Evaluation of LV function and CO via thermodilution or Fick method
  - Dx of cardiac tamponade, intracardiac shunt, MR
  - Evaluation of pulmonary HTN
- **Therapeutics**
  - Tailored therapy to optimize PCWP, SV, S_vO_2
  - Guide to vasodilator therapy for pulmonary HTN
  - Guide to perioperative management in high-risk Pt

Contraindications (*JACC* 1998;32:840)

- **Absolute**: right-sided endocarditis, thrombus, or mechanical heart valve
- **Relative**: coagulopathy (reverse), recent PPM or ICD implantation (place under fluoroscopy), LBBB (~3% risk of CHB, place under fluoro), bioprosthetic right-sided valve

Complications

- **Central venous access**: pneumo- or hemothorax (1-3%), arterial puncture, air embolism
- **Catheter advancement**: atrial or ventricular arrhythmias, RBBB (∴ CHB in ~3% of Pts w/ preexisting LBBB), catheter knotting, cardiac perforation and tamponade, PA rupture
- **Catheter maintenance**: infection (especially if catheter left in place for >3 d), thrombus, pulmonary infarction (≤1.3%), PA rupture, balloon rupture

Efficacy concerns

- In observational studies, use of PA catheter has *not* been shown to improve outcome and may be associated w/ ↑ adverse events & mortality (*JAMA* 1996;276:889 & 2001;286:309)
- Randomized studies in Pts s/p high-risk surgery or with septic shock ± ARDS showed no benefit to PA catheter-guided treatment (*NEJM* 2003;348:5; *JAMA* 2003;290:2713)
- Other series have shown clinical assessments of CO and PCWP incorrect ~50% of the time (*Chest* 1991;99:1451). ∴ may be reasonable to use PA catheter to answer a specific question that cannot be answered non-invasively, then remove ASAP to minimize complications.

Placement

- Insertion site of choice is either the **right internal jugular vein** or the **left subclavian vein** as flotation of the catheter into the pulmonary artery is easiest from these positions
- **Inflate** the balloon when **advancing** or when measuring PCWP
- Use resistance to inflation and pressure tracing to avoid overinflation
- **Deflate** the balloon when **withdrawing** and at all other times
- CXR should always be obtained post-placement to assess for catheter position and PTX
- If catheter cannot be successfully floated (typically in Pts with severe TR or RV dilatation) or if Pt has LBBB, consider fluoroscopic guidance

PA Catheter Waveforms				
Location	**RA**	**RV**	**PA**	**PCWP**
Pressure (mm Hg)	mean ≤6	syst 15-30 diast 1-8	syst 15-30 mean 9-18 diast 6-12	mean ≤12
Waves	simultaneous ECG; mm Hg 0–30; *a*, *c*, *v*, *x*, *y*			*a*, *v*, *x*, *y*
Comment	*a* = atrial contraction, occurs in PR interval *c* = bulging of TV back into RA at start of systole *v* = blood entering RA, occurs mid T wave *x* = atrial relaxation and descent of base of heart *y* = blood exiting RA after TV opens at start of diastole	RVEDP occurs right before upstroke and ≥ mean RA pressure unless there is TS or TR	Waveform should contain notch. Peak *during* T wave PA systolic = RV systolic unless there is a gradient (e.g., PS).	Similar to RA waveform except *dampened* and *delayed.* *a* wave *after* QRS, ± distinct *c* wave, *v* wave *after* T (helps distinguish PCWP w/ large *v* waves 2° MR from PA).

Relation to respiratory cycle

- Intrathoracic pressure (usually slightly ⊖) is transmitted to vessels and heart
- Transmural pressure (≈ preload) = measured intracardiac pressure - intrathoracic pressure
- **Always take measurements at end-expiration,** when intrathoracic pressure is closest to zero ("high point" in spont. breathing Pts and "low point" in Pts on ⊕ pressure vent.)
- When intrathoracic pressures are ↑ (lung disease, PEEP, auto-PEEP), measured PCWP will *overestimate* true transmural pressures. Can approximate by subtracting ½ PEEP.

Cardiac output

- **Thermodilution**: Fixed amount of saline injected in proximal injection port (usually in RA). Δ in temperature over time measured at thermistor (in PA) is used to calculate CO. May be inaccurate if low CO, severe TR, or intracardiac shunt.
- **Indocyanine green dye:** Fixed amount of dye is injected into central line. Concentration of dye in arterial line is sampled over time and CO is calculated from these data. May be inaccurate if low CO, severe valvular regurgitation, or intracardiac shunt.
- **Fick method**: O_2 consumption (L/min) = CO (L/min) × arteriovenous oxygen difference. ∴ derive CO by measuring O_2 consumption and calculating AV O_2 difference [10 x 1.34 ml O_2/g Hb x Hb g/dl x ($S_aO_2 - S_vO_2$)]. May be inaccurate in distributive shock (sepsis).

Tailored therapy

- **Goals**: optimize both MAP and CO while ↓ risk of pulmonary edema
  MAP = CO × SVR; CO = HR × SV (which depends on preload, afterload, and contractility)
  pulmonary edema when PCWP >20-25 (higher levels may be tolerated in chronic CHF)
- **Optimize preload** (= LVEDV ≈ LVEDP ≈ LAP ≈ PCWP) (*NEJM* 1973;289:1263)
  in MI LVEDP of 20-25 optimal → **PCWP of 15-20 optimal** (*a* wave boosts LVEDP)
  can determine in individual Pt by measuring SV w/ different PCWP (create Starling curve)
  give NS or diurese to achieve optimal filling pressure
- **Optimize afterload** (≈ MAP ∝ SVR)
  if SVR too high (→ ↓ SV & ↓ CO): vasodilators (e.g., nitroprusside, NTG, ACEI)
  if SVR too low (→ ↓ MAP): vasopressors (e.g., norepinephrine or phenylephrine)
- **Optimize contractility** (no direct measure; ∝ SV & CO for a given preload & afterload)
  if too low despite optimal preload & afterload: ⊕ inotropes (e.g., dobutamine)

• HEART FAILURE •

Definitions (Braunwald, *Heart Disease*, 6th ed., 2001)

- Failure of heart to pump blood forward at sufficient rate to meet metabolic demands of peripheral tissues or ability to do so only at abnormally high cardiac filling pressures
- "Low-output" (↓ cardiac output) vs. "high-output" (↑ stroke volume ± ↑ cardiac output)
- "Left-sided" (pulmonary edema) vs. "right-sided" (↑ JVP, hepatomegaly, peripheral edema)
- "Backward" (↑ filling pressures, congestion) vs. "forward" (impaired systemic perfusion)
- "Systolic" (inability to expel sufficient blood) vs. "diastolic" (failure to relax and fill normally)

Fig. 1-2. Approach to left-sided heart failure

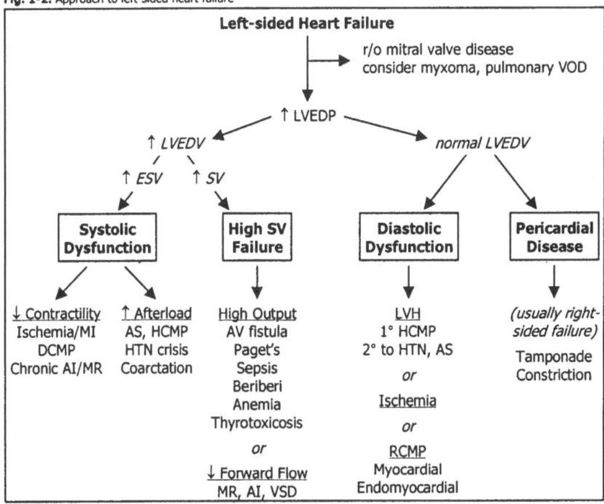

Symptoms

- Low output: fatigue, weakness, Δ MS, anorexia
- Congestive: left-sided → dyspnea, orthopnea, paroxysmal nocturnal dyspnea
  right-sided → peripheral edema, RUQ discomfort

Physical exam

- Hemodynamic profile
  Congestion ("dry" *vs.* "wet"): evidence for congestion includes
  ↑ JVP (~80% of the time JVP >10 → PCWP >22; *J Heart Lung Trans* 1999;18:1126)
  ⊕ abdominojugular reflex, Valsalva square wave (↑ SBP thru strain) (*JAMA* 1996;275:630)
  S_3 (in Pts w/ CHF, ⊕ S_3 → ↑ risk of hospitalization for CHF or death; *NEJM* 2001;345:574)
  rales, dullness at base 2° pleural effus. (often absent due to lymphatic compensation)
  ± hepatomegaly, ascites and jaundice, peripheral edema
  Perfusion ("warm" *vs.* "cold"): evidence for low perfusion includes
  narrow pulse pressure (<25% of SBP), cool and pale extremities, ↓ UOP, lethargy
- Other signs: ± Cheyne-Stokes respirations, abnormal PMI (diffuse, sustained, or lifting depending on the cause of heart failure), ± S_4 (diastolic dysfunction), ± murmurs (valvular disease, distorted MV annulus, displaced papillary muscles)

Diagnostic studies

- CXR: pulmonary edema, pleural effusions (usually R > L), ± cardiomegaly
- ↑ BNP may identify CHF as cause of dyspnea (*NEJM* 2002;347:161)
- Echocardiogram
  ↓ EF and ↑ chamber size → systolic dysfunction
  hypertrophy and/or abnormal inflow across the MV → ? diastolic dysfunction
- Pulmonary artery catheterization: ↑ PCWP, ↓ CO and ↑ SVR (low-output failure)
- Evidence of ↓ perfusion to vital organs: ↑ BUN, ↑ Cr, ↓ Na, abnormal LFTs

Recommended Therapy by CHF Stage			
Stage		**Pt Characteristics**	**Therapy**
A	High risk for HF ⊖ Structural heart disease Asx	HTN, DM, CAD Cardiotoxin exposure FHx of CMP	Treat HTN, hyperlipidemia d/c smoking, EtOH Encourage exercise ACEI if HTN, DM, CVD, PAD
B	⊕ Structural heart disease Asx	Prior MI, ↓ EF Asx valvular disease	All measures for stage A ACEI as in stage A β-blocker if CAD or ↓ EF
C	⊕ Structural heart disease ⊕ Symptoms of HF (prior or current)	Overt CHF	All measures for stage A ACEI, β-blocker Diuretics, digoxin Dietary salt restriction
D	Refractory HF requiring specialized interventions	Sx despite maximal medical Rx	All measures for stage A-C Mechanical assist devices Transplant Continuous IV inotropes

(*JACC* 2001;38:2101)

Drug/Intervention	Comments
Diet, exercise	Na <2g/d, fluid restriction, exercise training in ambulatory Pts
ACEI	40% ↓ mort. in NYHA IV (CONSENSUS, *NEJM* 1987;316:1429) 16% ↓ mort. in NYHA II/III (SOLVD-T, *NEJM* 1991;325:293) 20% ↓ mort. in asx, post-MI, EF ≤40% (SAVE, *NEJM* 1992;327:669) 20% ↓ reinfarction 20-30% ↓ rehospitalization for CHF (↑ amt of benefit w/ ↓ EF) 30% ↓ CHF in asx Pts w/ EF ≤35% (SOLVD-P, *NEJM* 1992;327:685) High-dose ACEI (>30 mg/d of lisinopril) more efficacious than low-dose (<5 mg/d) (ATLAS, *Circ* 1999;100:2312) Watch for azotemia, ↑ K (can ameliorate by low-K diet, diuretics, kayexalate), cough, angioedema
ATII receptor blockers (ARBs)	*Consider in Pts with ↓ EF and sx, in addition to ACEI or as alternative if cannot tolerate ACEI (e.g., b/c cough)* Non-inferior to ACEI (ELITE II, *Lancet* 2000;355:1582; OPTIMAAL, *Lancet* 2002;360:752; VALIANT, *NEJM* 2003;349:20) Good alternative if ACEI intol (CHARM-Alternative, Lancet 2003;362:772) 25% ↓ CHF (Val-HEFT, *NEJM* 2001;345:1667) and 15% ↓ mort. when *added* to ACEI (CHARM-Added, *Lancet* 2003;362:767)
Hydralazine + nitrates	*Consider if cannot tolerate ACEI or ARB* 25% ↓ mort. c/w placebo (V-HeFT I, *NEJM* 1986;314:1547) Not as good as ACEI (V-HeFT-II, *NEJM* 1991;325:303)
β-blocker	*EF will transiently ↓, then ↑. Contraindic in decompensated CHF.* 35% ↓ mort. in NYHA II-IV (U.S. Carvedilol, *NEJM* 1996;334:1349; MERIT, *Lancet* 1999;353:2001; CIBIS-II, *Lancet* 1999;353:9 ; COPERNICUS, *NEJM* 2001;344:1651; CAPRICORN, *Lancet* 2001;357:1385) ? Carvedilol superior to metoprolol (COMET, *Lancet* 2003;362:7) (*JAMA* 2002;287:883 & 890)
Diuretics	Loop ± thiazides diuretics
Aldosterone antagonists	*Consider in severe HF, preserved renal fxn; watch for ↑ K* 30% ↓ mort. in NYHA class III/IV (RALES, *NEJM* 1999;341:709) 15% ↓ mort. in Pts w/ CHF post-MI (EPHESUS, *NEJM* 2003;348:1309)
Digoxin	23% ↓ CHF hosp., no Δ mortality (DIG Trial, *NEJM* 1997;336:525) ? ↑ mort. in women, ? related to ↑ levels (*NEJM* 2002;347:1403) ? optimal dig concentration 0.5-0.8 ng/ml (*JAMA* 2003;289:871)
Anticoagulation	*Consider if AF, LV thrombus, lg akinetic LV segment, EF <30%*
Biventricular pacing	*Consider if refractory CHF and ↑ QRS* ↓ sx (MUSTIC, *NEJM* 2001;344:873; MIRACLE, *NEJM* 2002;346:1845) Meta-analysis suggests ↓ CHF mortality (*JAMA* 2003;289:730)
ICD	*Consider in 1° prevention if CAD + ↓ EF or for 2° prevention* ↓ mort. in Pts w/ MI and EF <30% (MADIT II, *NEJM* 2002;346:877) ↓ arrhythmic deaths in Pts w/ nonisch. DCMP (DEFINITE, AHA 2003)

(*Circ* 2002;105:2099 & 2223; *NEJM* 2003;348:2007)

Precipitants
- **Myocardial ischemia** or infarction
- **Hypertension**, volume overload, PE
- **Dietary or medical noncompliance**
- **Drugs** (β-blockers, CCB) or toxins (EtOH, chemotherapy)
- Myocarditis, endocarditis
- Arrhythmias
- Anemia, infection

Treatment of acute pulmonary edema (LMNOP)
- **L**asix
- **M**orphine (↓ sx of dyspnea + venodilator)
- **N**itrates (venodilator)
- **O**xygen
- **P**osition (sit Pt up & have legs dangling over side of bed → ↓ preload)

Treatment of advanced heart failure (*JAMA* 2002;287:628)
- Tailored therapy with PA catheter; goals of MAP >60, CI >2.2, SVR <800, PCWP <18 (see "Pulmonary Artery Catheter")
- Intravenous vasodilators and inotropes (e.g., nitroprusside and dobutamine; role of nesiritide to be elucidated; *NEJM* 2000;343:246)
- Mechanical circulatory support: intraaortic balloon pump (IABP), left ventricular assist device (LVAD, REMATCH, *NEJM* 2001;345:1435)
- Cardiac transplantation: survival rates of 85% at 1 year, 65-70% at 5 years

Functional classification (New York Heart Association)
- Class I: symptomatic only with greater than ordinary activity
- Class II: symptomatic with ordinary activity
- Class III: symptomatic with minimal activity
- Class IV: symptomatic at rest

Diastolic heart failure (*Circ* 2002;105:1387 & 1503; 2003;107:659)
- 33-50% of Pts w/ the clinical syndrome of CHF have normal or only minimally impaired systolic function and are thus said to have diastolic heart failure
- ~30% of population over age 45 w/ evidence of diastolic dysfunction (DD) on echo, ~20% mild, <10% moderate or severe (*JAMA* 2003;289:194)
  but only 50% of severe DD and 5% of moderate DD were symptomatic
- Etiologies
  causes of impaired relaxation: ischemia, LVH, HCMP, aging, hypothyroidism
  causes of ↑ passive stiffness: prior MI, LVH, RCMP
- Diagnosis: based on clinical symptoms/signs of CHF and echo evidence of impaired diastolic function (E/A reversal, ↑ deceleration time, LV hypertrophy, LA dilatation) and preserved systolic function
- Treatment (mostly guided by pathophysiologic rationale rather than RCT data)
  diuresis for volume overload
  HR & BP control w/ βB, CCB, ACEI, ARB (↓ rehosp., CHARM-Preserved, *Lancet* 2003;362:777)
  relief of ischemia

• CARDIOMYOPATHIES •

Myocardial dysfxn not due to ischemic, valvular, HTN, or congenital heart disease

DILATED CARDIOMYOPATHY (DCMP)

Definition and epidemiology

- Ventricular dilatation, normal to ↓ wall thickness, and ↓ contractility
- Incidence: 5-8 cases/100,000 population per yr; prevalence: 36 cases/100,000 population

Etiologies

- **Ischemia, valvular disease, HTN**: technically not CMP as not 1° diseases of heart muscle, *but* most common causes of ↓ EF and LV dilatation
- **Idiopathic** (25-50% of DCMP, ? undiagnosed infectious or alcoholic)
- **Infectious myocarditis** (usually due to immune rxn to infection; *NEJM* 2000;343:1388)
  viruses (coxsackievirus, echovirus), bacterial, fungal, rickettsial
  HIV: ~8% of asx HIV ⊕ ; due to HIV *vs.* other viruses *vs.* meds (*NEJM* 1998;339:1093)
  Lyme (often with AVB)
  Chagas: apical aneurysm ± thrombus, BBB, megaesophagus or colon (*NEJM* 1993;329:639)
- **Toxic**
  alcohol (7-8 drinks/d × >5 yrs)
  anthracyclines (risk ↑ as dose >550 mg/m^2, may manifest late); cyclophosphamide
  radiation
  cocaine
- **Infiltrative** (often mix of DCMP + RCMP): hemochromatosis, sarcoidosis, amyloidosis
- **Autoimmune**
  peripartum (last month → 3-4 mos postpartum): <0.1% of pregnancies; ↑ risk w/ multiparity & ↑ age; ~50% will improve; ? ↑ risk w/ next pregnancy (*JAMA* 2000;283:1183)
  collagen-vascular disease (rare): scleroderma, SLE, PAN, RA
  giant cell (idiopathic fulminant myocarditis)
- **Metabolic**: hypothyroidism, pheo, acromegaly, thiamine or selenium deficiency
- Tachycardia-induced (HR >140-160 × wks)
- Familial

Clinical manifestations

- **Heart failure**: both congestive symptoms and fatigue; signs of left- and right-sided CHF
  diffuse, lat.-displaced PMI, **S_3**, ± MR or TR (annular dilat., displaced pap. muscle)
- Embolic events (~10%)
- Arrhythmias
- Chest pain on exertion seen in up to one-third (even with no CAD)

Diagnostic studies

- CXR: cardiomegaly, pulmonary edema, pleural effusions
- ECG: may see PRWP, Q waves, or bundle branch block; low voltage; AF
- Echocardiogram: LV dilatation, ↓ EF, *regional or global* LV HK, ± RV HK, ± mural thrombi

Workup

- History: risk factors for or h/o CAD, HTN, drug or toxin exposure, viral prodrome, signs or symptoms c/w autoimmune diseases
- Stress test: completely ⊖ test useful to r/o ischemic etiology (low false ⊖ rate), but ⊕ test does not rule in ischemic etiology (high false ⊕ rate)
- Cardiac catheterization to r/o CAD if risk factors, h/o angina, Q waves on ECG
- Laboratory evaluation: TFTs, iron studies, HIV; other tests as indicated by clinical suspicion
- ? Endomyocardial biopsy (*Circ* 1989:79:971)
  yield 10% (of these, 75% show myocarditis, 25% show evidence of systemic disease)
  false ⊖ (patchy disease) and false ⊕ (necrosis → inflammation)
  no proven Rx for myocarditis; ∴ biopsy for *prognosis* or if *suspect systemic disease*

Treatment

- Standard CHF therapy
  ACEI, diuretics, digoxin, β-blockers (if not in decompensated CHF)
  anticoagulation (consider if EF ≤30%)
  ICD if EF <30-35% (MADIT II, *NEJM* 2002;346:877; DEFINITE, AHA 2003; SCD-HeFT, ACC 2004)
  ? biventricular pacing (if QRS >130-150 msec): ↑ exercise tolerance and quality of life (MUSTIC, *NEJM* 2001;344:873; MIRACLE, JAMA 2003;289:2685)
- Advanced, refractory CHF: tailored Rx, LVAD, cardiac transplantation
- Immunosuppression for myocarditis: no proven benefit; consider if fulminant/progressive

Hypertrophic Cardiomyopathy (HCMP)

Definition and epidemiology

- Inappropriate LV and/or RV hypertrophy
  in athletes, wall thickness usually <13 & usually symmetric (*NEJM* 1991;324:295)
- Prevalence: 1 case/500 population; 50% sporadic, 50% familial

Pathology

- Autosomal dominant mutations in genes encoding cardiac sarcomere proteins
- Myocardial fiber disarray
- 4 major morphologic variants: asymmetric septal hypertrophy; mid-cavity obstruction; concentric hypertrophy; apical obliteration

Pathophysiology

- Subaortic outflow obstruction: narrowed tract 2° hypertrophied septum + systolic anterior motion (SAM) of anterior leaflet of mitral valve 2° Venturi forces (may be fixed, variable, or nonexistent) and papillary muscle displacement; ↑'d with ↑ contractility (digoxin, β-agonists), ↓ preload, or ↓ afterload
- Mitral regurgitation: due to SAM (mid-to-late, post.-directed regurg. jet) and abnormal mitral leaflets and papillary muscles (pansystolic, ant.-directed regurg. jet)
- Diastolic dysfunction: ↑ chamber stiffness + impaired relaxation
- Ischemia: small vessel disease, perforating artery compression, ↓ coronary perfusion
- Syncope: Δs in load-dependent CO, arrhythmias

Clinical manifestations

- **Dyspnea**: due to ↑ LVEDP, MR, and diastolic dysfunction
- **Arrhythmias** (AF in 20-25%; VT/VF): palpitations, syncope, sudden cardiac death
- **Angina**

Physical exam

- Cardiac: sustained PMI, paradoxical splitting of S_2, ⊕ S_4
  systolic crescendo-decrescendo murmur (**↑ w/ Valsalva** & standing)
  ± mid-to-late or holosystolic murmur of MR
- Carotid pulse: bisferiens

Diagnostic studies

- CXR: cardiomegaly (LV and LA)
- ECG: LVH, anterolateral and inferior pseudo-Q waves, ± apical giant TWI (apical variant)
- **Echocardiogram**: no absolute cutoffs for degree of LVH but $\frac{\text{septum}}{\text{post wall}} \geq 1.3$ suggestive as is septum >15 mm; other findings include dynamic outflow obstruction, SAM, MR
- Cardiac catheterization: subaortic pressure ∇; *Brockenbrough sign* = ↓ in pulse pressure post-extrasystole

Treatment (*NEJM* 1997;336:775; *JAMA* 2002;287:1308)

- Heart failure
  Drug therapy: β-blockers, CCB, disopyramide. Avoid digoxin, diuretics, vasodilators unless systolic dysfunction.
  If refractory to drug therapy and there is *obstructive* pathophysiology (∇ >50 mm Hg)
    alcohol septal ablation (*Circ* 1997;95:2075; *JACC* 1998;31:252; *NEJM* 2002;347:1326)
      90% with acute benefit; ½ will have further improvement over 3 mos
      by 6 mos resting ∇ ~16 mm Hg & stress-induced ∇ ~45 mm Hg gradient
      ½ will develop 3° AVB, ¼ will need PPM
    surgical myotomy-myectomy (*Circ* 1975;52:88; *J Thorac Cardiovasc Surg* 1996;111:586)
    ? pacing, but improved sxs likely placebo effect (*JACC* 1997;29:435; *Circ* 1999; 99:2927)
  If refractory to drug therapy and there is *nonobstructive* pathophysiology: transplant
- AF: rate control with β-blockers, maintain SR with disopyramide, amiodarone, sotalol
- Sudden cardiac death: ICD (*NEJM* 2000;342:365). Risk factors: history of VT/VF/syncope, ⊕ FHx SCD, ⊕ Holter, massive LVH, hypotension w/ exercise, specific mutations
- Family screening
- Counsel to avoid dehydration, extreme exertion
- Endocarditis prophylaxis

RESTRICTIVE CARDIOMYOPATHY (RCMP)

Definition
- Impaired ventricular filling due to ↓ compliance

Etiology (*NEJM* 1997;336:267)
- **Myocardial processes**
  - idiopathic fibrosis
  - autoimmune (scleroderma, PM-DM)
  - diabetes mellitus
  - infiltrative diseases (amyloidosis, hemochromatosis, sarcoidosis)
  - storage diseases (Gaucher's, Fabry's, Hurler's, glycogen storage diseases)
- **Endomyocardial processes**
  - Löffler's endocarditis (temperate zone dis.; 2° Churg-Strauss or hypereos. synd.; ↑ eos.)
  - endomyocardial fibrosis (tropical zone dis.; normal eos.)
  - toxins (radiation, anthracyclines)
  - serotonin (carcinoid, serotonin agonists, ergot alkaloids)
  - cancer

Pathology
- Normal or ↑ wall thickness ± infiltration or abnormal deposition

Pathophysiology
- ↓ myocardial compliance → normal EDV but ↑ EDP → ↑ systemic and pulmonary venous pressures
- ↓ ventricular cavity size → ↓ SV and ↓ CO

Clinical manifestations
- **Right-sided > left-sided heart failure** with peripheral edema > dyspnea
- **Diuretic "refractoriness"**
- **Thromboembolic events**
- Poorly tolerated tachyarrhythmias

Physical exam
- ↑ JVP, ± Kussmaul's sign (classically seen in *constrictive pericarditis*)
- Cardiac: ± S_3 and S_4, ± murmurs of MR and TR
- Congestive hepatomegaly, ± ascites and jaundice, peripheral edema

Diagnostic studies
- CXR: normal ventricular chamber size, enlarged atria, ± pulmonary congestion
- ECG: low voltage, ± arrhythmias
- Echocardiogram
  - symmetric wall thickening + mural thrombi → cavity obliteration
  - diastolic dysfxn: ↑ early diastolic (E) and ↓ late atrial (A) filling, ↑ E/A ratio, ↓ decel. time
  - granular sparkling texture in amyloidosis
- Cardiac catheterization
  - atria: **M's** or **W's** (prominent *x* and *y* descents)
  - ventricles: **dip & plateau** or **square-root sign** (rapid ↓ pressure at onset of diastole, rapid ↑ to early plateau)
  - concordance of LV and RV pressure peaks during respiratory cycle (*vs.* discordance in constrictive pericarditis; *Circ* 1996;93:2207)
- Restrictive cardiomyopathy vs. constrictive pericarditis: see "Pericardial Disease"

Treatment
- Treat underlying disease
- Gentle diuresis
- Maintain sinus rhythm (important for filling)
- ? Anticoagulation
- ? CCB

• VALVULAR HEART DISEASE •

AORTIC STENOSIS

Etiologies

- **Degenerative heart disease** (i.e., calcific stenosis): cause in 50% of Pts >70 yrs
  inflammatory process ≈ atherosclerosis w/ common risk factors such as age, HTN, ↑ chol.
  ↑ CV mortality in Pts w/ aortic sclerosis (w/o stenosis) (*NEJM* 1999;341:142)
- **Congenital heart disease** (i.e., bicuspid AoV): cause in 50% of Pts <70 yrs
- **Rheumatic heart disease** (AS usually accompanied by AI)
- AS mimicker = hypertrophic cardiomyopathy

Pathophysiology

- Pressure overload → *concentric* LVH

Clinical manifestations (usually indicates AVA <1.0 cm^2)

- **Angina**: ↑ O_2 demand (hypertrophy) + ↓ O_2 supply (compression of subendocard.) ± CAD
- **Syncope** *(exertional):* peripheral vasodilatation (e.g., in the vascular supply to muscles) in the setting of a fixed CO → ↓ MAP → insufficient cerebral perfusion
- **Heart failure**: dyspnea or pulmonary edema if severe

Physical examination

- High-pitched **systolic crescendo-decrescendo murmur** at RUSB
  radiates to sternal notch, carotids, apex (where sounds holosystolic = Gallavardin effect)
  ↑ w/ passive leg raise, ↓ w/ standing & Valsalva, but not specific
- In contrast, dynamic outflow obstruction ↓ w/ passive leg raise & ↑ w/ standing & Valsalva
- Ejection click heard with *bicuspid* AoV
- Signs of severity: *late-peaking* murmur, paradoxically split S_2 or inaudible A_2, small and delayed carotid pulse ("pulsus parvus et tardus"), LV heave, ⊕ S_4 (occasionally palpable)

Diagnostic studies

- ECG: LVH, LAE, LBBB
- CXR: poststenotic dilation of aorta, AoV calcification, pulmonary congestion
- **Echocardiogram**: valve morphology, estimated pressure gradients, calculated AVA, EF
- **Cardiac catheterization**: gradient from simultaneous LV & Ao pressures, calculated AVA, but primarily to *r/o concomitant CAD* (seen in ~50% of Pts presenting with AS)

Classification of Aortic Stenosis			
Stage	**Mean gradients (mm Hg)**	**AVA (cm^2)**	**LVEF**
Normal	0	3.0-4.0	normal
Mild	<25	1.5-2.0	normal
Moderate	25-50	1.0-1.5	normal
Severe, compensated	>50	<1.0	normal
Severe, decompensated	variable	<1.0	↓

Treatment (*JACC* 1998;32:1486)

- **Surgery (AVR)**
  symptomatic AS
  asx **severe AS** *and* **↓ EF, AVA <0.6 cm^2, aortic jet >4 m/s**, or **↓ BP w/ exercise**
  asymptomatic mod-sev AS *and* undergoing CABG
- Medical therapy: indicated if Pt sx but not an operative candidate
  gentle diuresis, control of hypertension (? ACEI), digoxin, ? statin (*Circ* 2001;104:2205)
  avoid venodilators (e.g., nitrates) and ⊖ inotropes (e.g., β-blockers & CCB) in severe AS
- PAV: 50% ↑ in AVA and 50% ↓ peak AoV gradient, but 50% restenosis rate at 6-12 months (*NEJM* 1988;319:125), ∴ used as bridge to AVR or if Pt not a surgical candidate
- IABP: stabilization, bridge to surgery
- Endocarditis prophylaxis; avoid vigorous physical exertion once AS moderate-severe

Natural history (*Circulation* 1968;38 (Suppl. V):61)

- Usually *slowly progressive* until symptoms develop
- Follow with echocardiogram q 2 yrs or if Δ in sx; AVA ↓ ~0.1 cm^2 per yr (Circ 1997;95:2262)
- Angina → 5 yr mean survival; syncope → 3 yr mean survival; CHF → 2 yr mean survival

Aortic Insufficiency

Etiologies

- **Valve disease**
  - **rheumatic heart disease** (usually mixed AS/AI and concomitant MV disease)
  - **bicuspid AoV**: natural hx: 1/3 → normal, 1/3 → AS, 1/6 → AI, 1/6 → endocarditis → AI
  - **infective endocarditis**
  - valvulitis (RA, SLE, anorexigens)
- **Root disease**
  - **HTN**
  - aortic aneurysm or dissection, annuloaortic ectasia, Marfan's syndrome
  - large vessel vasculitis (giant cell, Takayasu's)
  - syphilis

Clinical manifestations

- Acute: pulmonary edema ± hypotension
- Chronic: clinically silent while LV dilates → LV decompensation & ↑ AI → CHF

Physical examination

- **Diastolic decrescendo murmur at LUSB** (RUSB if due to aortic root disease)
  - ↑ with sitting forward, expiration, handgrip
  - severity of AI proportional to duration of murmur (except in acute and severe late)
  - Austin Flint murmur: diastolic rumble at apex (AI jet interfering w/ mitral inflow)
- **Wide pulse pressure** due to ↑ stroke volume → many of classic signs (see table)
  - (pulse pressure narrows in late AI with ↓ LV function)
- Soft S_1, (early closure of MV); PMI diffuse and laterally displaced; ⊕ S_3 (≠ ↓ EF in AI)

Classic Eponymous Signs in AI	
Sign	**Description**
Corrigan's pulse	"water hammer" pulse (i.e., rapid rise and fall or collapsing)
Hill's sign	(popliteal SBP - brachial SBP) >60 mm Hg
Duroziez's sign	gradual pressure over femoral artery → systolic and diastolic bruits
Traube's sound	double sound heard at femoral artery when compressed distally
de Musset's sign	head-bobbing with each heartbeat (low sens.)
Müller's sign	systolic pulsations of the uvula
Quincke's pulses	subungual capillary pulsations (low spec.)

(*Southern Medical Journal* 1981;74:459)

Diagnostic studies

- ECG: LVH, LAD
- CXR: cardiomegaly ± aortic dilatation
- **Echocardiogram**: severity of AI (based on size of regurgitant jet and presence of flow reversal in descending aorta), and assess LV size & function

Treatment (*JACC* 1998;32:1486)

- **Surgery (AVR)**
  - **symptomatic severe AI** (if AI *not* severe, unlikely to be cause of sx)
  - asx **severe AI** *and* EF <50% or LV systolic diam. >55 mm or diastolic diam. >75 mm
  - asymptomatic severe AI *and* undergoing CABG
- Medical therapy
  - **vasodilators** (nifedipine, ACEI, hydralazine) if severe AI, HTN, or Pt not operative cand.
  - diuretics and digoxin if CHF
- Acute decompensation (consider ischemia and endocarditis as possible precipitants)
  - IV afterload reduction (nitroprusside) and inotropic support (dobutamine)
  - ± chronotropic support (↑ HR → ↓ diastole → ↓ time for regurgitation)
  - vasoconstrictors and IABP contraindicated
  - *surgery* usually needed for acute severe AI as poorly tolerated by LV
- Endocarditis prophylaxis

Natural history

- *Variable* progression (unlike AS, can be fast or slow)
- Once start to decompensate, prognosis poor
  - asx + normal EF → sx or LV dysfxn at <6%/yr and death at <0.2%/yr
  - asx but LV dysfxn → sx at 25%/yr
  - sx → death at 10%/yr

MITRAL STENOSIS

Etiologies

- **Rheumatic heart disease**: *fusion of the commissures* → "fish mouth" valve
- Congenital, myxoma, thrombus
- Valvulitis (e.g., SLE, amyloid, carcinoid) or infiltration (e.g., mucopolysaccharides)
- Functional MS secondary to severe MAC → encroachment on leaflets

Clinical manifestations

- **Dyspnea** and **pulmonary edema**
  if due to RHD, symptoms usually begin during 3rd-4th decades
  precipitants: tachycardia, volume overload, atrial fibrillation
- **Atrial fibrillation**
- **Embolic events** (especially in atrial fibrillation or endocarditis)
- Pulmonary symptoms: hemoptysis, frequent bronchitis (due to congestion), PHT

Physical examination

- **Low-pitched diastolic rumble at apex** with pre-systolic accentuation (if not in AF)
  appreciated best when patient in left lateral decubitus position, ↑ with exercise
  severity of MS proportional to *duration* of murmur (not intensity)
- **Opening snap** (high-pitched early diastolic sound at left sternal border and apex)
  MV area proportional to S_2-OS interval (i.e., tighter valve → shorter interval)
- Loud S_1 (unless MV calcified)
- Mitral facies = ruddy cheeks

Diagnostic studies

- ECG: **LAE** ("P mitrale"), ± atrial fibrillation, ± RVH
- CXR: **dilated left atrium** (straightening of left heart border, double density on right, left mainstem bronchus elevation)
- **Echocardiogram**: estimated pressure gradients, direct planimetry and calculated valve area, valve echo score (based on leaflet mobility, leaflet thickening, subvalvular thickening, calcifications)
- **Cardiac catheterization**: gradient from simultaneous PCWP and LV pressures, calculated valve area; LA pressure will have tall *a* wave and blunted *y* descent

Classification of Mitral Stenosis		
Stage	**Mean gradients (mm Hg)**	**MV area (cm^2)**
Normal	0	4.0-6.0
Mild	1-6	1.5-2.0
Moderate	6-12	1.0-1.5
Severe	>12	<1.0

Treatment

- Medical: Na restriction, cautious diuresis, β-blockers, anticoag. (if AF or prior embolism)
- Endocarditis prophylaxis (and if RHD, rheumatic fever prophylaxis as well)
- Surgical (MVR): **symptomatic MS**, pulmonary hypertension, ? onset of AF
- **Percutaneous mitral valvuloplasty** (PMV) → valve area doubles, gradient ↓ by 50%
  ≈ MVR *if* valve score <8, ≤ mild MR , ∅ AF or LA thrombus
  (*NEJM* 1994;331:961, *Circ* 2002;105:1465)

Mitral Regurgitation

Etiologies
- **Leaflet abnormalities**: **myxomatous degeneration**, **endocarditis**, **RHD**, valvulitis (collagen-vascular disease), congenital
- **Ruptured chordae tendinae**: myxomatous, spontaneous, endocarditis, collagen-vascular
- **Papillary muscle dysfunction**: ischemia/infarction (usually *posterior* papillary muscle b/c supplied by PDA alone while anterolateral papillary muscle supplied by diagonals & OMs), displacement due to cardiomyopathy, infiltration
- **Annulus dilatation**: any cause of LV dilatation

Clinical manifestations
- Acute: **pulmonary edema**, hypotension
- Chronic: progressive dyspnea on exertion, fatigue, atrial fibrillation, PHT

Physical examination
- **High-pitched, blowing, holosystolic murmur** at apex that radiates to the axilla
  ↑ with handgrip (sens. 68%, spec. 92%), ↓ with Valsalva (sens. 93%) (*NEJM* 1988 318:1572)
- Laterally displaced hyperdynamic PMI, obscured S_1, ± thrill, ± S_3

Diagnostic studies
- ECG: LAE, LVH, ± atrial fibrillation
- CXR: dilated LA, dilated LV, ± pulmonary congestion
- **Echocardiogram**: degree of MR (based on size of regurgitant jet) and LV function (EF *supernormal* in compensated states, ∴ EF <60% with severe MR = LV impairment)
- **Cardiac catheterization**: prominent PCWP *cv* waves, left ventriculography for degree of MR and LV EF

Treatment (*JACC* 1998;32:1486)
- **Surgery** (repair preferred over replacement)
  symptomatic severe MR
  asx **severe MR** *and* **EF <55-60%** and **LV systolic diam. >45-50 mm**, ? AF or PHT
- Medical: indicated if Pt not an operative candidate
  ↓ **afterload**: ACEI, hydralazine/nitrates (benefits unproven)
  ↓ **preload** (↓ CHF and ↓ amount of MR by ↓ MV orifice): diuretics, nitrates
  inotropy: digoxin
- Acute decompensation (consider ischemia and endocarditis as possible precipitants)
  IV afterload reduction (nitroprusside), inotropic support (dobutamine), IABP
  vasoconstrictors contraindicated
  surgery usually needed for acute severe MR as poorly tolerated by LV
- Endocarditis prophylaxis

Prognosis
- Asymptomatic: 5-yr survival with medical therapy = 80%
- Symptomatic: 5-yr survival with medical therapy = 45%

Mitral Valve Prolapse (MVP)

Definition
- Displacement of any part of either MV leaflet or their coaptation point beyond the plane of the MV in the *parasternal long axis view*
- Can be over-diagnosed in the four-chamber view
- Classic = ⊕ leaflet redundancy; nonclassic = no leaflet redundancy

Epidemiology
- Prevalence 2-4% of the general population

Etiologies
- Myxomatous involvement of the MV apparatus
- Associated with connective tissue diseases (e.g., Marfan's, Ehlers-Danlos)

Clinical manifestations
- Asymptomatic
- ? chest pain, AF, syncope or stroke (but not supported by recent data, *NEJM* 1999;341:1)

Physical exam
- Midsystolic click ± mid-to-late systolic murmur
  ↓ LV volume (standing, strain phase of Valsalva) → click & murmur heard earlier
  ↑ LV volume or ↑ impedance to LV ejection → click & murmur heard later & softer

Treatment
- Endocarditis prophylaxis if audible murmur or thickened leaflets
- Aspirin or anticoagulation if prior neurologic event
- β-blockers for symptomatic patients

PROSTHETIC HEART VALVES

Mechanical valves
- **Caged-ball** (e.g., Starr-Edwards)
- **Single-tilting disk** (e.g., Bjork-Shiley, Medtronic-Hall)
- Bileaflet-tilting disk (e.g., St. Jude Medical)
- Characteristics: very durable but thrombogenic and ∴ require anticoagulation
  consider if age <60-65 yrs or if already need for anticoagulation

Bioprosthetic
- **Heterograft** (e.g., Carpentier-Edwards)
- Pericardial
- Characteristics: less durable, but minimally thrombogenic
  consider if age >60-65 yrs, lifespan <10-12 yrs, or contraindication to anticoagulation

Physical examination
- Normal: **crisp sounds**, ± soft murmur during forward flow (normal to have small gradient across valve)
- Abnormal: regurgitant murmurs, absent mechanical valve closure sounds

Anticoagulation with Prosthetic Valves

Valve	Warfarin		ASA
	INR 2.0-3.0	INR 2.5-3.5	80-100 mg
Mechanical valves			
1st 3 months		⊕	⊕
After 3 months			
Aortic valve	⊕		±
Aortic valve + risk factor		⊕	⊕
Mitral valve ± risk factor		⊕	⊕
Bioprosthetic valves			
1st 3 months		⊕	⊕
After 3 months			
No risk factors			⊕
Aortic valve + risk factor	⊕		⊕
Mitral valve + risk factor		⊕	⊕
Risk factors: AF, ↓ EF, prior embolic event, hypercoagulable state, single-tilting disk & Starr-Edwards valves, ? multiple valves			

(*JACC* 1998;32:1486)

Management of Anticoagulation Peri-Procedure

Minor procedures (e.g., dental work)	Usually can continue anticoagulation
Major procedures (e.g., surgery)	d/c warfarin 72 hrs before surgery restart once hemostasis achieved
Major procedure but *risk factors* for *thromboembolism* (especially if mechanical valve in mitral position)	Preoperatively: d/c warfarin, start heparin 6 hrs preoperatively: d/c heparin Postop: restart heparin & warfarin ASAP

(*JACC* 1998;32:1486)

Endocarditis prophylaxis

Complications
- Valve thrombosis (especially with caged-ball valves) or pannus formation
- Embolization (r/o endocarditis); risk of thromboembolism 1-2%/yr even w/ warfarin Rx
- Structural failure
  mechanical valves: rare except for Bjork-Shiley
  bioprosthetic valves: 30% fail rate within 10-15 years
- Hemolysis (especially with caged-ball valves)
- Paravalvular leak (r/o endocarditis)
- Endocarditis

• PERICARDIAL DISEASE •

Pericarditis and Pericardial Effusion

Etiologies of Pericarditis	
Infectious	Viral: coxsackievirus, echovirus, adenovirus, EBV, VZV, HIV Bacterial (from endocarditis, pneumonia, or s/p cardiac surgery): *S. pneumococcus, S. aureus* Tuberculous (extension from lung or hematogenous) Fungal: histoplasmosis, coccidioidomycosis
Neoplastic	Primary cardiac & mesothelioma Metastatic (lung, breast, lymphoma, leukemia, renal cell)
Autoimmune	Connective tissue diseases (SLE, RA, scleroderma, Sjögren's) Vasculitides (PAN, Churg-Strauss, Wegener's) Drug-induced (procainamide, hydralazine) Dressler's syndrome (post-MI)
Systemic	Uremia (develops in 1/3 of Pts, especially if on HD) Hypothyroidism
Cardiovascular	Acute transmural MI (10-15%) Proximal aortic dissection Chest trauma or s/p cardiac procedure Post-irradiation (>4000 cGy to the mediastinum)
Idiopathic	
Effusions w/o pericarditis	CHF, cirrhosis, nephrotic syndrome

(*Lancet* 2004;363:717)

Clinical manifestations of pericarditis

- **Chest pain**: pleuritic, positional (lessened by sitting forward), radiates to trapezius may be *absent* in tuberculous, neoplastic, post-irradiation, and uremic pericarditis
- ± Fever

Physical exam

- **Pericardial friction rub** (leathery sound with up to 3 components: atrial contraction, ventricular contraction, ventricular relaxation) that is notoriously variable and evanescent
- If pericardial effusion: **distant heart sounds** (and rub may grow fainter); dullness over left posterior lung field (Ewart's sign) due to compressive atelectasis

Diagnostic studies

- ECG: diffuse ST elevations (*concave up*), PR depressions, TWI; 4 stages that evolve over hrs to wks; low voltage and *electrical alternans* may be seen if large is effusion present

Stage	PR	ST	T wave
1st	↓	↑	upright
2nd	isoelectric	isoelectric	flat
3rd	isoelectric	isoelectric	inverted
4th	isoelectric	isoelectric	upright

- CK-MB or troponin (⊕ in ~30%, *JACC* 2003;42:2144) if myopericarditis
- CXR: if effusion present, may see cardiomegaly or "water-bottle" heart (>250 cc of fluid); "oreo cookie" sign (radiolucency between heart and anterior pericardium on lateral view)
- Echocardiogram: may be normal or may see effusion ± stranding (fibrin or tumor)

Workup

- r/o infectious etiologies: usually apparent from Hx & CXR
  ? acute and convalescent serologies
- r/o non-infectious etiologies: BUN, Cr, ANA, RF, screen for common malignancies
- Pericardiocentesis if suspect effusion due to infection or malignancy
  ✓ cell counts, TP, LDH, glc, gram stain, cultures, cytology
  "exudate" criteria: TP >3 g/dl, TP_{eff}/TP_{serum} >0.5, LDH_{eff}/LDH_{serum} >0.6, or glc <60 mg/dl
  high sens. (~90%) but *very low* spec. (~20%) (*Chest* 1997;111:1213)

Treatment

- Anti-inflammatory drugs (e.g., ibuprofen 800 mg tid + colchicine 0.6mg bid)
  sx usually subside in 1-3 d, continue Rx for 7-14 d (*JAMA* 2003;289:1150)
  steroids for refractory idiopathic disease
- Avoid anticoagulants
- If infectious effusion → pericardial drainage + antibiotics
- If effusion likely to recur → consider pericardial window
- Large idiopathic effusions can be treated initially with pericardiocentesis; if recur (~60%), consider pericardiectomy (*NEJM* 1999;341:2054)

Pericardial Tamponade

Etiology

- Any cause of pericarditis but especially **malignancy**, **uremia**, **idiopathic**, proximal aortic dissection with rupture, myocardial rupture
- Rapidly accumulating effusions most likely to cause tamponade as no time for pericardium to stretch and accommodate fluid

Pathophysiology (*NEJM* 2003;349:684)

- ↑ intrapericardial pressure, compresses heart throughout cycle, ↓ venous return → ↓ CO
- Since diastolic pressures are ↑ and equal, when TV opens at start of diastole, pressure in RV = RA. ∴ no rapid exit of blood from RA, the *y* descent is *blunted*, and ↓ RV filling.
- Pulsus paradoxus
  Normally, inspiration → ↓ intrapericardial & RA pressures → ↑ venous return → ↑ RV size → septal shift to left. Also, ↑ pulmonary vascular compliance → ↓ pulm venous return. Result is ↓ LV filling → ↓ LV stroke volume & blood pressure (Δ SBP <10 mm Hg).
  Tamponade creates ↑ ventricular interdependence → ↑ pulsus (Δ SBP ≥10 mm Hg)

Clinical manifestations

- **Cardiogenic shock** (hypotension, fatigue) **without pulmonary edema**
- Dyspnea may be due to ↑ respiratory drive to augment venous return

Physical exam

- **Beck's triad: distant heart sounds, ↑ JVP, hypotension**
- Hypotension (50%; occasionally hypertensive), reflex tachycardia, cool extremities
- **Pulsus paradoxus** (75%) = ↓ SBP ≥10 mm Hg during inspiration
  Ddx = PE, hypovolemia, severe obstructive lung disease
- ↑ JVP with blunted *y* descent
- Distant heart sounds, ± pericardial friction rub (30%)
- Tachypnea but clear lungs

Diagnostic studies

- ECG: low voltage, electrical alternans, ± signs of pericarditis
- Echocardiogram: ⊕ **effusion**, **septal shift** with inspiration,
  diastolic collapse of RA (sens. >85%, spec. 80%) and/or RV (sens. <80%, spec. 90%)
  postsurgical tamponade may be localized and not easily visible
  respirophasic Δ's in transvalvular velocities (↑ across TV & ↓ across MV with inspir)
- Cardiac catheterization (right heart and pericardial): elevation (15-30) and equalization of intrapericardial and diastolic pressures (RA, RV, PCWP), blunted *y* descent on RA tracing

Treatment

- Volume resuscitation (do not diurese!) and ⊕ inotropes
- Pericardiocentesis (except if due to aortic or myocardial rupture)

Constrictive Pericarditis

Etiology

- Any cause of pericarditis but especially **post-viral**, **radiation**, **uremia**, **TB**, **post-cardiac surgery**, and **idiopathic**

Pathophysiology

- Rigid pericardium limits diastolic filling → ↑ systemic venous pressures
- Venous return is limited only after early rapid filling phase; ∴ rapid ↓ in RA pressure with atrial relaxation and opening of the tricuspid valve and *prominent x and y descents.*
- Kussmaul's sign: inspiration → ↑ venous return but negative intrathoracic pressure not transmitted to heart because of rigid pericardium → ↑ JVP

Clinical manifestations
- Right-sided > left-sided heart failure

Physical exam
- ↑ **JVP** with **prominent *y* descent**, ⊕ **Kussmaul's sign** (Ddx = TS, acute cor pulmonale, RV infarct, RCMP)
- Hepatomegaly, ascites, peripheral edema
- PMI usually not palpable, **pericardial knock**, usually no pulsus paradoxus

Diagnostic studies
- CXR: calcification, especially in lateral view (although does not *necessarily* = constriction)
- ECG: nonspecific
- Echocardiogram: ± thickened pericardium, **"septal bounce"** = abrupt displacement of septum during rapid filling in early diastole
- Cardiac catheterization
  atria: **M's** or **W's** (prominent *x* and *y* descents)
  ventricles: **dip-and-plateau** or **square-root sign** (rapid ↓ pressure at onset of diastole, rapid ↑ to early plateau)
  discordance between LV & RV pressure peaks during respiratory cycle (*Circ* 1996;93:2007)
- CT or MRI: thickened pericardium with tethering

Constrictive Pericarditis vs. Restrictive Cardiomyopathy		
Evaluation	**Constrictive pericarditis**	**Restrictive cardiomyopathy**
Physical exam	⊕ Kussmaul's sign Absent PMI ⊕ pericardial knock	± Kussmaul's sign Powerful PMI, ± S_3 and S_4 ± **Regurgitant murmurs of MR, TR**
ECG	± Low voltage	Low voltage ± **Conduction abnormalities**
Echocardiogram	Normal wall thickness **Septal bounce during early diastole** Inspiration → ↑ flow across TV and ↓ flow across MV	± **↑ wall thickness** **Biatrial enlargement** Inspiration → ↓ flow across TV & MV Slower peak filling rate Longer time to peak filling rate
CT/MRI	**Thickened pericardium with tethering**	Normal pericardium
Cardiac catheterization	Prominent *x* and *y* descents Dip-and-plateau sign LVEDP = RVEDP RVSP <50 mm Hg RVEDP > 1/3 RVSP **Discordance** of LV and RV pressure peaks during respiratory cycle	Prominent *x* and *y* descents Dip-and-plateau sign ± **LVEDP > RVEDP** (espec. with vol.) RVSP >60 mm Hg RVEDP < 1/3 RVSP Concordance of LV and RV pressure peaks during respiratory cycle
Endomyocardial biopsy	Usually normal	± **Specific etiology of RCM**

Treatment
- Pericardiectomy

• HYPERTENSION •

JNC VII Classification		
Category	**Systolic (mm Hg)**	**Diastolic (mm Hg)**
Normal	<120	<80
Pre-HTN	120-139	80-89
Stage 1 HTN	140-159	90-99
Stage 2 HTN	≥160	≥100

(*JAMA* 2003;289:2560)

Etiologies
- **Essential** (95%): 10-15% of white adults, 25% of black adults; onset 25-55 yrs; ⊕ FHx
- **Renal** (4%): renovascular (= RAS, 2%); parenchymal (= chronic Na retention, 2%)
- **Endocrine** (0.5%): pheochromocytoma; 1° hyperaldosteronism; Cushing's syndrome
- Coarctation of the aorta (0.2%)
- Other: sleep apnea, OCP, sympathomimetics, COX-2 inhibitors, epo, CsA

Standard workup
- Goals: (1) identify CV risk factors or other diseases that would modify prognosis or therapy
  (2) reveal 2° causes of hypertension
  (3) assess for target-organ damage
- History
  signs and symptoms of CAD, CHF, TIA/CVA, PAD, DM, renal insufficiency; ⊕ FHx for HTN
  diet, Na intake, smoking, alcohol, prescription and OTC medications, OCP
- Physical exam: ≥2 BP measurements separated by >2 mins; verify in contralateral arm
  funduscopic, cardiac (LVH, murmurs), vascular, abdominal (masses or bruits), neurologic
- Laboratory tests: electrolytes, BUN, Cr, glc, Hct, U/A, lipids, ECG (look for LVH)

Secondary causes workup
- *Consider if Pt <20 or >50 yrs; sudden onset, severe, refractory or ↑ HTN; suggestive H&P*
- Renovascular disease
  clinical clues: older, h/o atherosclerosis, renal artery bruits, ARF with ACEI, ↓ K
    unilateral RAS (70%) → normovolemic & normal Cr
    bilateral RAS (30%) → hypervolemic, ↑ Cr
  diagnostic studies
    captopril renal scan: 90% sens., 90% spec., may miss bilateral RAS
    duplex ultrasound: highly operator dependent
    MRA: 90% sens., 90% spec., may overestimate severity of stenosis
    renal vein renins + captopril (affected/unaffected > 1.5/1): >80% sens., 60% spec.
    angiography: gold standard
- Renal parenchymal disease: BUN, Cr, Cr clearance
- Endocrine etiologies → see "Adrenal Disorders"
- Coarctation: ↓ LE pulses, systolic murmur, radiofemoral delay, LVH, rib-notching on CXR
  diagnostic studies: echocardiogram, aortogram

Complications of HTN
- *Each ↑ 20 mm Hg SBP or 10 mm Hg DBP → 2× ↑ CV complications* (*Lancet* 2002;360:1903)
- Neurologic: **TIA/CVA**, ruptured aneurysms
- Retinopathy: I = arteriolar narrowing, II = copper-wiring, AV nicking, III = hemorrhages and exudates, IV = papilledema
- Cardiac: **CAD**, LVH, **CHF**
- Vascular: aortic dissection, aortic aneurysm
- Renal: proteinuria, **renal failure**

Treatment (*NEJM* 2003;348:610)
- Goal: <140/90 mm Hg; if diabetes or renal disease goal is <130/80 mm Hg
- *Treatment results in 50% ↓ CHF, 40% ↓ stroke, 20-25% ↓ MI* (*Lancet* 2000;356:1955)
- **Lifestyle modifications** (each ↓ SBP ~5 mm Hg)
  weight loss: achieve BMI 18.5-24.9
  diet: rich in fruits & vegetables, low in saturated and total fat
  sodium restriction: ≤2.6 g/d
  exercise: ≥30 min exercise/d, most days of week
  limit alcohol consumption: ≤2 drinks/d in men; ≤1 drink/d in women & lighter-weight Pts

- **Pharmacologic options** (if HTN *or* pre-HTN + diabetes or renal disease)
  - hypertension alone: thiazide-type diuretic (ALLHAT, *JAMA* 2002;288:2981)
  - concomitant CV disease may lead to compelling indications for specific drug classes:
    - + atherosclerosis: ACEI (HOPE, *NEJM* 2000;342;145)
    - + angina: β-blockers
    - + post-MI: β-blockers, ACEI (BHAT, *JAMA* 1982;247:1707; SAVE, *NEJM* 1992;327:669; HOPE)
    - + CHF: ACEI/ARB, β-blockers, diuretics (see "Heart Failure")
    - + diabetes mellitus: ACEI (UKPDS 39, *BMJ* 1998;317:713)
    - + chronic kidney disease: ACEI/ARB (*NEJM* 1993;329:1456; 2001;345:851 & 861)
  - most Pts with essential hypertension will require ≥2 anti-hypertensive drugs to reach goal
  - if not at goal BP → optimize dosages or add additional drugs
    (if on 2 drugs, one should almost always be a thiazide-type diuretic)
- Secondary causes
  - renovascular: angioplasty ± stenting, surgery
  - renal parenchymal: salt and fluid restriction, ± diuretics
  - endocrine etiologies → see "Adrenal Disorders"

HYPERTENSIVE CRISIS

Definitions

- **Hypertensive emergency**: ↑ BP + acute target-organ damage
  - neurologic damage: encephalopathy, hemorrhagic or ischemic stroke, papilledema
  - cardiac damage: ACS, CHF, aortic dissection
  - renal damage: proteinuria, hematuria, acute renal failure; scleroderma renal crisis
  - microangiopathic hemolytic anemia
  - preeclampsia-eclampsia
- **Hypertensive urgency**: SBP >210 or DBP >120 with minimal or no target-organ damage

Treatment

- Hypertensive emergency: ↓ MAP by 25% in *mins to 2 hrs* using IV agents
- Hypertensive urgency: ↓ BP in *hrs* using PO agents

Drugs for Hypertensive Crises			
Intravenous agents		**Oral agents**	
Agent	**Dose**	**Agent**	**Dose**
Nitroprusside	0.25-10μg/kg/min	Captopril	25-50 mg
Nitroglycerin	17-1000 μg/min	Labetalol	200-1200 mg
Labetalol	20-80 mg bolus q 10 min or 2.0-4.0 mg/min	Clonidine	0.2 mg load → 0.1 mg q hr
Hydralazine	10-20 mg q 20-30 min	Hydralazine	10-25 mg
Phentolamine	5-15 mg bolus prn		

• AORTIC DISSECTION •

Definition (*Circ* 2003;108:628)
- **Classic dissection**: intimal tear → extravasation of blood into and along aortic media
- **Intramural hematoma** (IMH): ruptured vaso vasorum → blood in aortic media. May extend retrograde or anterograde and provoke 2° tear & communication w/ aortic lumen.
- **Penetrating ulcer**: ulceration of aortic plaque (usually in descending aorta) can penetrate intima → medial hemorrhage. Extension rare, but rupture possible.

Classification
- **Proximal**: involves ascending aorta, regardless of origin (= Stanford A, DeBakey I & II)
- **Distal**: involves descending aorta only (= Stanford B, DeBakey III)

Risk factors (predispose to medial micro apoplexy or "cystic medial necrosis")
- **Hypertension** (h/o HTN in >70% of dissections)
- **Connective tissue disease**
  Marfan's (*fibrillin-1* gene): arachnodactyly, joint disloc., pectus, ectopia lentis, MVP
  Ehlers-Danlos type IV (type III procollagen): translucent skin; bowel or uterine rupture
  Annuloaortic ectasia and familial aortic dissection
- **Congenital aortic anomaly**: bicuspid aortic valve or coarctation
- **Aortitis**: Takayasu's, giant cell arteritis
- **Pregnancy** (3rd trimester)
- **Trauma**: blunt, IABP, cardiac or aortic surgery

Clinical Manifestations and Physical Examination		
Feature	**Proximal**	**Distal**
Pain (abrupt, severe, persistent, tearing)	**94% (chest, back)**	**98% (back, chest, abd)**
Syncope (often tamponade)	**13%**	4%
CHF (usually AI)	**9%**	3%
CVA	**6%**	2%
Hypertension	35%	**70%**
Hypotension/shock (tamp., AI, rupt.)	**25%**	4%
Pulse deficit	**19%**	**9%**
AI murmur	**44%**	12%

(IRAD, *JAMA* 2000;283:897)

Diagnostic studies (*NEJM* 1993;328:35)
- **CXR**: abnormal in 60-90% (↑ mediastinum, effusion), but *cannot* be used to r/o dissection
- **CT**: quick, non-invasive, good sens. (80% for proximal; 90-95% for distal); spiral & multislice may improve sens.; *however, if ⊖ & high clin. suspicion → additional studies*
- **TEE**: sens. >95% for proximal, 80% for distal; can assess coronaries, pericardium, AI
- **MRI**: sens. & spec. >98%, but time-consuming & not readily available
- **Aortography**: sens. <90%, time-consuming, cannot detect IMH; can assess coronaries

Treatment (*Circ* 2003;108:772)
- **Medical: ↓ dP/dt**
  ***first* with IV β-blockers** (blunt reflex ↑ HR & inotropy in response to vasodilators)
  ***then* ↓ SBP with IV vasodilators**
  titrate SBP 110 & HR 60; use short-acting agents (propranolol + nitroprusside; labetalol)
  control pain with MSO_4 prn
- **Surgery**
  proximal (root replacement): all acute; chronic if c/b progression, AI or aneurysm
  distal: if c/b progression, signif. branch artery involvement, uncontrolled HTN, aneurysm
  ? endovascular stenting ± fenestration (*NEJM* 1999;340:1539 & 1546)

Complications
- **Rupture**: pericardial sac → tamponade; pleural space; mediastinum; retroperitoneum
- **Obstruction of branch artery**
  coronary → AMI (usually RCA → IMI)
  innominate/carotid → CVA; intercostal/lumbar → spinal cord ischemia/paraplegia
  innominate/subclavian → upper extremity ischemia; iliac → lower extremity ischemia
  celiac/mesenteric → bowel ischemia; renal → acute renal failure
- **AI**: due to annular dilatation or disruption or displacement of leaflet by false lumen

Prognosis
- Acute proximal dissection: mortality 1%/hr × 48 hrs

• ARRHYTHMIAS •

BRADYCARDIAS, AV BLOCK, AND AV DISSOCIATION

Sinus bradycardia (SB)

- Etiologies: **medications** (βB, CCB, amiodarone, Li), ↑ **vagal tone**, **metabolic** (severe hypoxia, sepsis, myxedema), ↑ **ICP**
- Treatment: usually none required; atropine or pacing if symptomatic

Sick sinus syndrome (SSS)

- Features may include: periods of unprovoked SB, SA arrest, paroxysms of SB and atrial tachyarrhythmias ("tachy-brady" syndrome)
- Treatment: meds alone (? βB with ISA) usually fail and need **combination** of **meds** (βB, CCB, dig) for tachyarrhythmias and **PPM** for bradycardia

AV Block	
Type	**Features**
1°	Prolonged PR (>200 msec), but all impulses conducted.
2° Mobitz I (Wenckebach)	Progressive ↑ PR until impulse not conducted (→ "grouped beating"). Usually AV nodal in origin and transient. Seen in IMI, myocarditis. Classically (~50%), absolute ↑ in PR *decreases* over time (→ ↓ RR intervals, duration of pause <2× preceding RR interval). AVB usually worsens with CSM, improves with atropine. Often no Rx required.
2° Mobitz II	Occasional or repetitive blocked impulses w/o ↑ PR. Usually His-Purkinje in origin, chronic, and may precede 3° AVB. Seen in anteroseptal MI, degeneration of conduction system. AVB usually improves with CSM, worsens with atropine. Pacing wire or PPM often required.
3° (complete)	No conduction. Must distinguish from other forms of AV dissociation.

"High-grade" AVB usually refers to block of 2 or more successive impulses.

AV dissociation *(not a primary diagnosis, rather a manifestation of one of 3 processes)*

- *Default:* slowing of SA node allows subsidiary pacemaker (e.g., AV junction) to take over.
- *Usurpation:* acceleration of subsidiary pacemaker (e.g., nonparoxysmal AV jxnal tachycardia, VT w/o retrograde atrial capture).
- *AV Block:* prevention of normal pacemaker from capturing ventricles allows subsidiary pacemaker to take control of ventricle.

SUPRAVENTRICULAR TACHYCARDIAS (SVTs)

*Arise above the ventricles, ∴ **narrow QRS** unless aberrant conduction or preexcitation.*

Etiologies of SVT		
	SVT	**Description**
Atrial	Sinus tachycardia (ST)	Caused by pain, fever, hypovolemia, hypoxia, anemia, anxiety, β-agonists, etc.
Atrial	SA node reentrant tachycardia (SANRT)	Reentrant loop within SA node
Atrial	Atrial tachycardia (AT)	Originate at site in atria other than SA node Seen w/ CAD, COPD, ↑ catechols, EtOH, dig
Atrial	Multifocal atrial tachycardia (MAT)	↑ automaticity at multiple sites in the atria
Atrial	Atrial flutter (AFL)	Macroreentry within the right atrium
Atrial	Atrial fibrillation (AF)	Wavelets irregularly passing down AVN
AV Jxn	AV nodal reentrant tachycardia (AVNRT)	Reentry using dual pathways in AVN
AV Jxn	Atrioventricular reciprocating tachycardia (AVRT)	Reentry using accessory pathway
AV Jxn	Nonparoxysmal junctional tachycardia (NPJT)	↑ automaticity at AV junction Retrograde atrial capture or AV dissociation Seen in myo/endocarditis, card. surg, IMI, dig

(*NEJM* 1995;332:162)

Diagnosis (*Cardiol Clin* 1990;8:411; *Med Clin* 2001;85:193)

- **Onset**: abrupt onset/offset suggests AVNRT or AVRT; ST & AT tend to "warm up"
- **Rate**: not diagnostic as most SVTs can have a rate ranging from 140-250 bpm, *but:*
  ST is usually <150 bpm
  AFL often conducts with 2:1 AV block to give a ventricular rate of 150
  AVNRT and AVRT are usually >150 bpm
- **Rhythm**: if irregular, Ddx is limited to AF, AFL w/ variable block, and MAT
- **P wave morphology**: very helpful
  Upright P waves immediately before the QRS → ST (normal P), AT (P different from sinus, could be inverted and before QRS), MAT (≥3 different P wave morphologies)
  Retrograde P waves appear *inverted* in inferior leads and can appear in several locations:
  In AVNRT they are usually buried in or distort the terminal portion of the QRS (i.e., pseudo-S waves in the inferior leads and pseudo-R′ waves in lead V_1)
  In AVRT they are usually slightly after but distinct from the QRS
  Usually short RP interval, but atypical forms can have long RP
  No P waves or fine fibrillatory "f" waves → AF
  Saw-toothed "F" waves at a rate of ~300 bpm → AFL
- **Response to vagal maneuvers** (CSM, Valsalva) or **adenosine** (or β-blockers or CCB)
  Rhythms due to ↑ automaticity (ST, AT, MAT) → slowing of rate or ↑ AV block
  Rhythms due to reentry at AVN (AVNRT, AVRT) → abruptly terminate or no response
  AFL → ↑ AV block → unmasking of "F" waves

Fig. 1-3. Approach to SVT

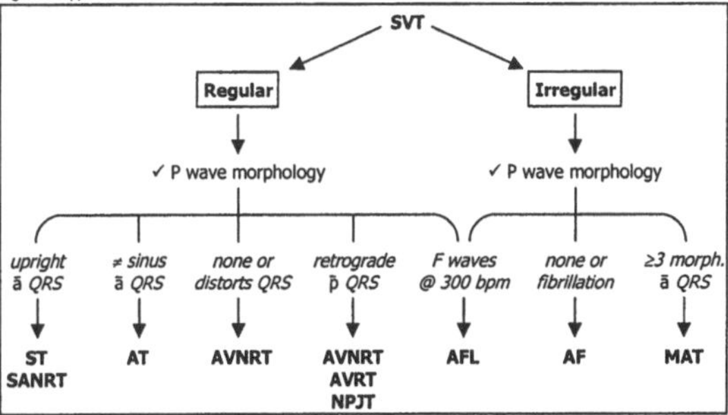

Treatment of SVT		
Rhythm	**Acute treatment**	**Long-term treatment**
Unstable	**Cardioversion** per ACLS	n/a
ST	n/a	n/a
AT	β-blockers or CCB	β-blockers or CCB ± anti-arrhythmics ? Radiofrequency ablation
AVNRT or AVRT	**Vagal maneuvers, adenosine** **CCB, β-blockers** (*Avoid IV verapamil & digoxin* if suspect accessory pathway)	**Radiofrequency ablation** CCB or β-blockers ± anti-arrhythmics
AF	**β-blockers, CCB, digoxin**	see "Atrial Fibrillation"
AFL	**β-blockers, CCB, digoxin**	Radiofrequency ablation β-blockers or CCB ± anti-arrhythmics
MAT	**CCB**	Treat underlying disease process ? AVN ablation + PPM

- Radiofrequency ablation has an overall success rate >95%. Complications include stroke, MI, bleeding, cardiac perforation, and conduction block.

Accessory Pathways (Wolff-Parkinson-White)

Definitions

- **Accessory pathway** (bypass tract) connecting atria to ventricles, allowing impulses to bypass AVN conduction delay
- **Preexcitation (WPW) pattern**: ↓ PR interval, ↑ QRS width w/ δ wave (slurred onset, *can be subtle*), ST & Tw abnormalities; only seen in pathways that conduct anterograde (if pathway only conducts retrograde then ECG is normal during SR and Pt has a "concealed" bypass tract)
- **WPW syndrome**: accessory pathway + tachycardia

Tachycardias

- **Orthodromic AVRT**: *narrow-complex* SVT conducting ↓ AVN & ↑ accessory pathway; requires retrograde conduction and ∴ can occur w/ concealed bypass tracts
- **Antidromic AVRT**: *wide-complex* SVT conducting ↓ accessory pathway & ↑ AVN; requires anterograde conduction and ∴ should see WPW pattern during SR
- **AF with rapid conduction** down accessory pathway, ∴ wide-complex irregular SVT; requires anterograde conduction and ∴ should see WPW pattern during SR

Treatment

- **AVRT**: vagal maneuvers, adenosine, β-blockers, (CCB); *always have defibrillator ready*
- **AF**: ↑ refractoriness of accessory pathway with procainamide *or* cardiovert
  digoxin can ↓ refractoriness of pathway → ↑ ventricular rate; *IV verapamil* → VF;
  as AF can develop during AVRT, *avoid these drugs*
- **Long-term**: Rx tachycardias with radiofrequency ablation or anti-arrhythmics (IA, IC)
  consider prophylactic ablation if asx but AVRT or AF inducible on EPS (*NEJM* 2003;349:1803)
  risk of SCD related to how short R-R interval is in AF

Wide-Complex Tachycardias (WCTs)

Etiologies

- **Ventricular tachycardia (VT)**
- **SVT conducted with aberrancy** (either fixed BBB, rate-dependent BBB, or an accessory pathway). Rate-dependent aberrancy usually presents with RBBB morphology.

Ventricular tachycardia

- **Monomorphic**
  Structurally *abnormal* heart: **prior MI**, **CMP**, arrhythmogenic RV dysplasia (ARVD, incomplete RBBB, right-sided TWI, ε wave on resting ECG, LBBB-type VT, dx w/ MRI)
  Structurally *normal* heart: RVOT VT (normal resting ECG, LBBB-type VT), idiopathic LV VT (responds to verapamil), Brugada syndrome (pseudo-RBBB w/ STE on resting ECG)
- **Polymorphic**: **ischemia**, **CMP**, **torsades de pointes** (= polymorphic VT + ↑ QT)

Diagnostic clues that favor VT

- Assume all WCT is VT until proven otherwise
- **Prior MI**, **CHF**, or **LV dysfunction** *best predictors* that WCT is VT (*Am J Med* 1998;84:53)
- Hemodynamic compromise and rate of tachycardia do *not* reliably distinguish VT from SVT
- Monomorphic VT is regular, but initially it may be slightly irregular, mimicking AF with aberrancy; *grossly* irregularly irregular rhythm suggests AF with aberrancy
- ECG features that favor VT (*Circ* 1991;83:1649)
  AV dissociation (independent P waves, capture or fusion beats) proves VT
  very wide QRS (>140 msec in RBBB-type or >160 msec in LBBB-type)
  extreme axis deviation
  QRS morphology atypical for BBB
  RBBB-type: absence of tall R′ (or presence of monophasic R) in V_1, r/S ratio <1 in V_6
  LBBB-type: onset to nadir >60-100 msec in V_1, q wave in V_6
  concordance (all precordial leads in same direction)

Long-term treatment

- Workup: **echo** to ✓ LV fxn, **cath** or **stress test** to r/o ischemia, ? MRI and/or RV bx to look for infiltrative cardiomyopathy or ARVD, **EP study** to assess for inducibility
- **Medications**: β-blockers, anti-arrhythmics (e.g., amiodarone)
- **Radiofrequency ablation** if isolated VT focus
- **ICD** (*NEJM* 2003;349:1836) potentially indicated in Pts with the following hx:
  SCD, VF, sx VT (AVID, *NEJM* 1997;337:1576; CASH, *Circ* 2000;102:748)
  non-sust. VT + CAD + ↓ EF + induc. (MADIT, *NEJM* 1996;335:1933; MUSTT, *NEJM* 1999;341:1882)
  CAD + EF <30% (MADIT II, *NEJM* 2002;346:877; high-risk Pts who benefit most remain undefined)
  nonischemic DCMP + *either* EF <35% (DEFINITE, SCD-HeFT) *or* unexplained syncope
  ? HCMP (*NEJM* 2000;342:365); congenital ↑ QT; Brugada syndrome

• ATRIAL FIBRILLATION •

Etiologies

- Acute
  - **Cardiac**: ischemia, MI, CHF, myocarditis/pericarditis, hypertensive crisis, cardiac surgery
  - **Pulmonary**: acute pulmonary disease or hypoxia (e.g., COPD flare, pneumonia), PE
  - **Metabolic**: high catecholamine states (stress, infection, post-op), thyrotoxicosis
  - **Drugs**: alcohol, cocaine, amphetamines, theophylline
- Chronic: older age, HTN, ischemia, valvular disease (MS, MR, AS), CMP, hyperthyroidism

Evaluation

- ECG, CXR, echocardiogram (LA size, presence of thrombus, valves, LV fxn, pericardium), r/o ischemia (but AF unlikely due to ischemia *in absence of other sxs*), TFTs

Fig. 1-4. Approach to acute AF

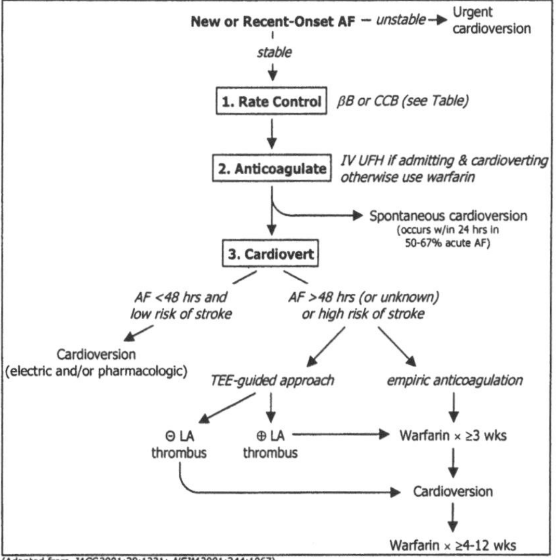

(Adapted from *JACC* 2001;38:1231; *NEJM* 2001;344:1067)

Rate Control for Acute AF			
Agent		**Dose**	**Side effects and comments**
CCB	**Verapamil**	5-10 mg IV over 2 min May repeat in 30 min	Hypotension (treat w/ Ca gluconate) *Contraindicated* in WCTs
CCB	**Diltiazem**	20 mg IV over 2 min May repeat in 15 min 5-15 mg/hr infusion	
βB	**Metoprolol**	5 mg IV over 2 min May repeat q 5 min × 3	Bronchoconstriction; hypotension
βB	**Propranolol**	1 mg IV q 2 min	
Digoxin		0.5 mg IV × 1, *then* 0.25 mg IV q 6 hrs × 2	Consider for patients in CHF

(Adapted from *NEJM* 2001;344:1067 & *Annals* 2003;139:1018)

Anti-Arrhythmics for AF			
Agent	Dose		Comments
	Conversion	Maintenance	
Ibutilide	1 mg IV over 10′ May repeat × 1	n/a	Contraindic. if ↓ K or ↑ QT 3-8% risk of torsades Mg 1-2 g IV to ↓ risk TdP
Dofetilide	0.5 mg PO bid	0.5 mg bid	✓ for ↑ QT Need to renally adjust
Flecainide	300 mg PO × 1	50-150 mg bid	*Contraindic. if struct. heart disease*
Propafenone	600 mg PO × 1	150-300 mg bid	Pretreat with AVN blocker
Amiodarone	150 mg IV over 10′ *then* 1 mg/min × 6 hrs *then* 0.5 mg/min	600 mg bid × 2 wks 200-400 qd	± Cardioversion efficacy Best drug to maintain SR Helps with rate control ✓ for ↑ QT Pulm, liver, thyroid toxicity
Procainamide	10-15 mg/kg IV over 1 hr	1000-2000 mg bid of slow release	Hypotension, ↓ inotropy ± PreRx with AVN blocker ✓ for ↑ QT
Sotalol	n/a	120-160 mg bid	✓ for ↓ HR, ↑ QT Need to renally adjust

(Adapted from *NEJM* 2001;344:1067 & *Annals* 2003;139:1018)

Cardioversion

- Consider in Pts with 1st episode of AF or in those with sx due to AF
- Likelihood of success dependent on AF duration and atrial size
- Consider pretreatment with anti-arrhythmic drugs (especially if 1st attempt fails)
- If duration of AF >48 hrs, cardioversion has 2-5% chance of *precipitating CVA*, ∴ must either visualize LA with TEE to r/o thrombus (ACUTE, *NEJM* 2001;344:1411) or empirically anticoagulate for ≥3 wks before
- Even if SR returns, atria are *mechanically stunned*. Also, greatest likelihood of recurrent AF in first 3 months after return to SR, ∴ must anticoagulate post-cardioversion ≥4-12 wks

Rate control (HR 60-80, 80-100 with exertion)

- β-blockers (especially if CAD)
- CCB (especially if COPD; n.b., that verapamil ↑ dig levels)
- Digoxin (poor efficacy for exertional HR control; consider in Pts with CHF)

Rhythm control

- Recent trial data suggest rhythm control offers no mortality benefit to rate control + anticoagulation in Pts with recurrent AF (AFFIRM, *NEJM* 2002;347:1825; *NEJM* 2002;347:1834)
- Anti-arrhythmic drug therapy: see above table
  CHF → dofetilide or amiodarone
  CAD → sotalol, dofetilide, amiodarone
- Radiofrequency ablation of foci at pulmonary veins (*NEJM* 1998;339:659; *JACC* 2003;42:185)
- Catheter-based or surgical "maze" procedure
- AV node ablation + PPM (*NEJM* 2001;344:1043 and 2002;346:2062)

Anticoagulation (*Archives* 1994;154:1449)

- Risk of stroke ↑↑ in valvular AF (i.e., 2° to MS, MR), ∴ anticoagulate all
- Risk of stroke ~4.5% per year in non-valvular AF; risk factors include:
  clinical: **prior stroke/TIA, diabetes, HTN, older age (≥65 yrs), CHF**, ? CAD
  echocardiographic: ↓ EF, ↑ LA size
- Risk of stroke in recurrent paroxysmal AF ≈ persistent AF
- "Lone AF" = AF in the absence of structural heart disease or any of the above risk factors
- Treatment options
  warfarin (INR goal 2-3, *NEJM* 1996;335:540 & 2003;349:1019) → 68% ↓ stroke
  aspirin: better than placebo (44% ↓ stroke) but inferior to warfarin
  ? ximelagatran ≈ warfarin (SPORTIF III, *Lancet* 2003;362:1691 & SPORTIF V, AHA 2003); ✓ LFTs
- Whom to treat
  valvular AF → warfarin
  non-valvular persistent or paroxysmal AF + ≥1 risk factor → warfarin
  (if age 65-74 and no other risk factors → ? aspirin)
  if Pt not good candidate for warfarin (↑ risk of bleeding/falling) → aspirin
  lone AF → aspirin or no Rx

• SYNCOPE •

Definition
- Sudden transient loss of consciousness due to cerebral hypoperfusion

Etiologies
- **Neurocardiogenic** (a.k.a. vasovagal, ~25%): ↑ sympathetic tone → vigorous contraction of LV → mechanoreceptors in LV trigger ↑ vagal tone (hyperactive Bezold-Jarisch reflex) → ↓ HR (cardioinhibitory) and/or ↓ BP (vasodepressor)
  related disorders: carotid hypersensitivity, cough, defecation, or micturition syncope
- **Orthostatic hypotension** (10%)
  hypovolemia, diuretics
  vasodilators (α-blockers, nitrates, ACEI, CCB, hydralazine)
  autonomic neuropathy (diabetes, EtOH, amyloid, renal failure, Shy-Drager)
- **Cardiovascular**
  Mechanical (5%)
    Endocardial: AS, MS, PS, prosthetic valve thrombosis, myxoma
    Myocardial: MI (but usually VT), HCMP (but usually VT)
    Pericardial: tamponade
    Vascular: aortic dissection, PE, PHT, subclavian steal
  Arrhythmia (15%)
    Bradyarrhythmias: SSS, high-grade AV block, PPM malfunction
    Tachyarrhythmias: VT, SVT (rare to cause syncope unless structural heart disease)
- **Neurologic** (10%): seizure (technically not syncope), TIA/CVA/VBI, migraine
- **Miscellaneous** (technically not syncope): hypoglycemia, hypoxia, anemia, psychogenic

Workup (etiology cannot be determined in ~35% of cases)
- **History** (from Pt and *witnesses* if available)
  activity and posture before the incident
  precipitating factors: exertion (AS, HCMP, PHT), positional Δ (orthostatic hypotension), stressors such as sight of blood, pain, emotional distress, fatigue, prolonged standing, warm environment, cough/micturition/defecation (neurocardiogenic)
  prodrome (e.g., diaphoresis, nausea, blurry vision): cardiac <5 sec, vasovagal >5 sec
  associated sx: chest pain, palp., neurologic, post-ictal, bowel or bladder incontinence
- **Past medical history**: prior syncope, previous cardiac or neurologic disease
- **Medications**
  vasodilators (e.g., α-blockers, nitrates, ACEI, CCB, hydralazine) and diuretics
  ⊖ chronotropes (e.g., β-blockers and CCB)
  ↑ QT: class IA or III antiarrhythmics, phenothiazines, TCAs, antihistamines, erythromycin, azoles
  psychoactive drugs: antipsychotics, TCA, barbiturates, benzodiazepines, EtOH
- **Family history**: CMP, SCD
- **Physical exam**
  VS including *orthostatics* (supine → standing results in >10-20 mmHg ↓ SBP or >10-20 bpm ↑ HR), BP in both arms
  cardiac exam: JVP, murmurs, LVH (S_4, LV heave), CHF (crackles, displaced PMI, S_3)
  vascular exam: ✓ for asymmetric pulses, carotid bruits
  fecal occult blood test
  neurologic exam: focal findings, evidence of tongue biting
- **ECG** (abnormal in ~50%, definitively identifies cause of syncope in ~10%)
  sinus bradycardia, sinus pauses, AVB, BBB, SVT, VT
  ischemic changes (new or old)
  atrial or ventricular hypertrophy
  markers of arrhythmia (ectopy, prolonged QT, preexcitation)

Other diagnostic studies (consider ordering based on results of H&P and ECG)
- Ambulatory ECG monitoring: if suspect arrhythmogenic syncope
  Holter monitoring (continuous ECG) yield (*Am J Med* 1991;90:91)
    arrhythmia + sx (4%); asx but signif. arrhythmia (13%); sx but no arrhythmia (17%)
  Event recorder (yield 20-50%)
    can be activated by Pt to record rhythm strip (problematic if no prodrome)
    loop recorders continuously save rhythm strip and ∴ can be activated *after* an event
    implantable loop recorders can be used for Pts with infrequent events

- Echocardiogram: if suspect structural heart disease based on cardiac exam or ECG
- Exercise stress test: r/o ischemia- or catecholamine-induced arrhythmias
- Cardiac catheterization: consider if non-invasive tests suggest ischemia
- Electrophysiologic studies (EPS)
  consider if arrhythmia on ECG, Holter or loop recorder or if structural heart disease
  50% abnl (inducible VT, conduction abnormalities) if heart disease, but ? significance
  3-20% abnl if abnl ECG; <1% abnl if normal heart and normal ECG (*Annals* 1997;127:76)
- Tilt table testing (provocative test for vasovagal syncope)
  ⊕ tests in 50% of Pts w/ recurrent unexplained syncope; spec. ≤90%; reproduc. ≤80%
- Neurologic studies (cerebrovascular studies, CT, MRI, EEG): if H&P suggestive

Fig. 1-5. Approach to syncope

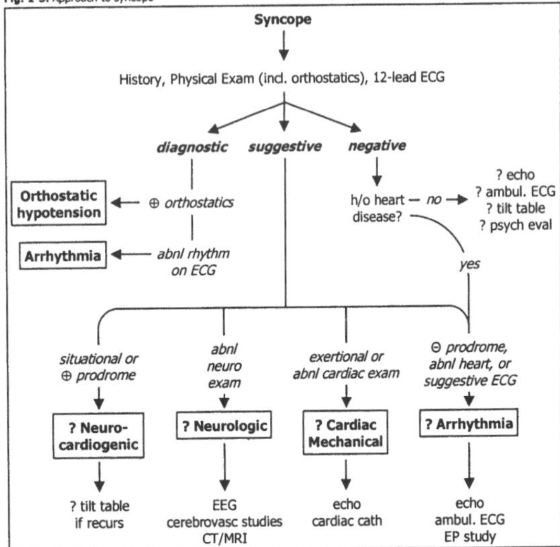

High-risk features (usually warrant admission with telemetry & further testing)
- Age >60 yrs, h/o CAD, CMP, valvular disease, congenital heart disease, arrhythmias
- Syncope c/w cardiac cause (lack of prodrome, exertional, resultant trauma)
- Abnormal cardiac exam
- Abnormal ECG

Treatment
- Cardiac or neurologic syncope: treat underlying disorder
- Orthostatic syncope: volume replete; if chronic → rise from supine to standing *slowly*, compressive stockings, midodrine, fludrocortisone
- Vasovagal syncope: ? β-blockers, disopyramide, midodrine, fludrocortisone, anticholinergics, theophylline; pacemaker of no benefit (VPS II, *JAMA* 2003;289:2224)

Prognosis (*NEJM* 1983;309:197, *Ann Emerg Med* 1997;29:459)
- Cardiac syncope: 20-40% 1-year SCD rate
- Noncardiac or unexplained syncope with normal ECG, no history of VT, no CHF, age <45 low recurrence rate and <5% 1-year SCD rate

• PACEMAKERS •

Pacemaker Code			
1st letter	**2nd letter**	**3rd letter**	**4th letter**
Chamber paced	Chamber sensed	Response to sensed beat	Programmable features

A = atrial, V = ventricular, I = inhibited, D = dual, R = rate-adaptive

Common Pacing Modes	
Mode	**Description**
VVI	Ventricular pacing on demand w/ single lead in RV. Sensed ventricular beat inhibits V pacing. Used in Pt w/ chronic AF and symptomatic bradycardia.
DDI	Atrial & ventricular sensing and pacing w/ leads in RA and RV. Sensed atrial beat inhibits A pacing; sensed ventricular beat inhibits V pacing. No tracking of intrinsic atrial activity. Used in Pts requiring atrial & ventricular pacing but who have frequent SVTs that might be inappropriately tracked by DDD PPM.
DDD	Atrial & ventricular sensing and pacing w/ leads in RA and RV. Sensed atrial beat inhibits A pacing *and triggers V pacing*, thereby allowing tracking of intrinsic atrial activity; sensed ventricular beat inhibits ventricular pacing. Used in Pts requiring atrial & ventricular pacing and AV synchrony.
Magnet	Magnet placed over generator Δ setting to DOO/VOO in which PPM paces ventricle at fixed rate regardless of ventricular activity. Use to check PPM's ability to capture when output inhibited by Pt's intrinsic rhythm. Use when Pt hemodynamically unstable due to bradycardia from inappropriate PPM inhibition or tachycardia that is pacemaker-induced.

Indications for Pacing	
Disorder	**Indications**
AV block	Symptomatic 3° or 2° AVB ? Asymptomatic 3° AVB or type II 2° AVB HR <40, pauses ≥3 sec while awake
Sinus node dysfunction	Sinus bradycardia or sinus pauses clearly associated with sxs ? SB or pauses in symptomatic Pt w/o clear association
Acute MI	See "STEMI"
Tachyarrhythmia	Symptomatic recurrent SVT that can be terminated by pacing after failing drugs and catheter ablation Sustained pause-dependent VT ? High-risk Pts w/ congenital long QT syndrome
Syncope	Hypersensitive carotid sinus syncope with asystole >3 secs ? Neurocardiogenic syncope w/ prominent cardioinhib. response
Cardiomyopathy	? Symptomatic HCMP with significant outflow obstruction

(*NEJM* 1996;334:89; *Circulation* 1998;97:1325; *JAMA* 2002;287:1848)

Complications		
Mode	**Manifestation**	**Description**
Failure to pace	Bradycardia	Battery depletion, lead fracture/dislodgment, ↑ pacing threshold due to local tissue rxn, or myopotential sensing → inappropriate inhibition. ✓ lead placement and settings.
Failure to sense	Inappropriate pacing	Lead dislodgment or sensing threshold set too high. Check lead placement and settings.
Pacemaker-mediated tachycardia	Tachycardia	Seen with DDD. Ventricular depolarization → retrograde atrial activation → sensed by atrial lead → triggers ventricular pacing → retrograde atrial activation, etc. Terminate with vagal maneuvers or magnet; usually requires Δ in settings.
Pacemaker syndrome	Syncope/presyncope, orthopnea, PND, CHF	Seen with VVI. Due to loss of AV synchrony → ↓ CO, ↑ atrial pressures. Change to DDD.

• CARDIAC RISK ASSESSMENT FOR NONCARDIAC SURGERY •

Goldman Criteria for General Surgery	
Risk factor	**Points**
History	
Age >70 yrs	5
MI within 6 mos	10
Physical exam	
S_3 or JVD on physical exam	11
Significant aortic stenosis	3
ECG	
Rhythm other than sinus rhythm on preop ECG	7
>5 PVCs/min at any time preop	7
General status (any of the following) PO_2 <60 mmHg, PCO_2 >50 mmHg, K <3.0 mEq/L, HCO_3 <20 mEq/L, BUN >50 mg/dl, Cr >3 mg/dl, ↑ AST, chronic liver disease, or bedridden due to noncardiac cause	3
Operation	
Intra-abdominal, intrathoracic, or aortic surgery	3
Emergency surgery	4

Risk Assessment				
Class	**Points**	**None/Minor Complic.**	**Serious Complic.**	**Cardiac Death**
I	0-5	99%	0.6%	0.2%
II	6-12	96%	3%	1%
III	13-25	86%	11%	2%
IV	>25	49%	12%	39%
Serious complication = perioperative MI, pulmonary edema, or VT				

(*NEJM* 1977;297:845, *Med Clin North Am* 1987;71:416)

Revised Cardiac Index for General Surgery	
Risk factor	**Points**
High risk surgery (intraperitoneal, intrathoracic, aortic)	1
Ischemic heart disease (prior MI, ⊕ ETT, angina, nitrate use, Qw)	1
History of CHF	1
History of cerebrovascular disease	1
Insulin therapy for diabetes	1
Preoperative serum Cr >2.0 mg/dl	1

Risk Assessment			
Class	**# Factors**	**Cardiac Complication Rate**	
		Derivation Set	**Validation Set**
I	0	0.5%	0.4%
II	1	1.3%	0.9%
III	2	3.6%	6.6%
IV	3-6	9.1%	11.0%
Cardiac complication = MI, CHF, VF, complete heart block			

(*Circ* 1999;100:1043)

Eagle Criteria for Vascular Surgery	
Clinical variables	**Stress testing**
Age >70 yrs Angina Diabetes requiring Rx Significant ventricular ectopy Q waves on ECG	Pts undergoing vascular surgery have high incidence of CAD. Claudication typically prevents Pts from displaying angina. Consider pharmacologic stress test (adenosine-MIBI or dobutamine stress echo) in Pts w/ 1-2 variables.

Risk Assessment				
# Variables	**0**	**1-2**		**≥3**
Stress test	n/a	⊖	⊕	n/a
Event rate	3.1%	3.2%	29.6%	50%

(*Annals* 1989;110:863)

ACC/AHA Guidelines (*Circ* 2002;105:1257)

Clinical Markers		
Major	**Intermediate**	**Minor**
• ACS • Decompensated CHF • Significant arrhythmia (e.g., high-grade AVB, VT, SVT w/ uncontrolled HR) • Severe valvular heart disease	• Mild angina pectoris • Prior MI • Compensated/prior CHF • Diabetes mellitus	• Advanced age • Abnormal ECG (e.g., LVH, LBBB, ST-T abnormalities) • Rhythm other than sinus • Low functional capacity • Prior CVA • Uncontrolled HTN

If possible, wait >4-6 wks after MI (even if ⊖ ETT or ⊕ ETT & revascularized). If Pt revascularized with a stent (especially a drug-eluting stent) avoid surgery until Pt can safely d/c anti-platelet medications; early d/c can lead to stent thrombosis. If not going to be revascularized, wait 6 months before elective surgery.

Functional Capacity		
1-4 METs	**4-10 METs**	**>10 METs**
ADLs	Climb a flight of stairs Heavy housework Exercise	Sports

Surgery-Specific Risk		
High	**Intermediate**	**Low**
• Emergent operation • Aortic or other major vascular • Peripheral vascular • Prolonged	• Carotid endarterectomy • Head and neck • Intraperitoneal • Intrathoracic • Orthopedic • Prostate	• Endoscopic • Superficial • Cataract • Breast

Noninvasive Testing Result		
High risk	**Intermediate risk**	**Low risk**
Ischemia at <4 METs and • ST ↓ ≥1 mm • ST ↑ ≥1 mm • ≥5 abnormal leads • Persistent ischemia >3 min after exertion • Typical angina	***Ischemia at 4-6 METs and*** • ST ↓ ≥1 mm • Typical angina • 3-4 abnormal leads • Persistent ischemia 1-3 min after exertion	***No ischemia or ischemia at >7 METs and*** • ST ↓ ≥1 mm • Typical angina • 1-2 abnormal leads

Fig. 1-6. Approach to preoperative cardiovascular evaluation

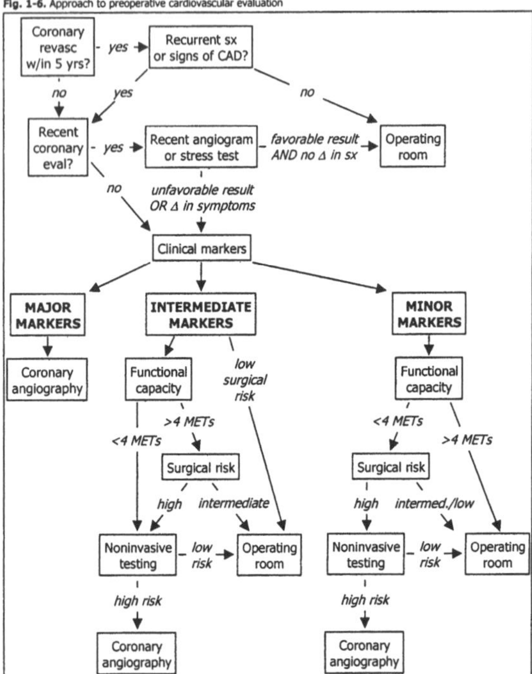

(Adapted from ACC/AHA Guideline Update for Perioperative Cardiovascular Evaluation for Noncardiac Surgery. *Circ* 2002;105:1257)

Preoperative and perioperative monitoring and therapy

- **Coronary revascularization** should be based on standard indications. If warranted, should *precede* intermediate or high-risk surgery. Given need for dual antiplatelet Rx after stenting, wait 4-6 wks after bare metal stent and ? >3 mos after drug-eluting stent.
- **β-blockers**: start before and continue after surgery, titrate to HR ~55 bpm; 65-90% ↓ cardiac death and MI (*NEJM* 1996;335:1713 & 1999;341:1789)
- **PA catheter**: consider in surgeries with large fluid shifts and in Pts with recent MI c/b CHF, h/o CHF, CMP, valvular disease, extensive CAD

• DYSPNEA •

Fig. 2-1. Causes of dyspnea

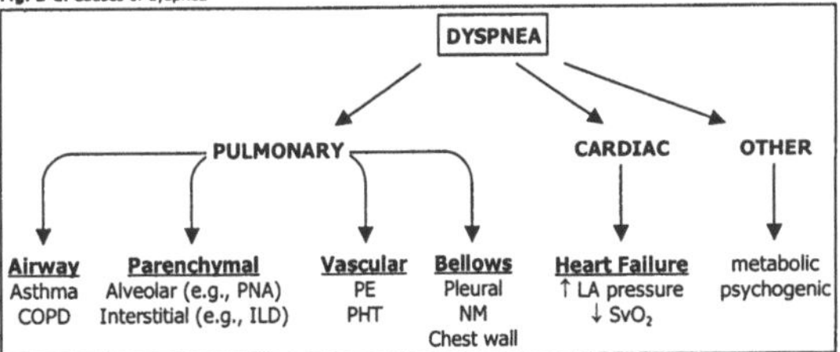

• PULMONARY FUNCTION TESTS (PFTs) •

Fig. 2-2. Approach to abnormal PFTs

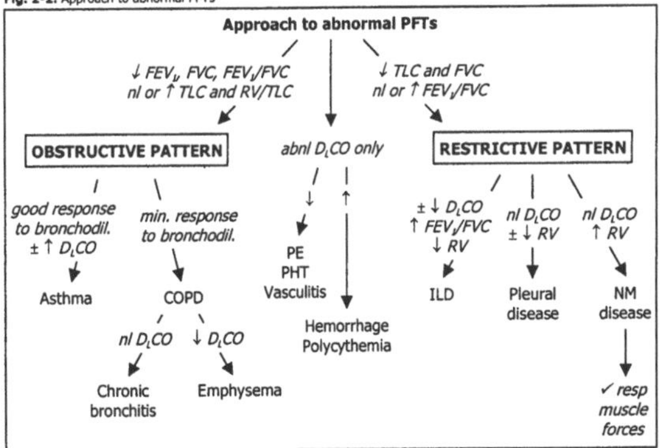

Utility of specific tests

- **Spirometry**: evaluate for obstructive disease
  - Flow-volume loops: diagnose and/or localize obstruction
  - Bronchodilator: indicated if obstruction present at baseline or asthma clinically suspected
  - Methacholine challenge: if spirometry *normal*, may use to diagnose asthma
- **Lung volumes**: evaluate for restrictive disease
- **D_LCO**: further differentiation of abnormal spirometry and volumes, evaluation for pulmonary vascular disease
- **Respiratory forces**: evaluate for neuromuscular causes of restrictive disease

• ASTHMA •

Definition and epidemiology
- Chronic inflamm. disorder w/ **airway hyperresponsiveness** + **var. airflow obstruction**
- Affects ~5% population; ~85% of cases by age 40; ? linked to ADAM-33 (*NEJM* 2002;947:936)

Clinical manifestations (*NEJM* 2001;344:350)
- Classic triad = **wheezing, cough, and dyspnea**; others include chest tightness, sputum; symptoms typically *chronic* with *episodic exacerbation*
- Precipitants (**"triggers"**)
  respiratory irritants (perfumes, smoke, laundry detergents, strong odors)
  allergens (house pets, carpets, dust mites, pollen)
  infections (URI, bronchitis, sinusitis)
  drugs (e.g., ASA via leukotrienes, βB via bronchospasm, morphine via histamine release)
  stress, cold air
- Exacerbations: important to note frequency, severity, duration, and required treatment including need for steroids, ED visits, hospitalizations, and intubations

Physical examination
- Wheezing and prolonged expiratory phase
- Presence of nasal polyps, rhinitis, rash → *allergic component*
- Exacerbation → pulsus paradoxus, use of accessory muscles of respiration

Diagnostic studies
- **PFTs**:
  ↓ peak expiratory flow rate (PEFR)
  spirometry: ↓ FEV_1, ↓ FEV_1/FVC ratio, coved flow-volume loop
  lung volumes: ± ↑ RV and ↑ TLC
  ⊕ bronchodilator response (↑ FEV_1 ≥12%) strongly suggestive of asthma
  methacholine challenge (↓ FEV_1 ≥20%) useful if asthma suspected but PFTs normal
  sens. >90%, NPV 95% (*AJRCCM* 2000;161:309)
- Allergy suspected → consider ✓ serum IgE, eosinophils, skin testing/RAST
- Sputum: *Curschmann's spirals* (mucus casts of distal airways), *Charcot-Leyden* crystals; normalization of sputum eosinophil count may help guide outPt Rx (*Lancet* 2002;360:1715)

Ddx ("all that wheezes is not asthma...")
- Mechanical airway obstruction or structural airway abnormalities (e.g., tumor)
- Laryngeal or vocal cord dysfunction (e.g., due to GERD or postnasal drip)
- COPD, CHF, vasculitis: consider in older Pts with new dx of "asthma"
- Other pulmonary causes: bronchiectasis, PE, aspiration, sarcoidosis, ILD
- "Asthma +" syndromes (*Lancet* 2002;360:1313)
  Atopy = asthma + allergic rhinitis + atopic dermatitis
  ASA-sensitive asthma (Samter's syndrome) = asthma + ASA sensitivity + nasal polyps
  ABPA = asthma + pulmonary infiltrates + allergic rxn to *Aspergillus*
  Churg-Strauss = asthma + eosinophilia + granulomatous vasculitis

"Quick-relief" medications
- *Short-acting* inhaled **β_2-agonists** (albuterol, pirbuterol, terbutaline): treatment of choice
- Inhaled **anticholinergics** (ipratropium) improve β_2-agonist delivery
- Systemic **corticosteroids**

"Long-term-control" medications
- Inhaled or systemic **corticosteroids**: treatment of choice (SOCS, *JAMA* 2001;285:2583)
- *Long-acting* inhaled **β_2-agonists** (salmeterol)
- **Nedocromil/cromolyn**: useful in young Pts, exercise-induced bronchospasm
- **Theophylline**: useful in hard to control Pts, PO convenience, but high side effect profile
- **Leukotriene modifiers**: some patients very responsive, especially aspirin-sensitive asthma (*AJRCCM* 2002;165:9); may consider trial in all patients

Other
- Behavior modification: identify and avoid triggers
- Immunotherapy (e.g., desensitization): may be useful if significant allergic component
- Omalizumab (SC anti-IgE) may be helpful in severe allergic asthma

Principles of treatment
- Use quick-relief rescue medication for all patients
- Persistent asthma requires long-term-control medication; anti-inflammatory meds preferred
- Step up treatment if control not maintained; step down if in control

Asthma Classification and Stepwise Therapy				
Severity	**Sx**	**Night Sx**	**FEV_1/PEFR (of predict.)**	**Control medications**
Mild intermittent	≤2×/wk	≤2×/mo	≥80% nl btw flares	Quick-relief prn
Mild persistent	>2×/wk but <1×/d	>2×/mo	≥80%	**Low-dose inhaled steroid** (START, *Lancet* 2003;361:1071) *or* Cromolyn/nedocromil *or* Theophylline *or* Anti-leukotriene
Moderate persistent	daily	>1×/wk	60-80%	**Low/med-dose inhaled steroid + long-acting bronchodilator** (β_2-agonist *or* theophylline)
Severe persistent	continual + flares	freq.	≤60%	**High-dose inhaled steroid + long-acting bronchodilator** (β_2-agonist *or* theophylline) + **systemic steroids** (if needed)

(Adapted from National Asthma Education and Prevention Project, Expert Panel Report-II, 2002 update)

EXACERBATION

Directed evaluation

- History
  - Previous asthma: baseline PEFR, steroid requirement, ED visits, hospital admissions; **previous need for intubation** a good predictor of risk of death (*Thorax* 1986;41:833)
  - Current exacerbation: duration, severity, potential precipitants, medications used
- Physical exam
  - Signs of severity: tachypnea, tachycardia, diaphoresis, cyanosis, fragmented speech, absent breath sounds, accessory muscle use, pulsus paradoxus, abdominal paradox
  - Assess for barotrauma: asymmetric breath sounds, tracheal deviation, subcutaneous air indicate pneumothorax, precordial (Hamman's) crunch → pneumomediastinum
- Diagnostic studies
  - ABG: not always considered essential because exam and S_aO_2 provide equivalent info; low P_aCO_2 usually seen initially, rises as patient tires
    - ∴ normal or high P_aCO_2 worrisome, but may respond to bronchodilator Rx
  - PEFR: used to follow clinical course
  - CXR: not essential unless suspicion for pneumonia, pneumothorax, etc.
  - ✓ theophylline levels

Classification of asthma exacerbation severity

- **Mild:** PEFR >80%, dyspnea on exertion, end-expiratory wheezes
- **Moderate:** PEFR 50-80%, dyspnea w/ talking, expiratory wheezes, accessory muscle use
- **Severe:** PEFR <50%, S_aO_2 <91%, P_aCO_2 >42, dyspnea at rest, inspiratory and expiratory wheezes, accessory muscle use, pulsus paradoxus >25 mm Hg

Acute Pharmacologic Treatment		
Agent	**Dose**	**Comments**
Oxygen	Titrate to achieve S_aO_2 >90%	
Albuterol	MDI 4-8 puffs q 20 min *or* nebulizer 2.5-5.0 mg q 20 min *continuous* if severe (*Ann Emerg Med* 1993;22:1842 & 1847)	First-line therapy
Corticosteroids	prednisone 60 mg PO *or* methylprednisolone 80 mg IV	IV not superior to PO (*JAMA* 1988;260:527)
Ipratropium	MDI 4-8 puffs q 30 min, *or* nebulizer 0.5 mg q 30 min × 3	↑ bronchodilation when combined with albuterol (*Ann Emerg Med* 1999;34:8)
Magnesium	2 g IV over 20 min	↑ PEFR & FEV_1 (*Lancet* 2003;361:2114)

Other treatments

- Aminophylline: high toxicity, little benefit shown in multiple trials
- Epinephrine (0.3-0.5 mL SC of 1:1000 dilution): no advantage over inhaled β_2-agonists
- Antibiotics: not needed unless evidence of bacterial infection
- IV montelukast: improves FEV_1 acutely; role to be defined (*AJRCCM* 2003;167:488)

Fig. 2-3. Initial assessment of asthma exacerbation

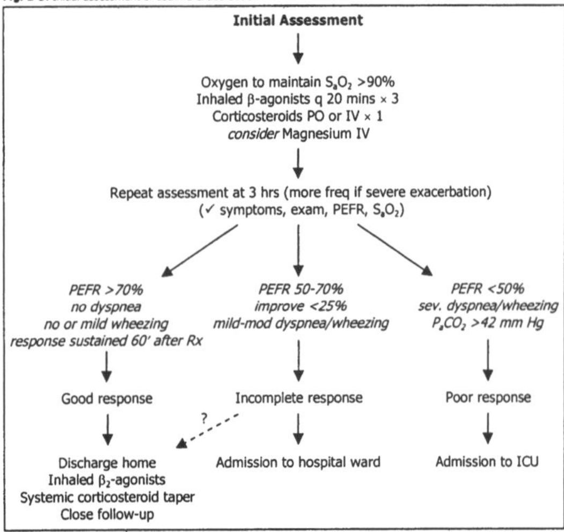

Hospital ward-level care

- ✓ PEFR q 8 hrs, S_aO_2 q 8 hrs (continuous if <90%), provide supplemental O_2
- **Bronchodilators and steroids usually sufficient**
  continue inhaled β_2-agonist as needed for sx, watch for *tachycardia* and *hypokalemia*
  start steroids at prednisone 60 mg qd or equivalent, begin taper when PEFR >50%

ICU-level care

- **High dose steroids**: methylprednisolone 125 mg IV q 6 hrs (*Archives* 1983;143:1324)
- **Non-invasive ventilation**: may ↓ need for intubation (*Int Care Med* 2001;27:486)
- Heliox: ? helpful in first hour, especially in more severe Pts (*Chest* 2003;123:882)
- **Invasive ventilation**
  large ET tube, permissive hypercapnia, allow increased expiratory time
  keep P_{plat} <30 (predicts barotrauma better than PIP), watch for auto-PEEP
  paralysis, inhalational anesthetics, bronchoalveolar lavage w/ mucolytic, and ECMO have been used with success

• CHRONIC OBSTRUCTIVE PULMONARY DISEASE •

Definition and epidemiology (*NEJM* 2000;343:269)
- Chronic respiratory disease with airflow limitation and impaired gas exchange → dyspnea

Emphysema vs. Chronic Bronchitis		
	Emphysema	**Chronic Bronchitis**
Definition	Dilation/destruction of airspaces (pathologic def'n)	Productive cough >3 mo/yr × ≥2 yrs (clinical def'n)
Pathophysiology	Parenchyma affected Matched V/Q defects Mild hypoxemia	Small airways affected V/Q mismatch Severe hypoxemia, hypercapnia PHT, cor pulmonale
Clinical manifestations	Severe, constant dyspnea Mild cough	Intermittent dyspnea Copious sputum production
Physical exam	"Pink puffer" Tachypneic, non-cyanotic, thin Diminished breath sounds	"Blue bloater" Cyanotic, obese, edematous Rhonchi & wheezes

Pathogenesis (*Lancet* 2003;362:1053)
- Caused by: **cigarette smoke** (centrilobular emphysema, affects 15-20% of smokers), α_1-antitrypsin deficiency (panacinar emphysema), recurrent airway infections

Clinical manifestations
- Cough, sputum production, dyspnea
- Exacerbation triggers: pollutants, bronchospasm, infection, other cardiopulmonary disease.
  Infection: overt tracheobronchitis/pneumonia from viruses, *S. pneumoniae*, *H. influenzae*, *M. catarrhalis*, or triggered by changes in strain of colonizers (*NEJM* 2002;347:465)
- Physical exam: ↑ AP diameter of chest ("barrel-chest"), hyperresonance, ↓ diaphragmatic excursion, ↓ breath sounds, ↑ expiratory phase, rhonchi, wheezes
  during exacerbation: tachypnea, use of accessory muscles, pulsus paradoxus, cyanosis

Diagnostic studies
- CXR: hyperinflation, flattened diaphragms, ± chronic interstitial marking and bullae
- PFTs
  Obstruction: ↓↓ FEV_1, ↓ FVC, ↓ FEV_1/FVC, expiratory scooping of flow-volume loop
  Hyperinflation: ↑↑ RV, ↑ TLC, ↑ RV/TLC
  Abnormal gas exchange: ↓ D_LCO (in emphysema)
- ABG: ↓ P_aO_2, ± ↑ P_aCO_2 (in chronic bronchitis, usually only if FEV_1 <1.5 L) and ↓ pH
- ECG: poor R wave progression, R-sided strain, RVH, ↑ P waves in lead II ("P pulmonale")

Chronic treatment (*JAMA* 2003;290:2301 & 2313)
("COPDer"): see table for when to initiate interventions
- **C**orticosteroids: benefit appears to be inversely proportional to FEV_1
  25% ↓ in exacerbations if FEV_1 <2.0 L (*Lancet* 1998;351:773; *BMJ* 2000;320:1297)
  no benefit if FEV_1 >2.0L (*NEJM* 1999;340:1948; *Lancet* 1999;353:1819)
  do not slow loss of FEV_1 (*NEJM* 2000;343:1902)
- **O**xygen: if P_aO_2 ≤55 mmHg or S_aO_2 ≤89% (rest, exercise, sleep) to prevent cor pulmonale
  only therapy proven to ↓ mortality (*Annals* 1980;93:391 & *Lancet* 1981;i:681)
- **P**revention: cigarette smoking cessation (can slow loss of FEV_1; *JAMA* 1994;272:1497), influenza prophylaxis/vaccine, Pneumovax
- **D**ilators: anticholinergics, β_2-agonists, theophylline
  anticholinergic + β_2-agonist may be more effective (*Chest* 1999;115:635)
  salmeterol + fluticasone → ↓ sx, ↑ FEV_1 (*Lancet* 2003;361:449)
- **E**xperimental
  Lung reduction surgery: improves exercise capacity, but no improvement in mortality, unless upper-lobe emphysema and low baseline exercise capacity (*NEJM* 1996;334:1095; 2001;345:1075; and NETT, 2003;348:2059)
  Lung transplant
- **R**ehabilitation: improves quality of life, subjective dyspnea, exercise tolerance

COPD Staging and Recommended Therapies by GOLD Criteria				
Stage	**PFTs (of predicted)**		**Therapies**	
0: ↑ risk	Normal but ± sx		Prevention	n/a
I: Mild	FEV_1/FVC <70%	FEV_1 ≥80%		**D**ilator prn
IIA: Mod		FEV_1 50-80%		Standing **D**ilator **C**orticosteroid if response **R**ehabilitation
IIB: Mod		FEV_1 30-50%		Above + **C**orticosteroid if ↑ exacerbations
III: Severe		FEV_1 <30% *or* respiratory failure *or* right heart failure		Above + **O**xygen if respiratory failure **E**xperimental as indicated

(Adapted from Global Initiative for Chronic Obstructive Pulmonary Disease, WHO/NHLBI 1998)

EXACERBATION

COPD Exacerbation Treatment		
Agent	**Dose**	**Comments**
Ipratropium	MDI 4-8 puffs q 1-2 hr *or* Nebulizer 0.5 mg q 1-2 hr	First-line therapy
Albuterol	MDI 4-8 puffs q 1-2 hr *or* Nebulizer 2.5-5.0 mg q 1-2 hr	Benefit if component of reversible bronchoconstriction
Corticosteroids	Methylprednisolone 125 mg IV q 6 hr × 72 hrs *then* Prednisone 60 mg PO qd × 4 d *then* Taper by 20 mg q 3-4 days *or* Prednisone 30 mg qd × 2 wks if pH >7.26 (*Lancet* 1999;354:456)	↑ FEV_1 (*Lancet* 1999;354:456) & ~30% ↓ in death, intubation, readmission for COPD or need for ↑ drug Rx (*NEJM* 1999;340:1941; *Archives* 2002;162:2527) OutPt Rx after ED visit ↓ relapse (*NEJM* 2003;348:2618)
Antibiotics	Amoxicillin, TMP-SMX, doxycycline, clarithromycin, anti-pneumococcal FQ, etc., all reasonable (no single antibiotic proven superior)	*H. influenzae, M. catarrhalis, S. pneumonia* most frequent precipitants ↑ PEFR & chance of clinical resolution (*JAMA* 1995;273:957)
Theophylline	Sustained release 100-300 mg PO bid (or IV aminophylline)	No utility in acute setting (*Cochrane* 2001;1:CD002168)
Oxygenation	↑ F_iO_2 to achieve P_aO_2 ≥55-60 *or* S_aO_2 90-93%	**Watch for CO_2 retention** (due to ↑ V/Q mismatch, loss of hypoxic respiratory drive, Haldane effect) *but must maintain oxygenation!*
Noninvasive positive-pressure ventilation	Early initiation → ↓ intubation, ↓ LOS, ↓ mortality Indic.: severe dyspnea/tachypnea, hypoxemia, hypercapnia/acidemia Contraindic.: Δ MS or inability to cooperate, hemodynamic instability, inability to clear respiratory secretions, UGIB (*NEJM* 1995;333:817; *Lancet* 1993;341:1555 & 2000;355:1931; *JAMA* 2002;288:932)	
Endotracheal intubation	Consider if P_aO_2 <55-60, ↑'ing P_aCO_2, ↓'ing pH, ↑ RR, respiratory fatigue, Δ MS, or hemodynamic instability	
Other measures	Chest physiotherapy, mucolytics *not* supported by data Monitor for cardiac arrhythmias	

(*NEJM* 2002;346:988)

Prognosis

- Prognosis worsens with declining FEV_1
  - FEV_1 <60% predicted → 5-year survival ~90%
  - FEV_1 <40% predicted → 5-year survival ~50%
  - FEV_1 <20% predicted → 5-year survival ~10%
- **Continued smoking**, frequent exacerbations also associated with poorer prognosis, smoking cessation retards progression of disease
- Lung transplant does not improve survival but may improve quality of life, symptoms COPD is leading reason for referral to transplant (*J Heart Lung Trans* 1999;18:611)

• INTERSTITIAL LUNG DISEASE •

Etiologies of ILD

Environmental & occupational exposures

- **Pneumoconioses** (inorganic dusts)
  Coal worker's (upper lobe coal macules; may progress to massive fibrosis)
  Silicosis (upper lobe opacities ± "eggshell calcification" of lymph nodes; ↑ risk of TB)
  Asbestosis (lower lobe fibrosis, calcified pleural plaques; ↑ risk of mesothelioma)
  Berylliosis (multisystemic granulomatous disease that mimics sarcoidosis)
- **Hypersensitivity pneumonitides** (organic dusts)
  Antigens: "farmer's lung" (spores of thermophilic actinomyces); "pigeon fancier's lung" (proteins from feathers and excreta of birds); "humidifier lung" (thermophilic bacteria)
  Pathophysiology: immunologic rxn; either acute (6 hrs after exposure) or chronic
  Pathology: loose, non-caseating *granulomas*

Sarcoidosis (*NEJM* 1997;336:1224; *AJRCCM* 1999;160:736; *Lancet* 2003;361:1111)

- Prevalent in African-Americans, northern Europeans, and females; onset in 3rd-4th decade
- Pathophysiology: depression of cellular immune system peripherally, activation centrally
- Clinical manifestations: **asx hilar LAN ± ILD** or fever, malaise, dyspnea, arthralgias, rash
  Stages: I = bilateral hilar LAN; II = LAN + ILD; III = ILD only; IV = diffuse fibrosis
  Extrathoracic: erythema nodosum and/or violaceous skin plaques (~25%); uveitis (~25%); hepatomegaly ± granulomatous hepatitis (~25%); BM & splenic granulomas in ~50%, but overt disease rare; CNS or peripheral neuropathy (~5%); cardiac conduction system disease (~5%); parotid enlargement classic but seen in <10%
  Löfgren's syndrome: erythema nodosum + hilar adenopathy + arthritis
  Ddx erythema nodosum: idiopathic (34%); infection (33%, Strep, TB); sarcoid (22%); drugs (OCP, PCNs); vasculitis (Behçet's); IBD; lymphoma (*Arthritis Rheum* 2000;43:584)
  Heerfordt-Waldenström syndrome: fever, parotid enlargement, uveitis, facial palsy
- Diagnostic studies: **LN bx → non-caseating granulomas** + multinucleated giant cells
  ↑ **ACE** (sens. 60%, 90% w/ active dis., spec. 80%, false ⊕ in granulomatous diseases)
  hypercalciuria and hypercalcemia (10%, due to vitamin D hydroxylation by Mϕ);
  lymphopenia, eosinophilia, ↑ ESR, polyclonal ↑ IgG, cutaneous anergy (70%)
- Treatment: corticosteroids if symptoms, hypercalcemia, or extrathoracic organ dysfunction, but indications controversial (*JAMA* 2002;287:1301)
- Prognosis: some spontaneously remit (60-80% of stage I, 50-60% stage II, 30% stage III); 40% improve on treatment; 20% go on to irreversible lung injury

Idiopathic interstitial pneumonias (IIPs) (*AJRCCM* 2002;165:277)

- Definitions: **interstitial lung diseases of unknown cause**, classified by pathology
- Usual interstitial pneumonia (**UIP**, also called **idiopathic pulmonary fibrosis, IPF**): inflammation, fibrosis and honeycombing, thought to be due to fibroblast proliferation, unrelenting progression and usually death in 5-10 yrs; rarely responds to steroids or immunosuppression; IFN-γ w/o effect on lung volumes, but ? 40%, non-stat. significant ↓ in mortality, better response in higher FEV_1 subgroup (*NEJM* 1999;341:1264 & 2004;350:125)
- Acute interstitial pneumonia (**AIP**, "Hamman-Rich syndrome"): similar to UIP but much more acute, rapidly progresses to respiratory failure and death, no treatment
- Cryptogenic organizing pneumonia (COP, also called bronchiolitis obliterans with organizing pneumonia, **BOOP**, if cause known): proliferation of granulation tissue in small bronchioles and inflammation of surrounding alveoli.
  Causes of **BOOP** include: post-infectious, drug-related (e.g., amiodarone, bleomycin), rheumatologic diseases, post-HSCT or XRT (*Archives* 2001;161:158)
  Progresses over 3-6 mos, most cases *steroid responsive* and prognosis good.
- Desquamative interstitial pneumonia (**DIP**): inflammatory infiltrate with "desquamated" (actually, migrated in) Mϕ in alveoli in *smokers* age 30-50, *steroid responsive,* d/c cigs
- Respiratory bronchiolitis-associated ILD (**RBILD**): *milder variant of DIP*, Mϕ + inflammation in 1st & 2nd order bronchioles, non-fatal, *steroid responsive,* d/c cigs
- Lymphocytic interstitial pneumonia (**LIP**): benign polyclonal infiltration of lung by lymphoid cells (usually B-cells), natural history poorly understood, may respond to steroids
- Nonspecific interstitial pneumonia (**NSIP**): ILD with pathologic changes sharing elements of DIP and UIP, with variable fibrosis, steroid responsive w/ good prognosis

Iatrogenic

- Chemo: bleomycin (triggered by hyperoxia), busulfan, cyclophosphamide, MTX, nitrosourea
- Other drugs: nitrofurantoin, sulfonamides, thiazides, amiodarone, INH, hydralazine, gold
- Radiation (→ BOOP): oftentimes with sharply linear, non-anatomic boundaries

Collagen vascular diseases

- **Rheumatologic disease**
  Scleroderma: fibrosis in ~67%; PHT also seen in ~10% of CREST Pts
  Polymyositis-dermatomyositis: ILD and weakness of respiratory muscles
  Mixed-connective tissue disease (MCTD): pulmonary hypertension & fibrosis
  SLE & RA: pleuritis and pleural effusions more often than ILD
- **Vasculitis** (can present with diffuse alveolar hemorrhage)
  Wegener's granulomatosis (⊕ c-ANCA) with necrotizing granulomas
  Churg-Strauss syndrome (⊕ c- or p-ANCA) with eosinophilia and necrotizing granulomas
  Microscopic polyangiitis (⊕ p-ANCA) without granulomas

Miscellaneous (a series of rare disorders, many with 3-letter abbreviations!)

- **Diffuse alveolar hemorrhage (DAH)**: infiltrates ≈ CHF, but fail to resolve with diuresis; ± hemoptysis; ± ↓ Hct; ± ↑ D_LCO; etiologies include:
  Goodpasture's syndrome = DAH + RPGN; typically in smokers; ⊕ anti-GBM in 90%
  idiopathic pulmonary hemosiderosis (IPH): a rare disease and a dx of exclusion
  other: ANCA ⊕ vasculitis; SLE; PM; APS; crack cocaine; HSCT; XRT
- **Pulmonary infiltrates with eosinophilia (PIE)** = eosinophils on BAL ± periph. blood
  allergic bronchopulmonary aspergillosis (ABPA): allergic reaction to *Aspergillus*
  criteria: asthma, pulmonary infiltrates (transient or fixed), skin rxn & serum precipitins to *Aspergillus*, ↑ IgE to Aspergillus & total (>1000), ↑ eos, central bronchiectasis
  Rx with steroids ± itraconazole for refractory cases (*NEJM* 2000;342:756)
  Löffler's syndrome: transient pulmonary infiltrates + cough, fever, dyspnea, eosinophilia due to parasites (*Ascariasis*, hookworm, *Strongyloides*) or drugs (nitrofurantoin, crack)
  acute eosinophilic pneumonia (AEP): acute febrile illness with severe hypoxia
  chronic eosinophilic pneumonia (CEP): "photonegative" of CHF, typically in women
  Churg-Strauss syndrome: see above
  hypereosinophilic syndrome: idiopathic, with bone marrow and multiorgan involvement
- Pulmonary alveolar proteinosis (PAP): accumulation of surfactant-like phospholipids, typically in male smokers; due to autoimmune targeting of GM-CSF (*NEJM* 2003;349:2527)
- Lymphangioleiomyomatosis (LAM): proliferation of immature smooth muscle cells seen in premenopausal women; also associated with PTX and chylous pleural effusions
- Langerhans cell granulomatosis (LCG): affects young male smokers; cysts; PTX in ~25%
- Graft versus host (GVH) disease: in setting of HSCT

WORKUP OF ILD

Rule-out non-primary pulmonary causes of interstitial pattern on CXR/Chest CT

- **Congestive heart failure**
- **Infection**
  viral (influenza, parainfluenza, adenovirus, coronavirus, RSV, CMV)
  bacterial (especially atypicals such as *Mycoplasma*, *Chlamydia*, and *Legionella*)
  fungal (PCP, histoplasmosis, coccidioidomycosis)
  mycobacterial (MTb and MAI)
  parasitic (see Löffler's syndrome above)
- **Malignancy**
  lymphangitic carcinomatosis: adenoCa (breast, pancreas, stomach, lung) > squamous
  bronchoalveolar cell carcinoma (although usually appears as air-space disease)
  lymphoproliferative disorders (leukemia and lymphoma)

History and physical exam

- Occupational, travel, exposure, and medications
- Tempo (acute → infection, CHF, hypersensitivity pneumonitis, eos PNA, AIP, COP)
- Extrapulmonary signs and symptoms (skin Δs, arthralgias/arthritis, neuropathies, etc.)

Diagnostic studies

- CXR and **high-resolution chest CT**: reticular, nodular, or ground glass pattern
  upper → coal, silicosis, hypersensitivity, sarcoid, TB, RA, LCG; lower → UIP, asbestosis
  adenopathy → sarcoidosis, berylliosis, silicosis, malignancy, fungal infections
  pleural disease → collagen-vascular diseases, asbestosis, infections, XRT, LAM
- PFTs: restrictive pattern (↓ volumes), ↓ D_LCO, ↓ P_aO_2 (especially w/ exercise)
- Serologies: ✓ ACE, ANA, RF, ANCA, anti-GBM, HIV
- Bronchoalveolar lavage: diagnostic in infections, hemorrhage, PIE syndromes, PAP
- Biopsy (transbronchial, CT-guided, VATS, or open): dx in granulomatous diseases (sarcoid, hypersensitivity, Wegener's, Churg-Strauss, LCG), pneumoconioses, IIPs, infection, malig
  ∴ consider if no clear precipitant and non-invasive workup unrevealing

• PLEURAL EFFUSION •

Pathophysiology
- **Systemic factors** (e.g., ↑ PCWP, ↓ oncotic pressure) → *transudative* effusion
- **Local factors** (i.e., Δ pleural surface permeability) → *exudative* effusion

Transudates
- **Congestive heart failure (40%)**: 80% bilateral, may be cardiomegaly
  may occasionally be exudative (especially after aggressive diuresis or if chronic), but ~75% of exudative effusions in CHF Pts found to have non-CHF cause (*Chest* 2002;122:1518)
- Constrictive pericarditis
- **Cirrhosis** ("hepatic hydrothorax"): often right-sided & massive (even w/o marked ascites)
- Nephrotic syndrome: usually small, bilateral, asymptomatic
- Other: PE (usually exudate), malignancy (lymphatic obstruction), myxedema, CAPD

Exudates
- **Infection (25%)**
  bacterial (parapneumonic)
  mycobacterial (tuberculous effusions almost always >50% lymphocytes)
  fungal, viral (usually small), parasitic (e.g., amebiasis, echinococcosis, paragonimiasis)
- **Malignancy (15%)**: primary lung cancer most common, metastases (especially breast, lymphoma, etc.), mesothelioma
- **Pulmonary embolism (10%)**: effusions in ~40% of PEs; exudate (75%) > transudate (25%); hemorrhagic – *must have high suspicion because presentation highly variable*
- **Collagen vascular disease**: RA (large), SLE (small), Wegener's, Churg-Strauss
- **Gastrointestinal diseases**: pancreatitis, esophageal rupture, abdominal abscess
- Hemothorax (Hct_{eff}/Hct_{blood} >50%): trauma, PE, malignancy, coagulopathy, leaking aortic aneurysm, aortic dissection, pulmonary vascular malformation
- Chylothorax (triglycerides >110): thoracic duct damage due to trauma, malignancy, LAM
- Other
  Post-CABG: left-sided; initially bloody, clears after several weeks
  Dressler's syndrome (pericarditis & pleuritis post-MI), uremia, post-radiation therapy
  Asbestos exposure (benign)
  Drug-induced (e.g., nitrofurantoin, methysergide, bromocriptine, amiodarone); ⊕ eos
  Meigs' syndrome = benign ovarian tumor → ascites & pleural effusion
  Yellow-nail syndrome = hypoplastic lymphatics → lymphedema, pleural effusion, yellow nails, bronchiectasis

Diagnostic studies
- **Thoracentesis**
  Indications: **all effusions >1 cm in decubitus view**
  if suspect due to CHF, can diurese and see if effusions resolve (75% do so in 48 hrs)
  asymmetry, fever, chest pain, or failure to resolve are indications for thoracentesis
  parapneumonics should be tapped ASAP (*cannot* exclude empyema clinically)
  Diagnostic studies: ✓ total protein, LDH, glucose, cell count with differential, gram stain + culture, pH; remaining fluid for additional studies as dictated by clinical scenario
  Complications: PTX (5-10%), hemothorax (~1%), re-expansion pulmonary edema (if >1.5 L removed), spleen/liver laceration; routine post-tap CXR not indicated if no suspicion of PTX, no air aspiration, 1 needle pass, no h/o chest XRT(*Annals* 1996;124:816)
- **Transudate vs. exudate** (*Annals* 1972;77:507)
  Light's criteria: exudate = TP_{eff}/TP_{serum} >0.5 *or* LDH_{eff}/LDH_{serum} >0.6 *or* LDH_{eff} >2/3 ULN of LDH_{serum}); 98% sens., 83% spec.
  other exudative criteria: serum-effusion alb gradient ≤1.2; $chol_{eff}$ >60; 92% spec for both
  effusions due to CHF: *TP may ↑ with diuresis or chronicity* → "pseudoexudate"; can use albumin gradient, cholesterol, or clinical judgment to distinguish (*Chest* 2002;122:1524)
- **Complicated vs. uncomplicated parapneumonic** (*Chest* 1995;108:299)
  complicated = ⊕ gram stain or culture *or* pH <7.2 *or* glucose <60
  complicated parapneumonic effusions usually require drainage to achieve resolution
  empyema = frank pus, also needs drainage to achieve resolution

- Additional pleural fluid studies (*NEJM* 2002;346:1971)
  - WBC & differential: exudates tend to have higher WBC than transudates but nonspecific
    - neutrophils → parapneumonic, PE, pancreatitis
    - lymphocytes (>50%) → cancer, TB
    - eosinophils (>10%) → blood, air, drug rxn, asbestos, paragonimiasis, Churg-Strauss
  - RBC: Hct_{eff} 1-20% → cancer, PE, trauma; Hct_{eff}/Hct_{blood} >50% → hemothorax
  - AFB: yield in TB 0-10% with stain, 11-50% with culture, 38-80% with pleural bx
  - adenosine deaminase (ADA): seen with granulomas, >70 suggests TB, <40 excludes TB
  - cytology: yield is 55% with 1 sample, 70% with 3 samples
  - amylase: seen in pancreatic disease and esophageal rupture
  - rheumatoid factor, C_H50, ANA: *limited utility* in diagnosing collagen vascular disease
  - triglycerides: >110 → chylothorax, 50-110 → ✓ lipoprotein analysis for chylomicrons
- Chest CT; pleural biopsy; VATS

Characteristics of Pleural Fluid (*not* diagnostic criteria)

Etiology	Appear	WBC *diff*	RBC	pH	Glc	Comments
CHF	clear, straw	<1000 *lymphs*	<5000	normal	≈ serum	bilateral, cardiomegaly
Cirrhosis	clear, straw	<1000	<5000	normal	≈ serum	right-sided
Uncomplicated parapneumonic	turbid	5-40,000 *polys*	<5000	normal to ↓	≈ serum (>40)	
Complicated parapneumonic	turbid to purulent	5-40,000 *polys*	<5000	↓↓	↓↓ (<40)	Need drainage
Empyema	purulent	25-100,000 *polys*	<5000	↓↓↓	↓↓	Need drainage
Tuberculosis	serosang.	5-10,000 *lymphs*	<10,000	normal to ↓	normal to ↓	⊕ AFB ⊕ ADA
Malignancy	turbid to bloody	1-100,000 *lymphs*	<100,000	normal to ↓	normal to ↓	⊕ cytology
Pulmonary embolism	*sometimes* bloody	1-50,000 *polys*	<100,000	normal	≈ serum	No infarct → transudate
Rheumatoid arthritis	turbid	1-20,000 *variable*	<1000	↓	↓↓↓	↑ RF, ↓ C_H50
Pancreatitis	serosang. to turbid	1-50,000 *polys*	<10,000	normal	≈ serum	left-sided, ↑ amylase
Esophageal rupture	turbid to purulent	<5,000 - >50,000	<10,000	↓↓↓	↓↓	left-sided, ↑ amylase

Treatment

- Symptomatic effusion: therapeutic thoracentesis, treat underlying disease process
- Parapneumonic effusion (*Chest* 2000;118:1158)
  - uncomplicated → antibiotics for pneumonia
  - **involves >½ hemithorax *or* complicated *or* empyema → tube thoracostomy**
  - loculated → tube thoracostomy + intrapleural thrombolytics or VATS
- Malignant effusion: serial thoracenteses vs. tube thoracostomy + pleurodesis (success rate ~80%); pH <7.2 *may* be associated with worse prognosis, more likely to fail pleurodesis

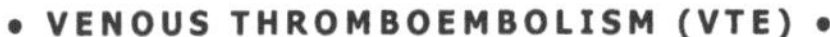

• VENOUS THROMBOEMBOLISM (VTE) •

Definitions

- Calf-vein thrombosis: less likely to cause significant thromboembolism, 80% resolve spont.
- Proximal deep venous thrombosis (DVT): thrombosis of popliteal, femoral, or iliac veins (n.b., "superficial" femoral vein is part of the deep venous system)
- Pulmonary embolism (PE): thrombosis that originates in the venous system and embolizes to the pulmonary arterial circulation; ~600,000 cases per yr

Risk factors

- Virchow's triad for thrombogenesis
  - **alterations in blood flow** (i.e., stasis): bed rest, inactivity, CHF
  - **injury to endothelium**: trauma, surgery
  - **thrombophilia** (40% ⊕): APC resistance, protein C or S deficiency, APLA, OCP, etc.
- Malignancy (found in 12% of "idiopathic" DVT/PE)
- History of thrombosis

Clinical manifestations

- Asymptomatic
- DVT: calf pain, edema, venous distention, pain on dorsiflexion
  - phlegmasia cerulea dolens: stagnant blood → edema, *cyanosis*, pain
  - 50% of patients with symptomatic DVT have asymptomatic PE
- PE: dyspnea (80%), pleuritic chest pain (70%), cough, hemoptysis
  - 33% of patients with PE have symptoms or signs of DVT
- Massive PE with acute cor pulmonale: syncope, hypotension, PEA

Physical exam

- DVT (sens. 60-88%, spec. 30-72%, *JAMA* 1998;279:1094): lower extremity swelling (>3 cm compared with unaffected side), edema, erythema, warmth, tenderness, palpable cord, ⊕ Homan's sign (calf pain on dorsiflexion, seen in <5% of patients)
- PE: tachypnea (>70%), tachycardia, fever, cyanosis, isolated crackles, pleural friction rub, loud P_2, right-sided S_3, pulmonary insufficiency murmur, elevated JVP

Pretest Probability of DVT	
Major points	**Minor points**
• Active cancer • Paralysis, paresis, immobilization of foot • Bed rest × >3 d or major surgery w/in 4 wks • Localized tenderness along veins • Swelling of thigh *and* calf • Swelling of calf >3 cm c/w asx side • ⊕ FHx of DVT (≥2 1° relatives)	• Trauma to symptomatic leg w/in 60 d • Pitting edema in symptomatic leg • Dilated superficial veins (non-varicose) in symptomatic leg only • Hospitalization w/in previous 6 mos • Erythema
High probability (~85% ⊕ DVT) ≥3 major + *no* alternative dx ≥2 major + ≥2 minor + *no* alternative dx **Intermediate prob** (~33% ⊕ DVT) neither high nor low probability	**Low probability** (~5% ⊕ DVT) 1 major + ≥2 minor + alternative dx 1 major + ≥1 minor + *no* alternative dx 0 major + ≥3 minor + alternative dx 0 major + ≥2 minor + *no* alternative dx

(*Lancet* 1995;345:1326 and *NEJM* 1996;335:1816)

Pretest Probability of PE			
Variable			**Point Score**
• Clinical signs or symptoms of DVT			3.0
• HR >100 bpm			1.5
• Immobilization (bed rest ≥3 d) or surgery w/in 4 wks			1.5
• Prior DVT or PE			1.5
• Hemoptysis			1.0
• Malignancy (Rx'd w/in past 6 mos or palliative)			1.0
• PE as likely or more likely than any alternative dx			3.0
	Low (0-2 points)	**Intermed. (2-6 points)**	**High (>6 points)**
Overall	**~3%**	**~20%**	**~60%**
⊖ D-dimer	~2%	~6%	~20%
⊕ D-dimer	~7%	~36%	~75%

(*Thromb Haemost* 2000;83:416; *JAMA* 2003;290:2849)

Diagnostic studies

- CXR: often normal, may show atelectasis, effusion, elevated hemidiaphragm, Hampton's hump (wedge-shaped density abutting pleura and projecting towards heart), Westermark's sign (avascularity distal to a PE); none sens. or spec. enough for diagnosis
- ECG: most often seen is RV strain w/ TWI V_1-V_3 (*Chest* 1997;111:537); also see sinus tachycardia, AF, RAD, RBBB, P pulmonale, $S_IQ_{III}T_{III}$; none sens. or spec. enough for dx
- ABG: hypoxemia, hypocapnia, respiratory alkalosis, ↑ A-a gradient (*Chest* 1996;109:78) (but $P_aO_2 \geq 80$ + $P_aCO_2 \geq 35$ + A-a gradient ≤20 → only ~70% NPV)
- D-dimer: high sens. but poor spec.; ∴ ⊖ ELISA has >95% NPV and can be used to *r/o PE in low risk Pts* (*JACC* 2002;40:1475); latex agglutination assay less useful with <90% NPV
- Compression ultrasonography: sens. >90%, spec. >90%
  70% of patients with PE have ⊕ venous ultrasonography
- V/Q scan: see PIOPED data below
- Helical CT: sens. ~85%, spec. ~95%, but vary widely in literature (*Annals* 2000;132:227)
  more sens. for proximal emboli; may demonstrate alternative dx (pneumonia, etc.)
  ⊖ CT & U/S → <2% rate of VTE in f/u, except if high clinical suspicion or inpatient (~5% rate of VTE in f/u) (ESSEP, *Lancet* 2002;360:1914 & ANTELOPE, *Annals* 2003:138:307)
- Pulmonary angiography: diagnostic gold-standard (morbidity 5%, mortality <0.5%)

Likelihood of PE Based on PIOPED Data

Scan category	Clinical Suspicion		
	High	**Intermediate**	**Low**
High	96%	88%	56%
Intermediate	66%	28%	16%
Low	40%	16%	4%

(*JAMA* 1990:263:2753)

Fig. 2-4. Approach to suspected PE

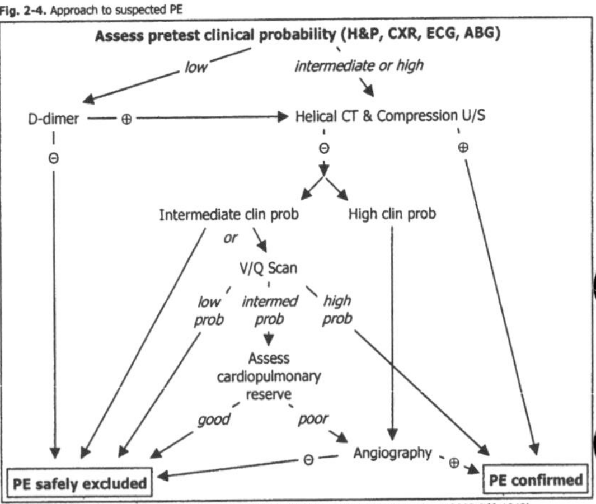

(*NEJM* 1998;335:1816 & 2003;349:1247, *Annals* 1998;129:997 & 2003;138:307, *Lancet* 2002;360:1949)

Other testing

- **Thrombophilia workup** indicated in recurrent DVT/PE or idiopathic DVT/PE + (age <50 *or* ⊕ family history *or* unusual location *or* massive)
- **Malignancy workup** (12% of patients with "idiopathic" DVT/PE will have a malignancy) adequate initial screening: H&P (incl. breast, abd, FOBT, pelvic, rectal), basic labs (SMA-20, CBC, U/A), CXR, up-to-date mammogram, colonoscopy, ? PSA

TREATMENT

Thromboprophylaxis		
Risk	**Patient & situation**	**Prophylaxis**
Low DVT 0.4%, PE 0.2%	• minor surgery, age <40, no RF	early ambulation
Moderate DVT 2-4% PE 1-2%	• minor surgery + age 40-60 *or* RF • major surgery, age <40, no RF	**LDUH** 5000 U q 12 hr LMWH dalteparin 2500 U qd enoxaparin 20 mg qd IPC + ES
High DVT 4-8% PE 2-4%	• minor surgery + age >60 *or* RF • major surgery + age >40 *or* RF • MI, CVA, bed rest, chronic illness	**LDUH** 5000 U q 8 hr **LMWH** dalteparin 5000 U qd enoxaparin 40 mg qd IPC + ES
Highest DVT 10-20% PE 4-10%	• orthopedic surgery, trauma • major surgery + age >40 *and* RF • acute spinal cord injury	**LMWH** dalteparin 5000 U qd enoxaparin 30 mg bid **fondaparinux** 2.5 mg qd (*NEJM* 2001;345:1298 & 1305) **ximelagatran** 24-36 mg d (*NEJM* 2003;349:1703) adjusted dose warfarin IPC + ES if bleed risk

RF = risk factor, and includes immobility, varicose veins, CHF, malignancy, thrombophilia, prior VTE.
ES = elastic stockings; IPC = intermittent pneumatic compression; LDUH = low-dose SC UFH.
For general surgery, administer 1st dose of LDUH or LMWH 1-2 hrs before operation. For orthopedic surgery, administer 1st dose of LMWH 8-12 hrs preop or 8-12 hrs postop. For trauma, administer 1st dose of LMWH 12 hrs postinjury or when deemed safe. For neurosurgery, IPC + ES. (Adapted from *Chest* 2001;119:132S)

Treatment of VTE (*Chest* 2001;119:176S)
- Calf-vein DVT (if symptomatic or extending), proximal DVT, and PE need anticoagulation
- **Acute anticoagulation** *(must achieve therapeutic levels ASAP!)*
  - **IV UFH**: 80 U/kg bolus → 18 U/kg/hr → titrate to goal PTT 46-70 sec (1.5-2.3 x cntl), *or*
  - **LWMH**: enoxaparin 1 mg/kg SC bid or dalteparin 200 IU/kg SC qd (*Annals* 1999;130:800)
  - *then* start **warfarin** (when PTT therapeutic on UFH or on day 1 of LMWH), overlap × 5 d (see Heme-Onc section in Appendix for rationale), titrate to INR 2.0-3.0
  - fondaparinux (pentasaccharide) 5-10 mg SC qd ≈ IV UFH (MATISSE, *NEJM* 2003;349:1695)
  - direct thrombin inhibitors (lepirudin, argatroban) useful in HIT
- **Thrombolysis** (TPA 100 mg over 2 hrs or 0.6 mg/kg over 3-15 min): *extensive DVT or massive PE* causing hemodynamic compromise; controversial in stable Pts with *RV dysfunction*; no mortality benefit (*NEJM* 2002;347:1143)
- IVC filter if anticoagulation contraindicated, but little data to support with ½ rate of PE, 2× rate of DVT, no difference in mortality (*NEJM* 1998;338:409; *Chest* 2002;122:963)
- Thrombectomy (surgical or catheter-based): limited data, may be beneficial in select Pts
- **Long-term anticoagulation** (*Chest* 2001;119:S176)
  - 1st event with reversible or time-limited risk factors: 3-6 mos of warfarin
  - Idiopathic PE/DVT: ≥6 months (DURAC, *NEJM* 1995:332;1661)
    - long-term warfarin (~5 yrs) appears superior to 6 mos (PREVENT, *NEJM* 2003;348:1425)
    - INR 2-3 appears better than INR 1.5-2.0 (ELATE, *NEJM* 2003;349:631)
    - ? ximelagatran 24 mg qd (THRIVE III, *NEJM* 2003;349:1713)
  - 2nd event, cancer, non-modifiable risk factor: 12 mos – lifelong (DURAC II, *NEJM* 1997;336:393)
    - in Pts w/ cancer, long-term Rx w/ LMWH superior to warfarin (*NEJM* 2003;349:146)

Complications
- Post-thrombotic syndrome (25%): pain, swelling; ↓ with compression stockings × 3 mos
- Recurrent DVT
  - D-dimer <250 after withdrawal of anticoag. → 1/3 risk of recurrence (*JAMA* 2003;290:1071)
  - ⊕ U/S at 3 months → 2.4× ↑ risk of recurrence (*Annals* 2002;137:955)

Prognosis (ICOPER Registry, *Lancet* 1999;353:1386)
- Mort. 17% @ 3 mos (PE, cancer, resp. failure); 75% of those will die during initial hosp.
- Mortality rate up to 50% in patients who are hemodynamically unstable
- ↑ troponin (*Circ* 2002;106:1263) and ↑ BNP (*Circ* 2003;107:1576) predict worse outcome
- <2% develop chronic pulmonary hypertension

• HEMOPTYSIS •

Definition

- Expectoration of blood or blood-streaked sputum
- **Massive hemoptysis**: >600cc/24-48 hrs, hemodynamic compromise, altered gas exchange, or respiratory failure

Etiologies	
Infection/ Inflammation	**Bronchitis** (most common cause of insignificant hemoptysis) **Bronchiectasis** (most common cause of significant hemoptysis; *NEJM* 2002;346:1383) Cystic fibrosis (due to bronchiectasis) Tuberculosis Pneumonia/lung abscess Aspergilloma
Neoplasm	Usually primary lung cancer, sometimes metastasis
Cardiovascular	Pulmonary embolism Congestive heart failure Mitral stenosis Pulmonary artery rupture (with instrumentation) Trauma/foreign body Bronchovascular fistula
Other	Vasculitis (Wegener's granulomatosis, Goodpasture's syndrome) AV malformation Idiopathic pulmonary hemosiderosis Excessive anticoagulation (with underlying lung disease) Catamenial (thoracic endometriosis)

Pathophysiology

- Most massive hemoptysis is due to bleeding from **bronchial arterial circulation** because of high arterial pressures. Most often, bronchial vessels become tortuous and vulnerable (bronchiectasis) or are directly invaded.

Diagnostic workup

- Localize bleeding site
  Rule out GI or ENT source by exam, history; may require endoscopy
  For pulmonary source: determine whether **unilateral or bilateral, localized or diffuse, parenchymal or airway** by CXR or chest CT, bronchoscopy if necessary
- PT, PTT, CBC to rule out **coagulopathy**
- Micro: sputum culture and stain for bacteria, fungi, and AFB
- Sputum cytology to **r/o malignancy**
- ANCA, anti-GBM, urinalysis to ✓ for **vasculitis** or **pulmonary-renal syndrome**

Treatment

- Reverse coagulopathy
- Suppress cough
- Treat underlying condition

Treatment of massive hemoptysis

- Position patient with bleeding side dependent to protect normal lung
- Selective intubation of normal lung
- Angiography: can be used for diagnosis and treatment – vascular occlusion balloons or **selective embolization of bronchial circulation** can be used
- Rigid bronchoscopy: allows more interventional options, including electrocautery, laser
- Surgical resection

• SOLITARY PULMONARY NODULE •

Principles

- Definition: single, <3 cm (>3 cm = "mass"), surrounded by normal lung, no lymphadenopathy or pleural effusion
- Often "incidentalomas", but may represent early localized (i.e., potentially *curable*) malignancy

Etiologies	
Benign (70%)	**Malignant (30%)**
Granuloma (80%): TB, histoplasmosis, coccidioidomycosis **Hamartoma** (10%) Bronchogenic cyst AV malformation Pulmonary infarct Wegener's granulomatosis Pneumonitis Lipoma, fibroma, amyloidoma Rheumatoid nodule Ascariasis, echinococcosis Aspergilloma	**Bronchogenic carcinoma** (75%): adenocarcinoma and large cell (peripheral) squamous and small cell (central) **Metastatic** (20%): breast, head & neck, colon, testicular, renal, sarcoma, melanoma Carcinoid Primary sarcoma

Initial evaluation

- **History**: age (<30 yrs = 2% malignant, + 15% for each decade >30), smoking history, ⊕ cancer history
- **CT**: size/shape, Ca, ✓ for LAN, effusions, bony destruction, **compare to old studies**
  Size: >3 cm usually malignant
  Shape: ill-defined border, irregular/spiculated edge
  Calcification: lack of calcification more likely to be malignant; granuloma has laminated pattern; hamartoma has "popcorn" pattern

Risk of Cancer			
Feature	**Low**	**Intermediate**	**High**
Diameter (cm)	<1.5	1.5-2.2	≥2.3
Nodule shape	smooth	scalloped	spiculated
Age (yr)	<45	45-60	>60
Smoking	never	current (≤1 ppd)	current (>1 ppd)
Smoking cessation	never or quit ≥7 yrs ago	quit <7 yrs ago	never quit

(*NEJM* 2003;348:2535)

Diagnostic studies

- **Positron-emission tomography** (PET): detects metabolic activity of tumors, 97% sens. and 78% spec. for detecting malignancy, also useful for surgical staging b/c may detect unsuspected metastatic lesions (*Chest* 2003;123:89S)
- **Transbronchial biopsy**: most lesions too small to sample reliably unless done with endobronchial ultrasound (*Chest* 2003;123:604); bronchoscopy with brushings is low-yield unless lesion intruding into bronchus
- **Transthoracic needle biopsy**: preferred if technically feasible, sens. 85-95% with CT guidance; helpful if confirms benign, if non-informative or malignant → resect
- **Video-assisted thorascopic surgery** (VATS): for percutaneously inaccessible lesions, highly sensitive and allows resection; has replaced thoracotomy
- PPD, fungal serologies, ANCA

Management

- **Low-risk**: observation with serial CT (q 3 mos × 4, then q 6 mos × 2)
- **Intermediate-risk**: PET, transthoracic needle biopsy or transbronchial biopsy depending on location; if non-informative → VATS
- **High-risk** (and surgical candidate): VATS → lobectomy if malignant

• PULMONARY HYPERTENSION (PHT) •

Definition

- PA mean pressure >25 mmHg at rest *or* >30 mmHg with exertion
- Primary pulmonary hypertension (PPH) has yearly incidence of 1-2 per million, ∴ assume secondary PHT until proven otherwise

Etiologies of Pulmonary Hypertension (WHO Classification)		
Pulmonary arterial HTN (PAH)	• Primary pulmonary HTN • Congenital shunts: ASD, VSD, PDA • Portal HTN	• Collagen-vascular disease • HIV • Anorexic agents/drugs • Cocaine/toxins
Pulmonary venous HTN	• Left-sided CHF • MS/MR • LA myxoma	• Pulmonary VOD • Extrinsic compression: mediastinitis, tumor, LAN
Respiratory system disorders or chronic hypoxia	• COPD • ILD • Hypoventilation • Cystic fibrosis	• Sleep apnea • Chronic hypoxemia (altitude) • Pneumonia
Chronic thrombotic or embolic disease	• Pulmonary embolism • Tumor emboli	• Chronic thromboembolic pulmonary HTN (CTEPH)
Disease directly affecting pulmonary vasculature	• Vasculitis • Sarcoidosis • Schistosomiasis	• Capillary hemangiomatosis

(www.who.int/ned/cvd/pph.html)

Clinical manifestations

- Average time from onset of symptoms to diagnosis is 2 yrs
- Dyspnea, exertional syncope (hypoxia, ↓ CO), exertional chest pain (RV ischemia)
- Symptoms of right-sided CHF (e.g., peripheral edema, RUQ fullness, abdominal distention)
- PPH: mean age of onset 36 (men older than women); female:male = 1.7-3.5:1 mutations in bone morphogenic protein receptor 2 (*BMPR2*; gene involved in proliferation & apoptosis) seen in ~50% familial and ~26% sporadic cases of PPH (*NEJM* 2001;345:319)

Physical exam

- Prominent P_2, right-sided S_4, RV heave, PA tap, PA flow murmur, PR, TR ± RV failure: ↑ JVP, hepatomegaly, peripheral edema

Diagnostic studies

- CXR: dilatation and pruning of pulmonary arteries, RA and RV enlargement
- ECG: RAD, RBBB, RAE ("P pulmonale"), RVH
- PFTs: ↓ D_LCO, mild restrictive pattern
- ABG: ↓ P_aO_2 and S_aO_2 (especially with exertion), ↓ P_aCO_2, ↑ A-a gradient
- Echocardiogram: right-sided pressure overload, abnormal septal motion, TR, PR
- Cardiac catheterization: ↑ RA, RV, and PA pressures, ↑ PVR, ↓ CO, normal PCWP

Workup (focus on ruling out secondary causes)

- CXR and high resolution chest CT: r/o parenchymal lung disease
- PFTs: r/o obstructive and restrictive lung disease, check D_LCO
- ABG & polysomnography: r/o hypoventilation
- V/Q scan ± pulmonary angiogram: r/o PE
- LFTs & HIV
- Vasculitis screening labs: ANA (commonly ⊕ in PPH), RF, anti-Scl-70, anti-centromere, ESR
- Echocardiogram: r/o myocardial, valvular, and congenital heart disease, evaluate LV function, estimate RV systolic pressure, visualize ventricular interdependence
- Cardiac catheterization: definitive evaluation of filling pressures, r/o shunt, r/o ↑ PCWP
- May require open lung biopsy

Treatment (*JAMA* 2000;284:3160 & *Lancet* 2003;361:1533)

- Oxygen: maintain S_aO_2 >90-92%, (reduces vasoconstriction)
- Diuretics: to relieve sx of right CHF, *gentle* because RV is preload dependent
- Digoxin: no evidence, but may counteract negative inotropic effects of CCB
- Anticoagulation: counteracts ↑ risk of thrombosis due to dilated heart, sluggish blood flow, low activity; ? mortality benefit (*Circ* 1984;70:580)
- Treat underlying causes of secondary PHT

• **Vasodilators**: most useful in PAH
  Vasodilator challenge (e.g., NO, adenosine, prostacyclin) to identify responders (↓ PA pressure and/or ↑ CO), which predicts Pts likely to respond to long-term oral therapy, no response → may be candidates for other vasodilators (*JAMA* 2000;284:3160)
  Oral CCB (e.g., nifedipine) in responders to vasodilator challenge (*NEJM* 1992;327:76):
    25% of Pts ↓ PA pressure & PVR, ↑ CO, unΔ'd SBP → improved survival
    50% of Pts unΔ'd PA pressure & PVR, ↑ CO → improved exercise tolerance, ? Δ survival
    25% of Pts unΔ'd PVR, ↓ SBP → "fixed" vascular disease, ∅ role for vasodilators
  Prostacyclin IV (e.g., *continuous* epoprostenol) in non-responders and in responders w/ refractory CHF (*NEJM* 1996;334:296 & 1998;338:273): ↓ PVR 21% acutely & 53% long-term; ↓ mortality (0% vs. 20%); may be beneficial even if ∅ acute hemodynamic response; complications include tolerance, infection, thrombosis, pump dysfunction
  Prostacyclin analogues including *oral* (e.g., beraprost; *JACC* 2002;39:1496), *inhaled* (iloprost; *NEJM* 2002;347:322) and *SC* (trepostinil) improve hemodynamics and symptoms
  Endothelin-1 receptor antagonist (e.g., bosentan PO; *NEJM* 2002;346:896): improves sx
  Phosphodiesterase inhibitors (e.g., sildenafil; *Lancet* 2002;360:895): ↓ PVR, ↑ P_aO_2
• Lung transplant: if severe symptoms refractory to medical therapy

Fig. 2-5. Treatment of PAH

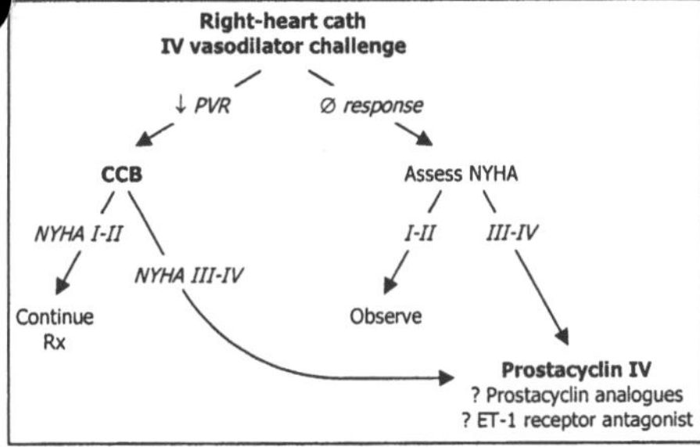

Prognosis
• Median survival after diagnosis ~ 2.5 yrs
  CCB responders = 94% survival at 5 yrs *vs.* CCB non-responders = 55% at 5 yrs
• Lung transplant: 5-yr survival 45-55%

• RESPIRATORY FAILURE •

Hypoxemia → $P_aO_2 = F_iO_2 \times (760 - 47) - \frac{P_aCO_2}{R}$ - Aa gradient

Fig. 2-5. Workup of hypoxemia

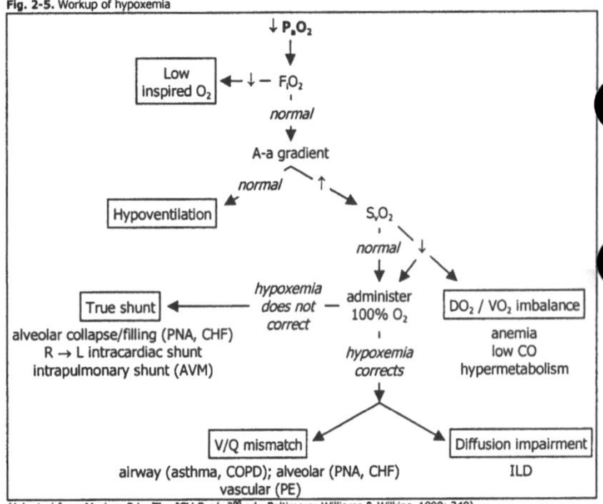

(Adapted from Marino, P.L. *The ICU Book*, 2nd ed., Baltimore: Williams & Wilkins, 1990: 349)

Hypercapnia → $P_aCO_2 = k \times \frac{\dot{V}_{CO_2}}{RR \times V_T \times \left(1 - \frac{V_D}{V_T}\right)}$

Fig. 2-6. Workup of hypercapnia

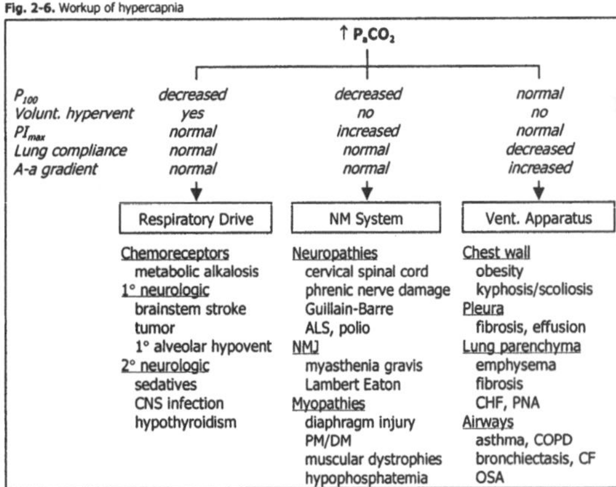

• MECHANICAL VENTILATION •

Indications

- Apnea
- Improve gas exchange
  - ↑ oxygenation
  - ↑ ventilation and/or reverse acute respiratory acidosis
- Relieve respiratory distress
  - ↓ work of breathing (can account for up to 50% of total oxygen consumption)
  - relieve respiratory muscle fatigue
- Airway protection
- Pulmonary toilet

Choosing settings (*NEJM* 2001;344:1986)

1) Pick ventilator mode
2) Choose volume-targeted or pressure-targeted
3) Set or ✓ remaining variables

Step 1: Pick Ventilator Mode	
Mode	**Description**
Assist control (AC)	Vent delivers a minimum number of supported breaths Additional Pt-initiated breaths trigger *fully-assisted* vent breaths ∴ Vent-triggered breaths identical to Pt-triggered breaths Tachypnea → ? respiratory alkalosis, breath-stacking, & auto-PEEP May be pressure-targeted (pressure-control vent, PCV) or volume-targeted (volume-cycled vent, VCV)
Synchronized intermittent mandatory vent (SIMV)	Vent delivers min. # of supported breaths (synch. to Pt's efforts) Additional Pt-initiated breaths → V_T determined by *Pt's efforts* ∴ Vent-assisted breaths ≠ spontaneous breaths Must overcome resp. circuit during spont. breaths → ? resp. fatigue SIMV = AC in patients who are not spontaneously breathing
Pressure support vent (PSV)	Vent supports Pt-initiated breaths with a set inspiratory pressure A mode of *partial* vent support because no set rate Can combine with SIMV to partially assist spontaneous breaths
Continuous positive airway pressure (CPAP)	Pt breathes spont. at their own rate while vent maintains constant positive airway pressure throughout respiratory cycle (7 cm H_2O overcomes 7 Fr ETT)
T-piece	No airway pressure, no rate set; patient breathes through ETT
Other (exp'tal)	Proportional assist vent (*Thorax* 2002;57:272) High-frequency vent (*AJRCCM* 2002;166:801)

Step 2: Choose Volume-Targeted or Pressure-Targeted	
Target	**Description**
Volume-targeted	Vent delivers a set V_T Airway pressures depend on airway resist. & lung/chest wall compliance Patient at risk for *↑ pressures* → barotrauma and volutrauma
Pressure-targeted	Vent delivers a set inspiratory pressure V_T depends on airway resistance and lung/chest wall compliance Patient at risk for *↓ volumes* → inadequate minute ventilation

Step 3: Set or ✓ Remaining Variables	
Variable	**Description**
F_iO_2	Fraction of inspired air that is oxygen
Positive end-expiratory pressure (PEEP)	Positive pressure applied during exhalation Generated by a resistor in exhalation port Benefits: prevents alveoli collapse, ↓ intrapulmonary shunt, ↑ O_2 Cardiac effects: ↓ preload by ↑ intrathoracic pressure and impeding venous return ↓ afterload by ↓ cardiac transmural pressure may ↑ or ↓ CO and may ↑ or ↓ oxygen delivery based on the above "Auto-PEEP" or "intrinsic PEEP": inadequate exhalation time → lungs unable to completely empty before the next breath (i.e., "breath stacking"); since there is flow at end-expiration there must be pressure = auto-PEEP Will ↓ preload and may ↓ CO just as ventilator-applied PEEP will do Will ↑ effort of breathing as must be overcome by Pt to trigger breaths Can be detected if end-expiratory flow ≠ 0 before next breath Can measure by occluding expiratory port of vent at end-expiration
Inspiratory time	Normally I:E ratio is ~1:2; however, can alter I time (and consequently flow rate, see below) – use in pressure control mode
Inspiratory flow rates	↑ flow rate → ↓ I time → ↑ E time → ∴ improved ventilation in obstructive disease (but ↑ PIPs) - use in volume control mode
Peak inspiratory pressure (PIP)	Dynamic measurement during inspiration Determined by airway resistance and lung compliance Set in pressure-targeted ventilation ↑ PIP w/o ↑ P_{plat} → ↑ airway resist (e.g., bronchospasm, secretions, plugging) ↓ PIP → ↓ airway resistance or air leak in the system
Plateau pressure (P_{plat})	Static measurement at the end of inspiration when there is no flow Determined by resp system compliance (resist. not a factor since ∅ flow) ↑ P_{plat} → ↓ lung or chest wall compliance (e.g., PTX, pulmonary edema, pneumonia, atelectasis), ↑ PEEP, or auto-PEEP

Initial Settings				
Mode	Tidal volume	Respiratory rate	F_iO_2	PEEP
Assist control Volume-targeted	~ 10 ml/kg IBW	10 breaths/min	1.0 (i.e., 100%)	? 5 cm H_2O

(Generally reasonable until settings can be tailored)

Noninvasive Ventilation	
Mode	**Description**
Continuous positive airway pressure (CPAP)	≈ PEEP No limit on O_2 delivered (i.e., can give hi-flow → F_iO_2 ≈ 1.0) Used in Pts whose primary problem is *hypoxemia* (e.g., CHF)
Bilevel positive airway pressure (BiPAP)	≈ PSV + PEEP Able to set both inspiratory (usually 8-10 cm H_2O) and expiratory pressures (usually <5 cm H_2O) May be limited in the amount of oxygen that can be delivered Used in patients whose primary problem is *hypoventilation*
Mask ventilation	Tight-fitting mask connecting patient to a standard ventilator Can receive pressure support of up to 20-30 cm H_2O, PEEP of up to 10 cm H_2O, F_iO_2 of up to 1.0 Used for short-term support (<24 hrs) for a reversible process (asthma, CHF, COPD)
Contraindications: altered mental status, vomiting, unable to protect airway, extrapulmonary organ failure, hemodynamic instability, severe upper GI bleeding, inability to fit mask (facial trauma/deformity or patient noncompliant)	

(*JAMA* 2002;288:932)

Tailoring the ventilator settings

- To improve oxygenation: ↑ F_iO_2, ↑ PEEP (optimize based on lung mechanics), ↑ I time
- To improve ventilation: ↑ V_T or inspiratory pressures, ↑ RR (may need to ↓ I time to accomplish Δs)
- **Permissive hypercapnia**: tolerating ↑ P_aCO_2 in order to avoid excessive barotrauma or volutrauma (see "ARDS")
  V_T = 4-6 ml/kg IBW (as long as P_aCO_2 <80 and pH >7.15)
  relative contraindications: cerebrovascular disease, hemodynamic instability, renal failure, pulmonary HTN

Acute ventilatory deterioration (usually ↑ PIP)

Fig. 2-7. Approach to acute ventilatory deterioration

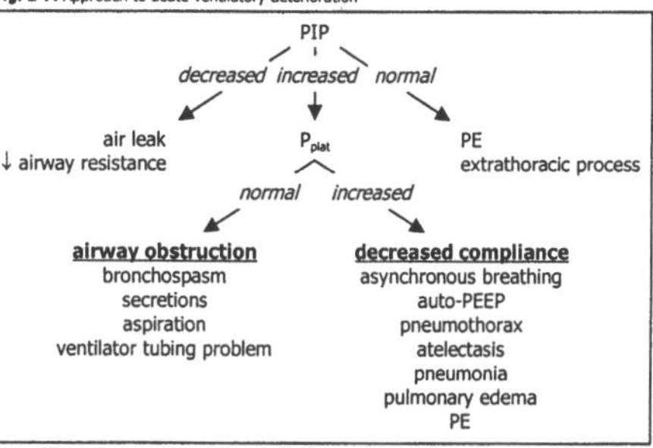

(Adapted from Marino, P.L. *The ICU Book*, 2nd ed., Baltimore: Williams & Wilkins, 1990:430)

- Response to ↑ PIP: disconnect Pt from ventilator, bag, auscultate, ✓ CXR and ABG

Weaning from the ventilator

- Weaning strategy: no single proven approach; ? easier from PSV (↓ 2-4 cm H_2O q 12 hrs) or using intermittent T-piece trials than from SIMV (↓ RR 2-4 breaths/min q 12 hrs + backup 5 cm H_2O PSV) (*AJRCCM* 1994;150:896; *NEJM* 332:345, 1995)
- Identify patients who can breathe spontaneously (*NEJM* 1991;324:1445 & 1996;335:1864)
  screening criteria: sedation reversed, VS stable, minimal secretions, adequate cough
  ventilator parameters: P_aO_2/F_iO_2 >200, PEEP ≤5, f/V_T <105, V_E <12 L/min, VC >10 ml/kg
  spontaneous breathing trial (e.g., CPAP × 1 to 2 hr)
    failure if: deteriorating ABGs, ↑ RR, ↑ or ↓ HR, ↑ or ↓ BP, diaphoresis, anxiety
    rapid shallow breathing index (f/V_T) >105 predicts failure (*NEJM* 1991;324:1445)
    if none of these events occurs → consider extubation

Complications

- Barotrauma and volutrauma (e.g., pneumothorax, pneumomediastinum)
  high PIPs are usually not harmful unless P_{plat} >35 cm H_2O → alveolar damage
- Oxygen toxicity (when F_iO_2 >0.6; proportional to duration and degree of toxic oxygen)
- Alterations in cardiac output
- Nosocomial pneumonia (1%/day, mortality rate ~30%)
  typical pathogens: MRSA, *Pseudomonas, Acinetobacter* and *Enterobacter* species
  preventive strategies (*NEJM* 1999;340:627)
    nonpharm: hand washing, semirecumbent position, non-nasal intubation, nutrition
    pharm: avoid unnecessary abx, ? sucralfate *vs.* H_2-blockers for stress-ulcer prophylaxis
- Laryngeal dysfunction (avoid by tracheostomy; consider after 2 weeks)
- Tracheal stenosis and tracheomalacia (softening of the tracheal cartilage)

• ACUTE RESPIRATORY DISTRESS SYNDROME •

Definition

- Acute respiratory distress syndrome (ARDS)
  - *clinical* = acute onset of severe hypoxemia refractory to O_2 and diffuse bilateral pulmonary infiltrates
  - *pathophysiological* = non-cardiogenic pulmonary edema
  - *pathological* = diffuse alveolar damage
- American-European Consensus Conference (1994): 4 criteria to define ARDS w/o bx
  - acute onset
  - bilateral patchy air-space disease
  - PCWP <18 mmHg or no clinical evidence of ↑ LVEDP
  - $P_aO_2/F_iO_2 \leq 200$; if $P_aO_2/F_iO_2 \leq 300$ → "acute lung injury" (ALI)

Etiologies			
Direct Injury		**Indirect Injury**	
• Aspiration	• Inhalation injury	• Sepsis	• Pancreatitis
• Pneumonia	• Lung contusion	• Shock	• Trauma/multiple fractures
• Near drowning		• DIC	• Hypertransfusion (TRALI)

Pathophysiology

- ↑ intrapulmonary shunt (∴ refractory to ↑ FiO_2)
- ↓ static compliance (V_T/P_{plat}-PEEP) <50 cc/cm H_2O
- Can develop 2° pulmonary hypertension as disease progresses

Diagnostic studies

- CXR: bilateral diffuse infiltrates developing w/in 24 hrs of appearance of air-space disease
- Chest CT: patchy infiltrate mixed w/ normal lung, densities greater in dependent areas

Treatment (primarily supportive)

- Mechanical ventilation strategies
  - *goals:* maintain adequate systemic O_2 delivery and minimize ventilator-induced lung injury from barotrauma/volutrauma, "atelectrauma", and hyperoxia
  - *strategies:*
    - **barotrauma/volutrauma**: avoid alveolar distention using low tidal volume protocol: goal $V_T \leq 6$ ml/kg, keep $P_{plat} \leq 30$ cm H_2O, tolerate permissive hypercapnia (keep pH >7.15), sedation/paralysis if needed (try to minimize); ↓ mortality (*NEJM* 2000;342:1301)
    - **atelectrauma** (tidal opening and collapse of alveoli): ideal PEEP controversial, may set PEEP > pressure needed to prevent end-expiratory alveolar collapse (i.e., set at lower point of maximal curvature on pressure-volume curve); or set lowest PEEP needed to maintain oxygenation; high-PEEP ("open-lung") strategies may benefit, but little data
    - **hyperoxia**: oxygen free radicals may potentiate lung injury, try to improve P_aO_2 by ↑ PEEP and ↑ inspiratory time rather than by ↑ F_iO_2; goal F_iO_2 <0.60
  - *rescue strategies* (little supportive data, but may try if conventional treatment failing)
    - **prone ventilation**: improve P_aO_2 but no benefit in outcomes (*NEJM* 2001;345:568)
    - **nitric oxide** (inhaled): selective pulmonary vasodilatation in ventilated lung units → improved V/Q matching, ↓ PA pressures, ↑ P_aO_2/F_iO_2 by 50 mmHg, but effect not sustained and no difference in mortality (*NEJM* 1993;328:399)
    - extracorporeal membrane oxygenation (ECMO), extracorporeal CO_2 removal ($ECCO_2R$)
    - inverse-ratio ventilation (prolonged inspiratory time to improve P_aO_2)
- PCWP as low as tolerated (*Chest* 1990;97:1176)
- **Steroids**: no benefit in the early phase; ? benefit in late fibroproliferative phase (*Chest* 1991;100:943, *JAMA* 1998;280:159). If no improvement by day 7 and no evidence of untreated infection (consider bronchoscopy, blood, urine and central line tip cultures, sinus and abdominal CT scans), consider methylprednisolone 2 mg/kg/d in divided doses q 6 hrs × 14 days, followed by gradual taper.
- Other strategies (little supportive data): surfactant, antioxidants, liquid ventilation, high frequency ventilation, prostacyclin

Prognosis

- Mortality: 35-40% overall, usually die of extrapulmonary complications
- Higher dead-space fraction $[(P_aCO_2\text{-}P_ECO_2)/P_aCO_2]$ predicts ↑ mortality (*NEJM* 2002;346:1281)
- Sequelae: PFTs nearly normalize but D_LCO remains low, muscle wasting, weakness persist (*NEJM* 2003;348:683)

• ESOPHAGEAL AND GASTRIC DISORDERS •

DYSPHAGIA

Definition

• Difficulty swallowing and passing food from the esophagus to the stomach

Etiologies (*BMJ* 2003;326:433)

Fig. 3-1. Etiologies of and approach to dysphagia

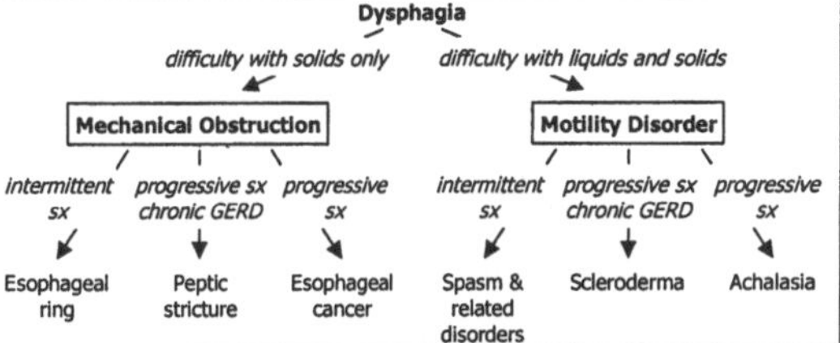

Diagnostic studies

• Barium swallow or EGD; ± manometry; rarely esophageal pH monitoring

DYSPEPSIA ("INDIGESTION")

Definition

• Discomfort centered in the upper abdomen

Etiologies

• Gastroesophageal reflux disease may be distinguished by its characteristic "heartburn"
• **Functional causes** ("non-ulcer dyspepsia" or NUD, ~60%): some combination of abnormal gastric motility, visceral afferent hypersensitivity, irritable bowel syndrome
• **Organic causes**: peptic ulcer disease (15-20%), gastric cancer (<2%), other causes (lactose intolerance, biliary colic, chronic pancreatitis, mesenteric ischemia)
• *Alarm factors* that suggest organic cause and warrant *EGD:* dysphagia, ⊕ FOBT or anemia, persistent anorexia or vomiting, weight loss, palpable mass or adenopathy, age >45 yrs

Treatment

• *H. pylori* eradication useful for PUD → ∴ empiric Rx reasonable if ⊕ serology; minimal data that eradication useful without PUD (*NEJM* 1998;339:1869, 1875 and 1999;341:1106)
• Functional dyspepsia: acid suppression with H_2-blockers, PPI, prokinetic agents, TCAs

Fig. 3-2. Workup and treatment of dyspepsia

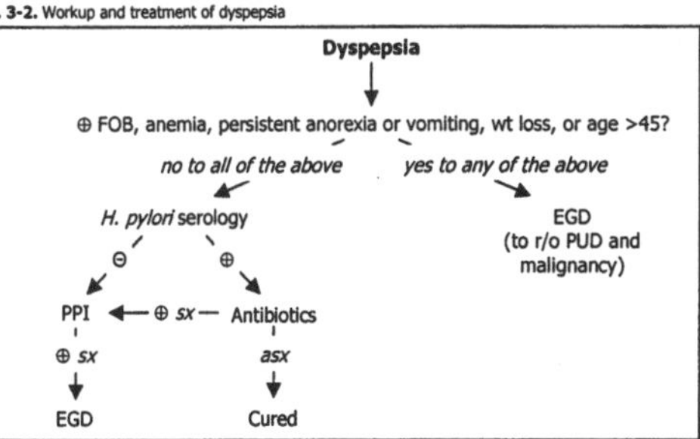

GASTROESOPHAGEAL REFLUX DISEASE (GERD)

Pathophysiology
- Excessive transient relaxations of lower esophageal sphincter (LES) or incompetent LES
- Esophageal mucosal damage (esophagitis) due to prolonged contact with acid, etc.
- Hiatal hernia: contributes to ↓ LES tone; acts as reservoir for refluxed gastric contents

Clinical manifestations
- **Heartburn**, atypical "angina"; regurgitation of stomach contents, water brash, dysphagia
- Cough (chronic nocturnal aspiration), asthma, hoarseness (vocal cord inflammation)
- **Precipitants**: large meals, supine position, fatty foods, caffeine, alcohol, cigarettes, CCB

Diagnostic tests
- Diagnosis often based on Hx, trial of PPI (e.g., omeprazole 40 mg q am + 20 mg PO q pm)
- EGD to detect esophagitis, ulcer, Barrett's esophagus, or stricture (*JAMA* 2002;287:1972)
- 24-hr ambulatory esophageal pH monitoring if diagnosis is uncertain

Treatment
- Conservative measures: avoid precipitants, elevate head of bed, avoid late meals
- Medical: antacids, H_2-blockers, proton pump inhibitors (PPI), prokinetic agents
- Surgical: fundoplication (often laparoscopic), success rate >90% (*NEJM* 1992;326:786)
- Endoscopic (under study, *Lancet* 2003;361:1119): suture fundoplication, radiofrequency ablation, microsphere injection of LES

Complications
- Esophagitis, *Barrett's esophagus* (specialized intestinal metaplasia with ~40× ↑ risk of adenocarcinoma, ~0.8% per yr, *NEJM* 1999;340:825 & 2002;346:846), stricture
- If Barrett's is found, endoscopic surveillance (e.g., q 2-3 yrs) for *dysplasia* is warranted

GASTROPATHY AND GASTRITIS

Acute gastropathy
- Etiologies: **NSAIDs, alcohol**, stress-related mucosal disease (critical illness)
- Clinical manifestations: often asymptomatic; anorexia, N/V, epigastric pain; UGIB

Chronic antral gastritis ("Type B")
- Etiology: ***H. pylori* infection**
- Clinical manifestations: most asx; *H. pylori* gastritis does *not* account for most cases of non-ulcer dyspepsia; can → atrophic gastritis w/ *↑ risk of gastric adenocarcinoma*
- Treatment: see below for *H. pylori* treatment

Chronic fundal gastritis ("Type A")
- Etiology: **pernicious anemia**
- Pathogenesis: autoantibodies against parietal cells (∴ lack of acid and intrinsic factor)
- Clinical manifestations: atrophic gastritis, achlorhydria, and hypergastrinemia; pernicious anemia; increased risk of gastric carcinoid tumors and adenocarcinoma

PEPTIC ULCER DISEASE (PUD)

Epidemiology
- **Duodenal ulcer (DU)**: ~300,000 cases per yr
- **Gastric ulcer (GU)**: ~75,000 cases per yr
- Lifetime prevalence ~10%

Principal etiologies (*Lancet* 2002;360:933)
- ***H. pylori* infection**: 90% of DU and 70% GU
  however, ~30% population colonized with *H. pylori* but only 15% will develop an ulcer
- **NSAIDs** (15-30% GU, 0.1-4% UGIB) and **ASA**
- Gastrinoma and other hypersecretory states (consider if multiple recurrent ulcers)
- Malignancy (5-10% of gastric ulcers)

Clinical Manifestations
- **Epigastric abdominal pain**, relieved with food (duodenal) or worsened by food (gastric)
- **Complications** include UGIB, perforation & penetration (6-7%), gastric outlet obstruction

Diagnostic studies

- Tests for *H. pylori*
  - serology (90% sens., 70-80% spec., not useful in confirming eradication)
  - urea breath test (UBT, sens. and spec. >95%)
  - stool antigen (HpSA, 94% sens., 86-92% spec., useful in confirming eradication)
  - EGD + rapid urease testing (e.g., CLOtest™, sens. and spec. >95%) or bx and histology
- EGD more sensitive (>95%) than UGI series to detect PUD
  - bx GU to r/o gastric carcinoma

Treatment

- ***H. pylori* eradication**: **clarithromycin** 500 mg bid + **amoxicillin** 1 g bid + **PPI** bid × 10-14 d has >90% success rate (*NEJM* 1995;333:984)
  - metronidazole 500 mg bid can be substituted for amoxicillin in penicillin allergic Pts
  - ? document eradication with UBT or HpSA (consider if Pt would not tolerate recurrence)
- If *H. pylori* negative, acid suppression with PPI
- **Discontinue NSAIDs**; if must continue, consider:
  - adding PPI (*NEJM* 1998;338:719 & 727)
  - adding misoprostol (*Annals* 1995;123:241)
  - Δ to COX-2 selective inhibitor (~80% ↓ in PUD, ~50% ↓ in UGIB, *JAMA* 1999;282:1921 & 2000;284:1247, *NEJM* 2000;343:1520; but not in all studies, *NEJM* 2002;347:2104)
- Lifestyle changes: discontinue smoking and ? EtOH; diet irrelevant
- Endoscopy: acutely to control UGIB; to document resolution of GU after 8 wks of Rx
- Surgery: usually reserved for rare cases refractory to medical management (rule out surreptitious NSAID use) or for complications (see above)

• GASTROINTESTINAL BLEEDING •

Definition
- Intraluminal blood loss anywhere from the oropharynx to the anus
- Classification: **upper** = above the ligament of Treitz; **lower** = below the ligament of Treitz
- Signs: **hematemesis** = blood in vomitus (UGIB); **hematochezia** = bloody stools (LGIB or rapid UGIB); **melena** = black, tarry stools from digested blood (usually UGIB, but can be anywhere above and including the right colon)

Etiologies of upper GI bleed (UGIB)
- Oropharyngeal bleeding and epistaxis → swallowed blood
- **Erosive esophagitis** (10%)
  - immunocompetent host: GERD/Barrett's esophagus, XRT
  - immunocompromised: CMV, HSV, Candida
- **Varices** (10%)
- **Mallory-Weiss tear** (10%; GE junction tear due to retching against closed glottis)
- **Gastritis/gastropathy** (15%; NSAIDs, alcohol, stress-related mucosal disease)
- **Peptic ulcer disease** (PUD) (50%)
- **Vascular malformations** (5%)
  - Dieulafoy's lesion (superficial ectatic artery usually in cardia → sudden, massive UGIB)
  - AVMs (isolated or with Osler-Weber-Rendu syndrome)
  - aorto-enteric fistula (AAA or aortic graft erodes to 3rd portion of duodenum; presents with "herald bleed")
  - vasculitis
- Neoplastic disease (esophageal or gastric)

Etiologies of lower GI bleed (LGIB)
- Diverticular disease
- Angiodysplasia
- Neoplastic disease
- Colitis: infection, ischemic, radiation, inflammatory bowel disease (UC >> CD)
- Hemorrhoids

Clinical manifestations
- UGIB > LGIB: nausea, vomiting, hematemesis, coffee-ground emesis, epigastric pain, vasovagal reactions, syncope, melena
- LGIB > UGIB: diarrhea, tenesmus, BRBPR or maroon stools

Workup
- **History**
  - acute or chronic GIB, number of episodes, most recent episode
  - hematemesis, vomiting *prior* to hematemesis, melena, hematochezia
  - abdominal pain, Δ in stool caliber
  - use of aspirin, NSAIDs, anticoagulants, or known coagulopathy
  - alcohol abuse, cirrhosis
  - prior GI or aortic surgery
- **Physical exam**
  - tachycardia at 10% volume loss; orthostatic hypotension at 20% loss; shock at 30% loss
  - pallor, telangectasias (alcoholic liver disease or Osler-Weber-Rendu syndrome)
  - signs of chronic liver disease: jaundice, spider angiomata, gynecomastia, testicular atrophy, palmar erythema, caput medusae
  - localizable abdominal tenderness or peritoneal signs, masses, signs of prior surgery
  - rectal exam: appearance of stools, presence of hemorrhoids or anal fissures
- **Laboratory studies: Hct** (*may be normal* early in acute blood loss before equilibration, which may take 24 hrs; ↓ 2-3% → loss of 500 cc blood), **platelet count, PT, PTT**, BUN/Cr (ratio >36 in UGIB due to GI resorption of blood *and/or* prerenal azotemia), LFTs
- **Nasogastric tube**: Useful for localization (presence of non-bloody bile in lavage excludes active bleeding proximal to the ligament of Treitz), can also clear GI contents prior to EGD and detect continued bleeding
- Diagnostic studies in UGIB: EGD (and potentially therapeutic)

- Diagnostic studies in LGIB (r/o UGIB before attempting to localize presumed LGIB)
  bleeding spontaneously stops → **colonoscopy** (identifies cause in >70%, potential Rx)
  stable but continued bleeding → colonoscopy after rapid purge or **bleeding scan** (^{99m}Tc-tagged RBC/albumin): detects bleeding rates ≥0.1 ml/min, but localization difficult
  unstable → **arteriography** (detects bleeding rates ≥0.5 ml/min and potentially therapeutic (intraarterial vasopressin infusion or embolization)
  exploratory **laparotomy**

<u>Treatment</u>

- ***Acute treatment of GIB is hemodynamic resuscitation with IV fluid and blood***
  establish **access** with 2 large-bore (18-gauge or larger) intravenous lines
  volume resuscitation with normal saline or lactated Ringer's solution
  transfusion therapy (blood bank sample for type & cross; O-neg if Pt exsanguinating)
  correct coagulopathies (FFP to normalize PT, platelets to keep count >50,000/mm^3)
  nasogastric tube lavage if hematemesis
  airway management as needed
  consult GI and surgical services as needed

Etiology	Options
Varices	*Pharmacologic* **octreotide** 50 μg IVB → 50 μg/hr infusion (84% success; *Lancet* 1993;342:637) β-blockers (non-selective) ± nitrates once stable *Non-pharmacologic* **endoscopic** band ligation (>90% success) has replaced sclerotherapy (88% success) (*Semin Liver Dis* 1999;19:439) octreotide + endoscopic therapy (>95% success; *NEJM* 1995;333:555) balloon tamponade (Sengstaken-Blakemore) if bleeding severe embolization or TIPS if endoscopy fails (*NEJM* 1994;330:165)
PUD	*Pharmacologic* High dose PPI (*NEJM* 1997;336:1054) ? octreotide 50 μg IVB → 50 μg/hr infusion *Non-pharmacologic* **endoscopic therapy** (injection, thermal, laser) arteriography with infusion of vasopressin or embolization surgery if endoscopic and pharmacologic therapy fails
Mallory-Weiss	*Usually stops spontaneously; endoscopic therapy if active*
Esophagitis Gastritis	PPI, H_2-antagonists
Diverticular disease	*Usually stops spontaneously* Endoscopic therapy (e.g., epinephrine injection), arterial vasopressin or embolization, surgery
Angiodysplasia	Arterial vasopressin, endoscopic therapy, surgery, hormonal Rx (*Am J Gastroenterol* 1998;93:1250)

<u>Poor prognostic signs in UGIB</u>

- Demographics: age >60, comorbidities, variceal or neoplastic etiology
- Severity: bright red blood in NGT, ↑ transfusion requirement, hemodynamic instability
- Appearance of ulcer (from best to worst prognosis): clean base → oozing without visible vessel → adherent clot → active bleeding

<u>Obscure GIB</u>

- Etiologies: angiodysplasia, small intestinal tumors, Meckel's diverticulum, Crohn's disease, mesenteric ischemia, vasculitis
- Workup: push enteroscopy, enteroclysis, bleeding scan, angiography (to look for abnormal "vascular blush"), ^{99m}Tc-pertechnetate scan ("Meckel's scan"), wireless capsule endoscopy

• DIARRHEA •

Stool output > 200 g/day or ↑ frequency and ↓ consistency of stool

ETIOLOGIES

Infections (*NEJM* 2004;350:38)
- **Acute**
  - **Pre-formed toxins** ("food poisoning", <24 hrs): *S. aureus, C. perfringens, B. cereus*
  - **Viruses**: rotavirus, Norwalk
  - **Non-invasive bacteria**
    - enterotoxin-producing (no fecal WBC or blood): enterotoxigenic *E. coli, Vibrio cholera*
    - cytotoxin-producing (⊕ fecal WBC and blood): *E. coli* O157:H7, *C. difficile*
  - **Invasive bacteria** (⊕ fecal WBC and blood): enteroinvasive *E. coli* (EIEC), *Salmonella, Shigella, Campylobacter, Yersinia, V. parahemolyticus*
  - **Parasites**: *Giardia, E. histolytica*
  - **Opportunistic**: *Cryptosporidia, Isospora, Microsporidia, Cyclospora*, MAC, CMV
- **Chronic**: *Giardia, E. histolytica, C. difficile*, opportunistic organisms
- Clues as to etiology
  - Travel: *E. coli*, parasites (*Giardia* with ingestion of water from streams)
  - Shellfish: Norwalk, *Vibrio* sp.
  - Undercooked hamburger: E. coli O157:H7
  - Poultry: *Campylobacter, Salmonella*
  - Antibiotic use: *C. difficile*

Malabsorption (↓ diarrhea with fasting, ↑ osmotic gap & fecal fat, defic. in fat-soluble vit.)
- **Bile salt deficiency**
  - bacterial overgrowth (e.g., blind loops) → deconjugation of bile salts
  - ileal disease (e.g., Crohn's, surgery) → interruption of enterohepatic circulation
- **Pancreatic insufficiency**
- **Mucosal abnormalities**
  - *Celiac sprue:* intestinal reaction to α-gliadin in gluten → loss of villi & absorptive area
    - diagnostic studies: ⊕ IgA or anti-transglutaminase or endomysial Abs; small bowel bx
    - treatment: gluten-free diet (*Lancet* 2003;362:383)
  - *Tropical sprue:* occurs in residents of the tropics; treatment with antibiotics, folate, B_{12}
  - *Whipple's disease:* due to infection with *Tropheryma whippelii* (gram ⊕ bacilli)
    - typically affects middle-aged white men
    - other s/s: fever, LAN, edema, arthritis, CNS Δs, gray-brown skin pigmentation, murmur
    - treatment: prolonged course of antibiotics
  - *Intestinal lymphoma*

Other osmotic (↓ diarrhea with fasting, ↑ osmotic gap, normal fecal fat)
- **Medications**: antacids, lactulose, sorbitol
- **Lactose intolerance**: 1° or 2° mucosal abnormality, viral/bacterial enteritis, s/p resection
  - clinical manifestations: bloating, flatulence, discomfort, diarrhea
  - diagnostic studies: lactose hydrogen breath test or empiric lactose-free diet
  - treatment: lactose-free diet, use of lactaid milk and lactase enzyme tablets

Inflammatory (fever, hematochezia, abdominal pain)
- **Inflammatory bowel disease**
- Radiation enteritis

Secretory (normal osmotic gap, large volume, no Δ in diarrhea after NPO)
- **Hormonal**: VIP (VIPoma, Verner-Morrison), serotonin (carcinoid), calcitonin (medullary cancer of the thyroid), gastrin (Zollinger-Ellison), glucagon, substance P, thyroxine
- **Laxative abuse**
- Villous adenoma
- Idiopathic bile salt malabsorption
- Lymphocytic colitis, collagenous colitis

Motility
- **Irritable bowel syndrome** (10-22% of adults; *NEJM* 2001;344:1846): abd pain & Δs in bowel habits; pain relief with bowel action; loose, freq. stools, incomplete evacuation
  - treatment: constipation → fiber; diarrhea → anti-diarrheals; pain → anti-spasmatics
- Scleroderma (pseudo-obstruction)
- Endocrinopathies: diabetes mellitus; hyperthyroidism (hyperdefecation)

Diarrhea workup

Fig. 3-3. Workup of acute diarrhea (<3 wks duration)

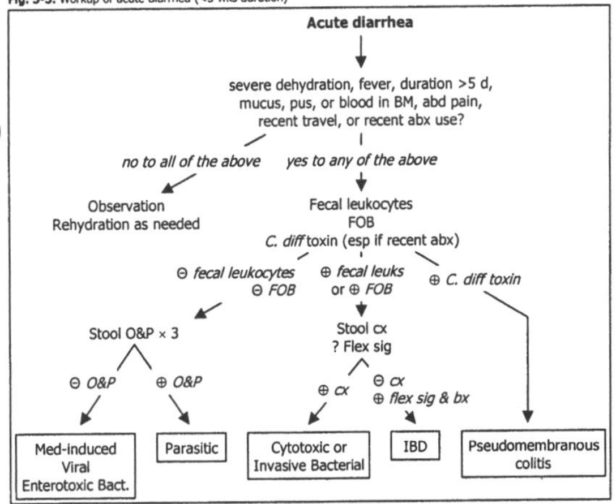

Fig. 3-4. Workup of chronic diarrhea (>3 wks duration)

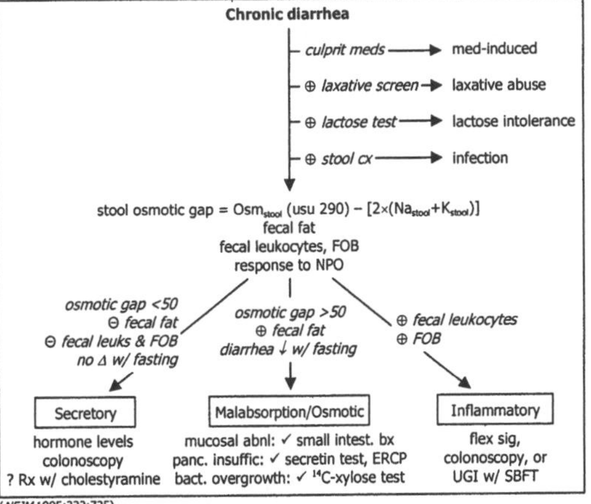

(*NEJM* 1995;332:725)

Empiric treatment for acute, likely infectious diarrhea

- Mild: bismuth subsalicylate & loperamide prn
- Moderate-severe *or* fever, blood or pus: empiric fluoroquinolone × 3 d

• DIVERTICULAR DISEASE •

DIVERTICULOSIS

Definition and Pathology (*Lancet* 2004;363:631)
- Acquired herniations of colonic mucosa and submucosa through the colonic wall
- More common on the **left side** than the right side of the colon
- May be a consequence of a **low-fiber diet** → colonic musculature contracting against small, hard stools

Epidemiology
- Affects 20-50% of persons over the age of 50

Clinical manifestations
- Usually asx, but can be complicated by **diverticulitis** or **bleeding**

DIVERTICULITIS

Pathophysiology (*NEJM* 1998;338:1521)
- Retention of undigested food and bacteria in diverticulum → fecalith formation → obstruction → compromise of diverticulum's blood supply, infection, perforation
- Microperforation (→ localized infection) or macroperforation (→ abscess and/or peritonitis)

Clinical manifestations
- **LLQ abdominal pain, fever**, nausea, vomiting, constipation

Physical exam
- Mild: LLQ tenderness, ± palpable mass, ± positive FOBT (~25%)
- Severe: peritonitis, septic shock

Diagnostic studies
- **Plain abdominal radiographs** to r/o free air, ileus, or obstruction
- Abdominal CT may show thickening of bowel wall; usually reserved for Pts who fail to respond to therapy or if suspect pericolic abscess
- Sigmoidoscopy/colonoscopy *contraindicated* in acute setting because of ↑ risk of overt perforation; colonoscopy recommended 2-6 wks after resolution to rule out neoplasm

Treatment
- **Mild**: PO antibiotics (FQ + MNZ) and liquid diet × 7-10 d
- **Severe**
  NPO, IV fluids, NGT (if ileus)
  IV antibiotics (GNR & anaerobic coverage): cefotetan/MNZ or amp/gent/MNZ
- Abscess drainage percutaneously or surgically
- Surgery if medical therapy fails, free perforation, large abscess that cannot be drained percutaneously, recurrent disease (≥2 episodes)

DIVERTICULAR BLEEDING (ALSO SEE "GASTROINTESTINAL BLEEDING")

Pathophysiology
- Erosion of blood vessel feeding diverticulum by a fecalith
- Diverticula more common in left colon; *but bleeding diverticula are usually in right colon*

Clinical manifestations
- Usually sudden onset of abdominal cramping followed by voluminous hematochezia
- Usually stops spontaneously (80%) but may follow a stuttering course for hours to days

Physical exam
- Usually benign

Diagnostic studies
- Colonoscopy (after acute bleeding has stopped and following oral lavage) or, for severe bleeding, mesenteric arteriography (usually after a bleeding scan)

Treatment (see "Gastrointestinal Bleeding" for persistent bleeding)
- Endoscopy → epinephrine injection ± electrocautery, hemoclip placement, or banding
- Arteriography → intraarterial vasopressin infusion
- Surgery

• INFLAMMATORY BOWEL DISEASE •

Definition (*NEJM* 2002;347:417)
- **Ulcerative colitis (UC)**: idiopathic inflammation of the colonic *mucosa*
- **Crohn's disease (CD)**: idiopathic *transmural* inflammation of the GI tract, *skip areas*
- In 5-10% of patients with chronic colitis a clear distinction between UC and CD cannot be made even with mucosal biopsy ("indeterminate colitis")

Differential diagnosis
- Infectious: bacterial (SSCY, *E. coli* O157:H7), pseudomembranous, amebic, CMV, STDs
- Ischemic colitis
- Intestinal lymphoma or carcinoma; collagenous colitis
- Irritable bowel syndrome
- Drugs (NSAIDs, OCP, gold, allopurinol)

ULCERATIVE COLITIS

Epidemiology
- Prevalence 1:1000
- Age of onset 20-25 yrs; ↑ incidence in Caucasians, especially Jews; familial in ~10%
- Appendectomy prior to age 20 for appendicitis (*NEJM* 2001;344:808) and tobacco use (*NEJM* 1987;316:707) have been reported to be protective against the development of UC

Pathology
- Extent: involves rectum (95%) and extends proximally and *contiguously*
  50% of patients have proctosigmoiditis, 30% left-sided colitis, and 20% extensive colitis
- Appearance: granular, friable mucosa with diffuse ulceration; *pseudopolyps*
  on barium enema → hazy margins, loss of haustra ("lead pipe")
- Microscopy: superficial microulcerations; crypt abscesses (PMNs)

Clinical manifestations
- **Grossly bloody diarrhea**, lower abdominal cramps and urgency
- **Fulminant colitis**: progresses rapidly over 1-2 weeks with ↓ Hct, ↑ ESR, fever, hypotension, >6 bloody BMs per day, distended abdomen with absent bowel sounds
- **Toxic megacolon**: colon dilatation (≥6 cm on KUB), colonic atony, and systemic toxicity
- Perforation → pneumoperitoneum, peritonitis
- Extracolonic (25%)
  erythema nodosum, pyoderma gangrenosum, aphthous ulcers, iritis, episcleritis
  thromboembolic events
  seronegative arthritis, chronic hepatitis, cirrhosis, primary sclerosing cholangitis (PSC) with ↑ risk of cholangiocarcinoma
- Serologies: p-ANCA in 60-70% (associated with pancolitis and PSC)

Complications
- Stricture (rare, occurs in rectosigmoid)
- **Colon cancer**: risk in patients with *pancolitis* is greatest (7-16% cumulative risk at 20 yrs), patients with left-sided colitis and PSC are also at increased risk; the risk of colorectal cancer is not increased with ulcerative proctitis
- Surveillance: yearly *colonoscopy* with random biopsies after 8 yrs of pancolitis or 15 yrs of left-sided colitis to look for dysplasia → colectomy

Prognosis
- Intermittent exacerbations in 80%; continual active disease in 10-15%; severe initial attack requiring urgent colectomy in 5-10%
- Mortality rate for severe attack of ulcerative colitis is <2%
- No difference in life expectancy compared to individuals without ulcerative colitis

CROHN'S DISEASE

Epidemiology
- Prevalence 1:3000
- *Bimodal* with peaks in 20s and 50-70; ↑ incidence in Caucasians, Jews, and smokers
- Mutation of the *NOD 2/CARD 15* gene found in 20% of patients (*Nature* 1996;379:821)

Pathology

- Extent: can affect any portion of GI tract from mouth to anus, with *skip lesions*
  30% of Pts have ileitis, 50% ileocolitis, and 20% colitis; isolated upper tract disease rare
- Appearance: non-friable mucosa, cobblestoning, deep & long **fissures**
  on barium enema → sharp lesions, long ulcers & fissures
- Microscopy: **transmural inflammation** with mononuclear cell infiltrate, non-caseating **granulomas** (seen in <25% of mucosal biopsies), fissures

Clinical manifestations

- **Smoldering disease with abdominal pain**
- Mucus-containing **non-grossly bloody diarrhea**
- Fevers, malaise, weight loss
- ↓ albumin, ↑ ESR, ↓ Hct due to Fe, B_{12}, folate deficiency, or chronic disease
- Extracolonic: same as UC, plus *gallstones* (due to malabsorption of bile salts) and *kidney stones* (Ca oxalate stones due to binding of intraluminal Ca^{++} by unabsorbed bile salts allowing ↑'d oxalate absorption)
- Serologies: anti-*Saccharomyces cerevisiae* antibodies (ASCA) in 60-70%

Complications

- Perianal fissures, perirectal abscesses
- **Stricture**: postprandial bloating, distention, borborygmi
- **Fistulas**: abscesses, bacterial overgrowth & malabsorption
- **Abscess**: fevers, chills, tender abdominal mass, ↑ WBC
- **Cancer**: small intestinal and colorectal; risk of colorectal cancer is in CD is similar to that in UC; recommendations for colonoscopic surveillance are the same as those for UC

TREATMENT

General measures

- Avoid NSAIDs (both UC and CD) & tobacco (CD)
- Antidiarrheals only in *mild* disease
- Rule out infection before treating with immunosuppressants

Acute Flare Treatment	
Severity	**Options**
Mild	**5-ASA compounds (oral)** Sulfasalazine (5-ASA + sulfa): bacterial reductases release 5-ASA in *colon* Mesalamine (5-ASA in pH-sensitive or time-dependent capsules) Asacol: dissolves at pH 7.0 → 5-ASA released in *terminal SI & colon* Pentasa: 5-ASA released throughout the *small intestine & colon* Olsalazine & Balsalazide (5-ASA dimer): cleaved in the *colon* **Other useful agents** budesonide: oral steroid useful in *ileocecal* CD; low systemic absorption rectal 5-ASA (enemas, suppositories) for distal UC, proctitis metronidazole: useful in perianal, fistulizing and active colonic CD ciprofloxacin: useful in combination with metronidazole in active CD
Moderate	**Oral steroids**
Severe	**Intravenous steroids** ± cyclosporine for UC (*NEJM* 1994;330:1841) ± infliximab for CD (*NEJM* 1997;337:1029 & 1999;340:1398) Bowel rest, d/c antidiarrheals, TPN, IV antibiotics Serial abdominal exams and radiographs/CTs to r/o dilatation, perforation, or abscess

Maintenance of remission

- 5-ASA compounds (? UC only): appropriate formulation to treat affected areas
- Immunomodulators: azathioprine, 6-MP, methotrexate (CD, *NEJM* 2000;342:1627), infliximab (CD)

Indications for surgery

- UC (25% of all patients): failed medical therapy, hemorrhage, perforation, stricture, fulminant colitis or toxic megacolon that fails to respond within 48-72 hrs of medical therapy, confirmed high grade dysplasia or carcinoma
- CD (75% of all patients): failed medical therapy, ? chronic steroid requirement, stricture, fistula, abscess, carcinoma

• MESENTERIC ISCHEMIA •

Small Bowel

Etiologies

- **SMA embolism** (50%): from LA (AF) or LV (↓ EF)
- **SMA thrombosis** (10%): usually at site of atherosclerosis, often at origin of artery
- **Focal segmental ischemia of the small bowel** (5%): vascular occlusion to small segments of the small bowel (vasculitis, atheromatous emboli, strangulated hernias, XRT)
- **Non-occlusive mesenteric ischemia** (25%): low cardiac output ± high doses of vasoconstrictors
- **Venous thrombosis** (10%): due to hypercoagulable states, portal hypertension, malignancy, inflammation (pancreatitis, peritonitis), trauma, surgery

Clinical manifestations

- Sudden onset of abdominal pain out of proportion to abdominal tenderness on exam
- "Intestinal angina": postprandial abdominal pain & early satiety occurring weeks to months prior to the onset of acute pain may be seen with superior mesenteric arterial thrombosis
- Abdominal distension without pain (usually with non-occlusive disease)
- GIB (the right colon is supplied by the superior mesenteric artery)

Physical exam

- May be unremarkable
- Bowel infarction suggested by peritoneal signs

Diagnostic studies

- Laboratory evaluation: may be normal; ↑ WBC; ↑ amylase, LDH and CK; metabolic acidosis and ↑ lactate (late), ⊕ FOBT (75% of cases)
- Imaging studies
  - plain radiograph: normal prior to infarction, "thumbprinting" & ileus in later stage disease
  - Doppler U/S: useful for identifying venous and proximal arterial occlusion
  - **abdominal CT**: early signs nonspecific; bowel wall thickening, pneumatosis of bowel wall; best test to detect mesenteric venous thrombosis
  - **angiography**: gold standard

Treatment

- Volume resuscitation, optimization of hemodynamics, discontinue pressors if possible
- **Antibiotics** for infarction, sepsis
- Intraarterial infusion of **thrombolytic** agent for acute arterial embolism
- **Anticoagulation**: for arterial and venous thrombosis, embolic disease
- Intraarterial infusion of **papaverine** for non-occlusive mesenteric ischemia
- Surgery: **embolectomy** for acute arterial embolism; revascularization for acute superior mesenteric arterial thrombosis; resection of infarcted bowel

Prognosis

- Mortality 20-70%
- Diagnosis prior to onset of intestinal infarction is the strongest predictor of survival

Ischemic Colitis

Definition and pathophysiology

- Usually a non-occlusive disease with unclear pathophysiology
- Predisposing factors: ↑ age and Δs in systemic circulation and local mesenteric vasculature
- "Watershed" areas (splenic flexure → sigmoid) are most susceptible

Clinical manifestations, diagnosis, and treatment

- Disease spectrum: reversible colopathy (35%), transient colitis (15%), chronic ulcerating colitis (20%), stricture (10%), gangrene (15%), fulminant colitis (<5%)
- Usual clinical presentation is crampy LLQ pain associated with guaiac ⊕ or overtly bloody stool; fever and peritoneal signs should raise clinical suspicion for infarction
- Diagnosis: **flexible sigmoidoscopy** or **colonoscopy** within 48 hours if no peritonitis
- Treatment: bowel rest, IV fluids, ? broad spectrum antibiotics, serial abdominal exams; **surgery** for infarction, fulminant colitis or obstruction due to ischemic stricture
- Resolution within 48 hrs with conservative measures occurs in over 50% of cases

• ACUTE PANCREATITIS •

Etiologies

- Common
  - **alcohol** (30% of cases, typically in men): usually chronic, with acute flares
  - **gallstones** (35% of cases, typically in women): usually small (<5 mm) stones are culprit
- Rare
  - Obstructive: ampullary or pancreatic tumors, pancreas divisum
  - Metabolic: hypertriglyceridemia (TG need to be >750; for type I and type V familial hypertriglyceridemia, TG usually ~4500), hypercalcemia
  - Drugs: furosemide, thiazides, sulfa, didanosine, protease inhibitors, estrogen, azathioprine, 6-MP, ACE inhibitors
  - Infection: echovirus, Coxsackievirus, mumps, rubella, EBV, CMV, HIV, HAV, HBV, Ascaris
  - Trauma: blunt abdominal trauma, post ERCP (35-70% with ↑ amylase, ~5% with clinical, overt pancreatitis)
  - Scorpion sting (in Trinidad)

Clinical manifestations

- **Epigastric abdominal pain**, radiating to the back, constant, little change with position
- Nausea and vomiting; fever is common
- Ddx: biliary disease, perforated viscus, intestinal obstruction, mesenteric ischemia, IMI, AAA leak, distal aortic dissection

Physical exam

- Abdominal tenderness and guarding, ↓ bowel sounds (adynamic ileus)
  ± palpable abdominal mass; ± jaundice if biliary obstruction
- Signs of retroperitoneal hemorrhage (Cullen's = periumbilical; Grey Turner's = flank) rare
- ± hypotension or shock

Diagnostic studies

- Laboratory
  - ↑ **amylase**: levels >3× ULN very suggestive of pancreatitis, but level ≠ severity
    - false ⊖: acute on chronic (e.g., alcoholic); hypertriglyceridemia (↓ amylase activity)
    - false ⊕: other abd. or salivary gland process, acidemia, renal failure, macroamylasemia (amylase binds to other proteins in serum, cannot be filtered out)
  - ↑ **lipase**: may be more specific than amylase
  - ALT >3× ULN → gallstone pancreatitis (*Am J Gastroenterol* 1994;89:1863); Aϕ, bili not helpful
  - other labs depending on severity: ↑ WBC, ↓ Hct, ↑ BUN, ↓ Ca, ↑ glucose
- Imaging studies
  - **abdominal CT** to diagnose pancreatitis, exclude other abdominal processes, stage severity, and look for complications; performed with oral and IV contrast, although latter is generally avoided for 1st few days b/c theoretical concern of ↑ necrosis (and necrosis may not be radiographically apparent for 48-72 hrs)
  - **abdominal ultrasound** to evaluate for gallstones, CBD dilatation, ascites, pseudocyst pancreas often obscured by bowel gas, if seen → enlarged, hypoechoic
  - **abdominal plain films** may show "sentinel loop" or Ca 2° to chronic pancreatitis
- CT-guided abscess drainage or fine-needle aspiration if pancreatic necrosis present on CT to r/o infection (96% sens., 99% spec.) and Pt w/ persistent fevers, ↑ WBC, organ failure

Treatment (*Lancet* 2003;361:1447)

- Supportive therapy
  - **fluid resuscitation** (may need up to *10L/day* if hemodynamically severe pancreatitis)
  - **NPO**; NG suction if protracted vomiting; **nutritional support** & electrolyte repletion consider feeding by day 3 if non-severe with no pain and near normal amylase
  - **analgesia** with meperidine
- Antibiotics
  - gut decontamination w/ oral nonabsorbable abx may be efficacious (*Ann Surg* 1995;222:57)
  - **systemic abx** w/ imipenem in Pts w/ severe necrotizing pancreatitis (>30% necrosis by CT) may ↓ mortality (*J Gastrointest Surg* 1998;2:496)
- ERCP: ↓ biliary sepsis in gallstone pancreatitis (*NEJM* 1993;328:228), no effect on local or systemic pancreatitis complications; only effective in those with obstructive jaundice (*NEJM* 1997;336:237)

Complications

- Systemic: shock, ARDS, renal failure, GI hemorrhage
- Metabolic: hypocalcemia, hyperglycemia, hypertriglyceridemia
- **Acute fluid collection** (30-50%): seen early, low attenuation, no capsule, no Rx required
- **Pseudocyst** (10-20%): fluid collection that persists for 4-6 wks & becomes encapsulated
  suggested by persistent pain or persistent elevation of amylase or lipase
  most resolve spont.; if >6 cm or persists >6 wks + pain → internal/precutan. drainage
- **Sterile pancreatic necrosis** (20%): area of non-viable pancreatic tissue
  Rx conservatively with prophylactic antibiotics (e.g., imipenem; *NEJM* 1999;340:1412) & supportive measures for as long as possible; surgery if Pt unstable
- **Infection** (5% of all cases, 30% of severe): fever and ↑ WBC; usually 2° enteric GNR
  pancreatic abscess: circumscribed collection of pus (usually w/o pancreatic tissue) treat with antibiotics + drainage (CT-guided if possible)
  infected pancreatic necrosis (aspiration → ⊕ bacterial culture): antibiotics + surgical debridement (100% mortality w/o debridement; *Hepatogastroenterology* 1991;38:116)
- Pancreatic ascites or pleural effusion: indicates disrupted pancreatic duct; consider ERCP with stent placement across duct
- Scarring of pancreatic duct → stricture → chronic pancreatitis

Prognosis

- Severe pancreatitis = organ failure *or* local complications (necrosis, abscess, pseudocyst) *or* ≥3 Ranson's criteria

Ranson's Criteria	
At diagnosis	**At 48 hours**
age >55	Hct ↓ >10%
WBC >16,000/mm^3	BUN ↑ >5 mg/dl
glucose >200 mg/dl	base deficit >4 mEq/L
AST >250 U/L	Ca <8 mEq/L
LDH >350 U/L	P_aO_2 <60 mmHg
	fluid sequestration >6 L
Prognosis	
# of criteria	**Mortality**
≤2	<5%
3-4	15-20%
5-6	40%
≥7	>99%

(*Am J Gastroenterol* 1982;77:633)

CT Grade	Description
A	Normal pancreas consistent with mild pancreatitis
B	Focal or diffuse enlargement of the gland, including contour irregularities and inhomogeneous attenuation but without peripancreatic inflammation
C	Grade B + peripancreatic fluid collections
D	Grade C + associated single fluid collection
E	Grade C + ≥2 peripancreatic fluid collections or gas in the pancreas or retroperitoneum

(*Radiology* 1990;174:331)

• ABNORMAL LIVER TESTS •

Tests of hepatic function

- **Albumin**: general marker for liver protein synthesis, ↓ slowly in liver failure ($t_{½}$ ~20 d)
- **Prothrombin time** (PT): depends on synthesis of coagulation factors; because $t_{½}$ of some of these factors (e.g., V, VII) is short, ↑ PT can occur within hrs of liver dysfunction
- **Bilirubin**: product of heme metab. in liver; unconjugated (indirect) or conjugated (direct)

Abnormal liver tests in hepatocellular injury or cholestasis

- **Aminotransferases** (AST, ALT): intracellular enzymes released 2° necrosis/inflammation
  ALT relatively specific for liver
  AST found in liver, heart, skeletal muscle, kidney, and brain
  ALT > AST → viral hepatitis or fatty liver/nonalcoholic steatohepatitis (pericirrhotic)
  AST:ALT > 2:1 → alcoholic hepatitis; ↑↑↑ LDH → ischemic or toxic hepatitis
- **Alkaline phosphatase** (Aϕ): enzyme bound in hepatic canicular membrane
  besides liver, also found in bone, intestines, and placenta
  confirm liver origin with: ↑ 5′-NT, ↑ GGT, or heat fractionation
  ↑ levels seen with biliary obstruction or intrahepatic cholestasis (e.g., hepatic infiltration)

Patterns in liver injury

- **Hepatocellular**: ↑↑ aminotransferases, ± ↑ bilirubin or Aϕ
  ↑↑↑ aminotransferases (>1000): severe viral hepatitis, acetaminophen, and ischemia
- *Jaundice* is a clinical sign seen when bilirubin >2.5 mg/dl (especially in sclera); part of either cholestatic pattern or isolated hyperbilirubinemia; if conjugated → ↑ urine bilirubin
- **Cholestasis**: ↑↑ Aϕ and bilirubin, ± ↑ aminotransferases
- **Isolated hyperbilirubinemia**: ↑↑ bilirubin, near normal Aϕ and aminotransferases
- **Infiltrative**: ↑ Aϕ, ± ↑ bilirubin or aminotransferases

Fig. 3-5. Approach to abnormal liver tests with hepatocellular pattern

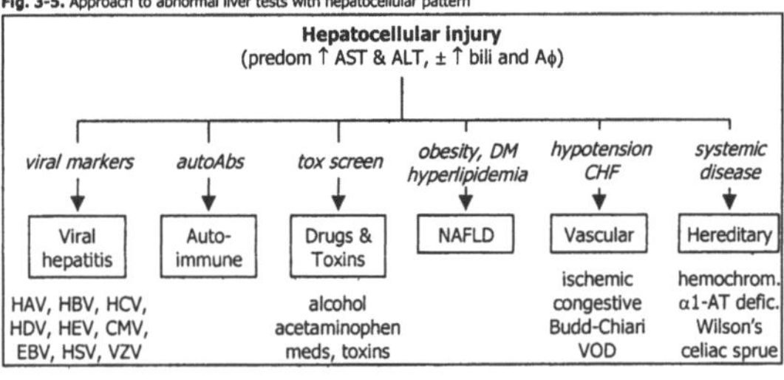

Fig. 3-6. Approach to abnormal liver tests with cholestatic pattern

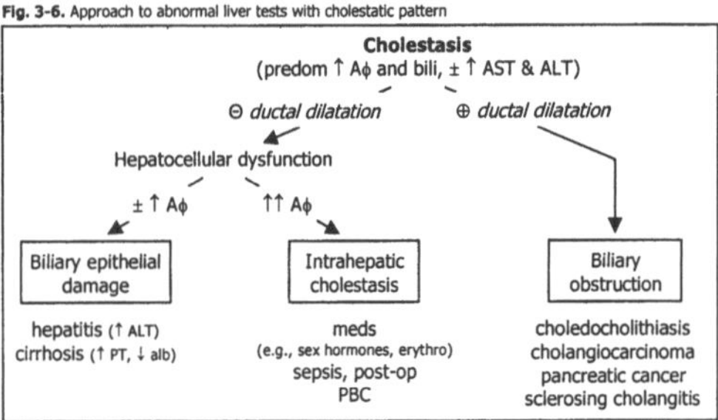

Fig. 3-7. Approach to abnormal liver tests with isolated hyperbilirubinemia

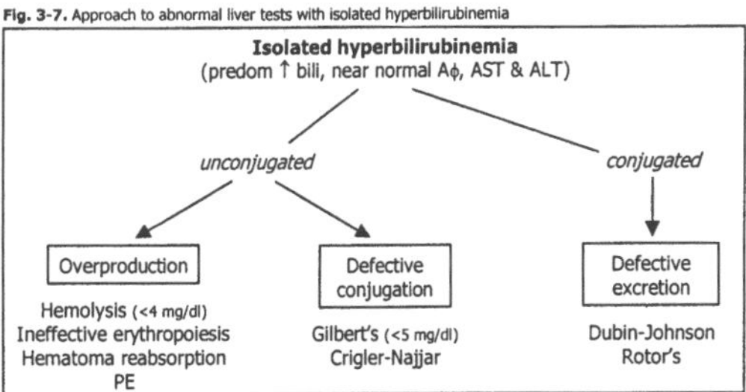

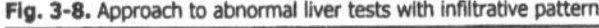

Fig. 3-8. Approach to abnormal liver tests with infiltrative pattern

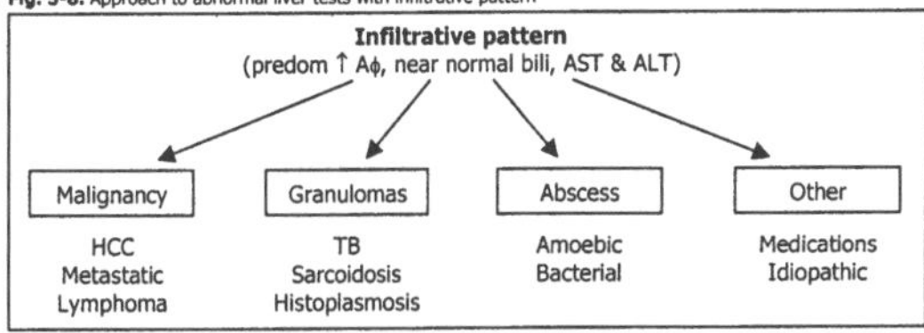

Abnormal liver tests in asymptomatic patients (*NEJM* 2000;342:1266)

- **Hepatocellular**: usually alcohol, NAFLD, HBV/HCV, meds (e.g., NSAIDs, abx, statins) review meds, ✓ HBC & HCV serologies, RUQ U/S; consider globulin, Fe studies
- **Cholestatic**: ✓ 5′-NT, if ↑ → ✓ RUQ U/S, AMA

• HEPATITIS •

VIRAL

Hepatitis A

- Transmission: fecal-oral route; contaminated food, water, shellfish; day-care ctr outbreaks
- Incubation: 2-6 wks
- Chronicity: none
- Diagnosis: acute hepatitis = ⊕ IgM anti-HAV; past exposure = ⊕ IgG anti-HAV (⊖ IgM)

Hepatitis B (*Lancet* 2003;362:2089)

- Transmission: percutaneous, sexual, perinatal
- Incubation: 2-6 months
- Extra-hepatic syndromes: polyarteritis nodosa (<1%), MPGN
- Natural history
  - acute infection: 70% subclinical, 30% jaundice, <1% fulminant hepatitis
  - chronic: <5% (adult-acquired), >90% (perinatally-acquired)
    - can be divided into *replicative* and *non-replicative* phases (see below)
- Serologic and virologic tests
  - HBsAg: appears before symptoms; used to screen blood donors
  - HBeAg: evidence of viral replication and ↑ infectivity (not seen in "precore mutants")
  - IgM anti-HBc: first Ab to appear; indicates acute infection
    - window period = HBsAg become ⊖, anti-HBs not yet ⊕ , anti-HBc only clue to infection
    - ∴ workup for suspected acute, symptomatic HBC is HBsAg & anti-HBc
  - IgG anti-HBc: indicates previous (HBsAg ⊖) or ongoing (HBsAg ⊕) HBV infection
  - anti-HBe: indicates waning viral replication, ↓ infectivity
  - anti-HBs: indicates resolution of acute disease & immunity (sole marker after vaccination)
  - HBV DNA: presence in serum correlates with active viral replication in liver

Fig. 3-9. Serologic course of acute HBV infection with resolution

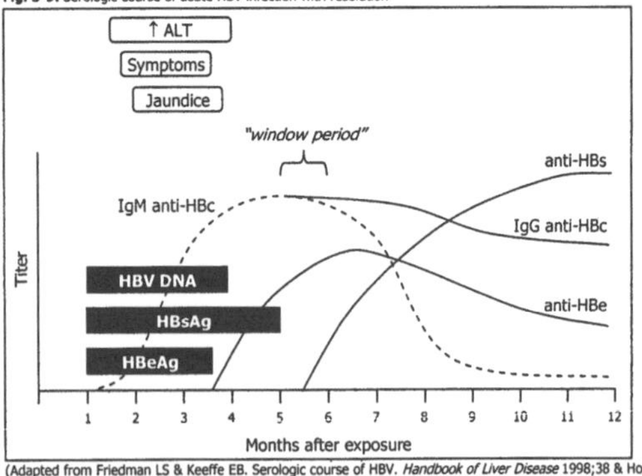

(Adapted from Friedman LS & Keeffe EB. Serologic course of HBV. *Handbook of Liver Disease* 1998;38 & Hoofnagle JH & DiBisceglie AM. Serologic diagnosis of acute and chronic viral hepatitis. *Semin Liver Dis* 1991;11:73.)

Diagnosis	HBsAg	anti-HBs	anti-HBc	HBeAg	anti-HBe
Acute hepatitis	⊕	⊖	IgM	⊕	⊖
Window period	⊖	⊖	IgM	±	±
Recovery	⊖	⊕	IgG	⊖	±
Immunization	⊖	⊕	⊖	⊖	⊖
Chronic hepatitis *replicative*	⊕	⊖	IgG	⊕	⊖
Chronic hepatitis *non-replicative*	⊕	⊖	IgG	⊖	⊕

(Precore mutant: eAg not generated, but anti-HBe can develop due to cross-reactivity with cAg.)

- Treatment for acute HBV: supportive
- Treatment for chronic HBV (⊕ HBsAg & DNA) if ↑ ALT or inflammation on bx, ? ⊕ HBeAg
  options: **IFN-α-2b** (*NEJM* 1990;323:295) or **lamivudine** (*NEJM* 1999;341:1256) or **adefovir dipivoxil** (*NEJM* 2003;348:800 & 808)
  loss of viral markers of replication and normalization of LFTs in 20-40%
  longer Rx → ↑ anti-HBe, but development of lamivudine-resist. mutants (YMDD variant)
  liver transplantation: 80-100% reinfection; poor outcome unless HBIG and/or lamivudine
- Risk of hepatocellular carcinoma: 10-390x increased risk (highest: perinatal acquired and HBeAg ⊕); screen with serum AFP and hepatic ultrasound

Hepatitis C (*Lancet* 2003;362:2095)
- Transmission: percutaneous >> sexual; ~20% without a clear precipitant
- Incubation: 1-3 months
- Extra-hepatic syndromes: cryoglobulinemia, porphyria cutanea tarda, MPGN, lymphoma
- Natural history
  acute infection: 75% subclinical; 25% jaundice; fulminant hepatitis very rare
  chronic: 50-80% → chronic hepatitis, 20-30% of whom develop cirrhosis (after ~20 yrs), hepatocellular carcinoma develops in 2-5% of cirrhotics/year (usually after 20-30 yrs)
- Serologic and virologic tests
  anti-HCV (ELISA): ⊕ in 6 wks, does *not* imply recovery, may become ⊖ after recovery
  HCV RNA: ⊕ in 2 wks, marker of active infection
  HCV RIBA: used to confirm ⊕ anti-HCV ELISA in patients with undetectable HCV RNA (i.e., resolved infection)
- Diagnosis
  acute hepatitis = ⊕ HCV RNA, ± anti-HCV
  resolved hepatitis = ⊖ HCV RNA, ± anti-HCV
  chronic hepatitis = ⊕ HCV RNA, ⊕ anti-HCV
- Treatment if ↑ ALT & active inflammation and some fibrosis on biopsy (*JAMA* 1998;280:2088)
  IFN-α-2b → ~20% sustained response rate (*NEJM* 1989;321:1501 & 1506)
  IFN + ribavirin → ~44% sustained response rate (*NEJM* 2002;347:975)
  PEG-IFNα-2a→ ~29% sustained response rate (*NEJM* 2002;347:975)
  PEG-IFNα-2a + ribavirin → ~56% sustained response rate (*NEJM* 2002;347:975)
  liver transplantation: 100% reinfection rate; some with rapidly progressive disease
- Predictors of response: low HCV RNA, absence of cirrhosis, female gender, age <40 yrs; viral genotype other than 1 (for genotypes 2 and 3, sustained response rates with PEG-IFNα + ribavirin are ~80%)

Hepatitis D
- Transmission: percutaneous or sexual
- Pathogenesis: requires HBV to cause either simultaneous or superimposed infection
- Natural history: more severe hepatitis, faster progression to cirrhosis
- Diagnosis: anti-HDV
- Follow during treatment with IFN-α: HDV RNA (by PCR) (high relapse rate)

Hepatitis E
- Transmission: fecal-oral; travelers to Pakistan, India, SE Asia, Africa, and Mexico
- Natural history: acute hepatitis with ↑ mortality (10-20%) during pregnancy
- Diagnosis: IgM anti-HEV (through CDC)

Other viruses (CMV, EBV, HSV, VZV)

AUTOIMMUNE HEPATITIS

Hepatitis + ↑ globulins + AutoAbs

Classification (*NEJM* 1996;334:897; *Gastroenterology* 2001;120:1502)
- Type 1: anti-smooth muscle Ab (ASMA), ANA; 2/3 female; ± autoimmune thyroiditis or RA
- Type 2: anti-liver/kidney microsome type 1 (anti-LKM1)
- ? Type 3: anti-soluble liver antigen (anti-SLA) (clinically similar to type 1)
- Diagnosis: Combination of autoimmune serologies, ↑ globulin, exclusion of other causes of liver disease, and liver biopsy (plasma cell infiltrate with interface hepatitis)

Overlap syndromes
- Autoimmune hepatitis + primary biliary cirrhosis or primary sclerosing cholangitis

Treatment

- Indications: ALT/AST 10× ULN or ALT/AST 5× ULN + globulins 2× ULN)
- **Prednisone** ± azathioprine → 65% remission within 3 years; 50% relapse on withdrawal of meds at 6 mos; up to 90% by 3 years; ∴ most will require long-term Rx

OTHER CAUSES OF HEPATITIS OR HEPATOTOXICITY

Alcoholic hepatitis

- Aminotransferases usually <300-500 w/ AST:ALT > 2:1, in part b/c concomitant B_6 defic.
- Treatment: when discriminant function >32 or encephalopathy (w/o GIB or infection)
  discriminant function = [4.6 × (PT-control)] + total bilirubin (mg/dl)
  prednisolone or prednisone 40 mg PO qd × 1 month then taper over 4-6 weeks (*NEJM* 1992;326:507); mortality 12% prednisolone vs 55% placebo at day 66
  pentoxifylline 400 mg PO tid x 1month (*Gastroenterology* 2000;119:1637) mortality 25% pentoxifylline vs 46% placebo at 4 weeks; ↓ hepatorenal syndrome

Acetaminophen hepatotoxicity

- Normal metabolism via glucuronidation and sulfation → non-toxic metabolites
- Overdose (usually >10 g): N-hydroxylation by CYP2E1 → reactive electrophilic compounds (NAPQI) that are scavenged by glutathione until reserves exhausted → hepatotoxicity
- CYP2E1 *induced* by fasting and alcohol (allowing for "therapeutic misadventure" in malnourished alcoholics taking even low-doses (2-6 g) of acetaminophen)
- Liver dysfunction may not be apparent for 2-6 days
- Treatment = **N-acetylcysteine**: administer up to 36 hrs after ingestion if acetaminophen level above "no-risk" zone *or* if time of ingestion unknown and ↓'ing levels (∴ peak unknown) *or* if level unknown but reliable history of major poisoning (>10 g)
  regimen: 140 mg/kg loading dose → 70 mg/kg q 4 hr × 17 additional doses

Fig. 3-10. Acetaminophen toxicity nomogram

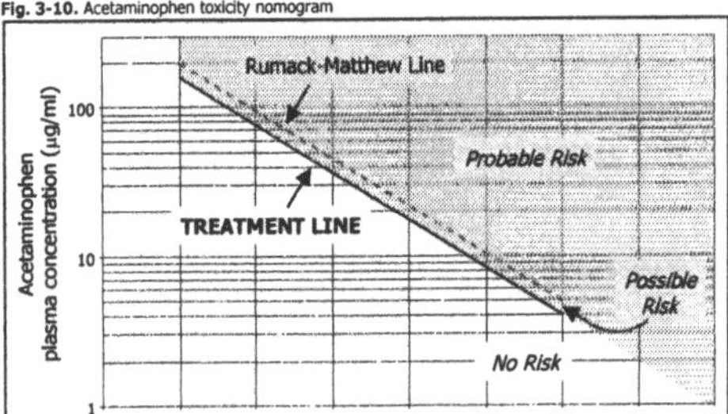

(If acetaminophen level determined ≥ 4 hrs after overdose falls above treatment line, administer entire course of acetylcysteine. Adapted from *Archives* 1981;141:382 & *Guidelines for the Management of Acute Acetaminophen Overdose*. McNeil, 1999.)

Other drugs and toxins that may cause hepatitis (*NEJM* 2003;349:474)

- Amiodarone, azoles, statins (rare), INH, methyldopa, phenytoin, PTU, rifampin, sulfonamides, minocycline
- Halothane, CCl_4
- Toxic mushrooms (*Amanita phalloides*)

Ischemic hepatitis: "shock liver" with aminotransferases > 1000 and ↑↑ LDH

Non-alcoholic fatty liver disease (NAFLD) (*Annals* 1997;126:137; *JAMA* 2003;289:3000)

- Spectrum of fatty infiltration ± inflammation ± fibrosis *not* in setting of EtOH abuse
- Prevalence 7-9%; associated with diabetes mellitus, hyperinsulinemia, obesity, hyperlipidemia, HAART, medications (tamoxifen, amiodarone)
- Clinical manifestations: usually asx 2-3× ↑ in ALT and AST; ± RUQ pain; may → cirrhosis
- Diagnosis: exclusion of other causes of hepatitis or cirrhosis; U/S → hyperechoic liver; ⊕ bx
- Treatment: weight loss, glycemic/lipid control
  possible roles for vitamin E, ursodeoxycholic acid, metformin, thiazolidinediones

• ACUTE LIVER FAILURE •

Definition
- Acute hepatic disease + coagulopathy + encephalopathy
- Fulminant = develops within 8 wks; subfulminant = develops between 8 wks and 6 mos

Etiology
- **Viral**
  HAV, HBV, HCV (rare), HDV + HBV, HEV (especially if pregnant)
  HSV (immunocompromised hosts), EBV, CMV, adenovirus, paramyxovirus, parvovirus B19
- **Drugs/Toxins**
  acetaminophen (most common cause; ~40% of all cases)
  other drugs: phenytoin, INH, rifampin, sulfonamides, tetracycline, amiodarone, PTU
  toxins: fluorinated hydrocarbons, CCl_4, *Amanita phalloides*
- **Vascular**: ischemic hepatitis, Budd-Chiari syndrome, hepatic VOD, malignant infiltration
- **Autoimmune hepatitis**
- **Miscellaneous**: Wilson's disease, acute fatty liver of pregnancy, HELLP syndrome, Reye's syndrome
- Idiopathic (~20%)

Clinical manifestations
- Neurologic
  asterixis
  encephalopathy: stage I = ΔMS; stage II = lethargy, confusion; stage III = stupor; stage IV = coma
  cerebral edema → Cushing's reflex (hypertension + bradycardia), pupillary dilatation, decerebrate posturing, apnea
- Cardiovascular: **hypotension** with low SVR
- Pulmonary: **respiratory alkalosis**, impaired peripheral O_2 uptake, ARDS
- Gastrointestinal: GIB, pancreatitis
- Renal: ATN, **hepatorenal syndrome**, hyponatremia, hypokalemia, hypophosphatemia
- Hematology: **coagulopathy** (due to ↓ synthesis of clotting factors ± DIC)
- **Infection**: seen in 90% of patient, especially with gram + organisms and fungi; SBP in 32% of patients; fever and leukocytosis may be absent
- Endocrine: **hypoglycemia**

Workup
- Viral serologies
- Toxicology screen (acetaminophen levels q 1-2 hr until peak determined)
- Imaging studies (RUQ U/S or abdominal CT, doppler studies of portal and hepatic veins)
- Other tests: autoimmune serologies, ceruloplasmin and urine copper
- Liver biopsy (unless precluded by coagulopathy → in which case consider transjugular)

Treatment
- ICU-level care at a liver transplant center potentially including monitoring and treating ICP, hemodynamic and ventilatory support, reversing coagulopathies, aggressive monitoring for and treatment of infection, D_{10} drip for hypoglycemia, etc.
- Treatment of specific causes (N-acetylcysteine for acetaminophen, corticosteroids for autoimmune hepatitis, chelation therapy for Wilson's disease, penicillin + silymarin for *Amanita phalloides*)
- Liver transplantation if poor prognosis (see below)

Prognosis
- Survival 10-50%
- Predictors of poor outcome (*Gastroenterology* 1989;97:439):
  age >40; cause other than acetaminophen, HAV and HBV
  grade III or IV encephalopathy (onset >7 days after onset of jaundice)
  PT >50, bilirubin >17.5
- Liver transplantation 1-year survival rate >60%
- Extracorporeal liver assist devices now under evaluation as "bridge" to transplant

• CIRRHOSIS •

Definition
- Definition: **fibrosis and nodular regeneration** resulting from hepatocellular injury

Etiologies
- **Alcohol**
- **Viral hepatitis** (chronic HBV, HCV, HDV infection)
- **Autoimmune hepatitis** (female, ↑ IgG, ⊕ ANA, anti-smooth muscle Ab)
- **Metabolic diseases**: hemochromatosis, Wilson's disease, α_1-antitrypsin deficiency
- **Biliary tract diseases**: primary biliary cirrhosis, secondary biliary cirrhosis (calculus, neoplasm, stricture, biliary atresia), primary sclerosing cholangitis
- **Vascular diseases**: Budd-Chiari syndrome, R-sided heart failure, constrictive pericarditis
- **Cryptogenic**: may reflect terminal progression of nonalcoholic fatty liver disease

Clinical manifestations
- Subclinical or may present as progressive liver dysfunction (jaundice, coagulopathy, encephalopathy) and/or portal hypertension (ascites, varices)

Physical exam
- Liver: enlarged, palpable, firm, nodular → shrunken and nodular
- Signs of liver failure: jaundice, spider angiomata, palmar erythema, Dupuytren's contractures, white nail lines (Muehrcke's lines) & proximal nail beds (Terry's nails), ↑ parotid & lacrimal glands, gynecomastia, testicular atrophy, asterixis, encephalopathy, fetor hepaticus
- Signs of portal hypertension: splenomegaly, ascites, dilated superficial abdominal veins (caput medusae), epigastric "Cruveilhier-Baumgarten" venous hum

Laboratory studies
- **↑ bilirubin**, **↑ PT**, **↓ albumin**, ± ↑ aminotransferases and ↑ Aϕ (variable)
- ↓ Na
- Anemia (marrow suppression, hypersplenism, Fe and/or folate deficiencies), neutropenia (hypersplenism), thrombocytopenia (hypersplenism, ↓ TPO production by liver)

Workup
- Abdominal U/S with Doppler: liver size, r/o HCC, ascites, assess patency of portal, splenic and hepatic veins
- Hepatitis serologies (HBsAg, anti-HBs, anti-HCV), autoimmune hepatitis studies (IgG, ANA, anti-smooth muscle Ab), Fe and Cu studies, α_1-AT, anti-mitochondrial Ab, echocardiogram (if concerned about right-sided heart failure)
- ± Liver biopsy (percutaneous or transjugular)
- AFP to screen for hepatocellular carcinoma

Complications
- **Portal hypertension**
  - **ascites** (50% within 10 yrs) ± spontaneous bacterial peritonitis (19%)
  - **gastroesophageal varices** (if hepatic venous pressure ∇ >12 mmHg) ± **UGIB**
    - *1° prevention* UGIB (indicated in Pts with mod-large varices):
      - non-selective β-blockers (titrate to 25% ↓ HR): ~50% ↓ bleeding (*NEJM* 1991;324:1532)
        - addition of nitrates may further ↓ bleeding (*Lancet* 1996;348:1677)
      - band ligation: greater ↓ bleeding c/w βB, but no Δ in mortality, ∴ reserve for Pts intolerant of βB (*Hepatology* 2001;33:802)
    - *2° prevention* UGIB (indicated in all Pts): β-blocker & nitrates (*NEJM* 2001;345:669), oftentimes plus band ligation; if rebleed → TIPS or transplant
- **Hepatic encephalopathy**: failure of liver to detoxify noxious agents (NH_3 and others)
  - precipitated by ? excess dietary protein, constipation, GIB, medication non-compliance, infection, azotemia, hypokalemia, hepatic failure, HCC, portosystemic shunt, hypotension, alkalosis
  - treatment: restrict dietary protein acutely, but only modestly (60-80 g/d) long-term, lactulose (acidification of colon leading to $NH_3 \rightarrow NH_4^+$; Δ gut flora → ↓ NH_3-producing organisms), gut decontamination with neomycin or MNZ
- **Hepatorenal syndrome:** progressive azotemia (note, often *overestimate* renal function in cirrhotics b/c low muscle mass, ↑ Cr renal tubular secretion, and ↓ conversion of creatine → creatinine) and oliguria, U_{Na} <10 mEq/L, no response to volume challenge, exclusion of other causes of renal failure (drugs, ATN, obstruction) (*Lancet* 2003;362:1819)
  Precipitants: GIB, overdiuresis, paracentesis, aminoglycosides, NSAIDs

Treatment: octreotide (200 mcg sq tid) + midodrine (12.5 mg po tid) beneficial (*Hepatology* 1999;29:1690), IV norepinephrine + albumin, TIPS may be beneficial

- **Hepatopulmonary syndrome:** hypoxemia (± platypnea-orthodeoxia) due to pulmonary AV shunts; initial diagnosis by contrast echocardiography (R → L shunt)
- **Liver failure:** precipitated by progressive hepatic damage or stressors (infection, surgery)
- **Infections**
- **Hepatocellular carcinoma** (*Lancet* 2003;362:1907): consider if ↑ liver size, ↑ ascites, abdominal pain, ↑ encephalopathy, ↓ weight, ↑ AFP, or hepatic mass on U/S, CT, MRI
- **Prognosis:** correlates with Child-Turcotte-Pugh class (A>B>C)

Modified Child-Turcotte-Pugh Classification			
	Points scored		
	1	**2**	**3**
Ascites	none	easily controlled	poorly controlled
Encephalopathy	none	grade I or II	grade III or IV
Bilirubin (mg/dl)	<2.0	2.0-3.0	>3.0
Albumin (g/dl)	>3.5	2.8-3.5	<2.8
PT (sec > control)	<4	4-6	>6
	Classification		
	A	**B**	**C**
Total points	5-6	7-9	10-15

(*Brit J Surg* 1973;60:646)

MELD: Model for End Stage Liver Disease: Used to stratify Pts on liver transplant list; based on Cr, INR, & total bilirubin to predict 3-mo survival in Pts with a variety of underlying forms of liver disease; to calculate: www.mayo.edu/int-med/gi/model/mayomodl.htm

Liver transplantation

- Evaluate ± list when Child class B or C
- Indications: MELD score ≥26; recurrent or severe encephalopathy, refractory ascites, SBP, recurrent variceal bleeding, bili >10 mg/dl, albumin <3 g/dl, PT >3 sec above control
- Contraindications: advanced HIV, active substance abuse, sepsis, malignancy (extrahepatic), severe comorbidity
- Survival: 1-year survival up to 90%, 5-year survival up to 80%

Less Common Etiologies of Cirrhosis

Hemochromatosis

- Definition: autosomal recessive inherited disorder of **iron overload**
- Epidemiology: 1 in 300; usually manifests in middle-age and in men
- Manifestations of advanced disease: bronzing of the skin (melanin + iron), hypogonadism, diabetes mellitus, arthritis (2nd & 3rd MCPs), CHF, infections (*Vibrio, Listeria, Yersinia*)
- Diagnosis: ↑ iron saturation (>45%), ↑ ferritin, "black liver" on MRI, hepatic iron index >1.9, *HFE* gene mutation (C282Y/C282Y or C282Y/H63D)

Condition		Fe sat	Ferritin	Iron index
Normal		≤45%	<200	<1.0
Alcoholic liver disease		≤60%	<500	<2.0
Hemochromatosis	*Heterozygotes*	variable	<500	<2.0
	Asx homozygotes	>50%	>500	>2.0
	Sx homozygotes	>50%	>900	>2.0

(Adapted from *Harrison's Principles of Internal Medicine*, 15th ed., 2001)

- Treatment: phlebotomy q wk until Fe parameters normal, then prn to keep in range; deferoxamine if can't undergo phlebotomy; genetic counseling

Wilson's disease

- Definition: autosomal recessive inherited disorder of **copper overload**
- Epidemiology: 1 in 40,000, usually manifests before age 30; almost always before 40
- Additional manifestations: neuroΨ disorders, Kayser-Fleischer rings, hemolytic anemia
- Diagnostic studies: ↑ serum & urinary copper, ↓ serum ceruloplasmin, hepatic copper content >250 μg/g dry wt, Aϕ often low in fulminant Wilson's disease, AST/ALT >1 because of hemolysis
- Treatment: chelation therapy with penicillamine + pyridoxine; trientine if intolerant of penicillamine; oral zinc if asx (not to be given with chelators as rendered ineffective)

α1-antitrypsin deficiency (α1-AT)
- Abnormal α_1-AT → polymerization in liver (cirrhosis) & uninhibited protease activity in lung (emphysema)
- Additional clinical manifestations: emphysema
- Diagnostic studies: absence of α_1-AT globulin on SPEP, ⊕ PAS inclusion bodies on liver bx, abnormal protease inhibitor (Pi) type (usually Z/Z, null/null, or null/Z)
- Treatment: liver transplantation (for cirrhosis); α_1-AT replacement (for emphysema)

Primary biliary cirrhosis (PBC) (*NEJM* 1996;335:1570; *Lancet* 2003;362:53)
- Definition: autoimmune destruction of *intrahepatic* bile ducts
- Epidemiology: middle-aged *women*, concomitant autoimmune diseases
- Clinical manifestations: fatigue, pruritus, fat malabsorption, xanthomas, xanthelasma
- Diagnostic studies: ↑ Aϕ, ↑ bilirubin, ⊕ anti-mitochondrial Ab (AMA) in 95%, ↑ cholesterol
- Treatment: ursodeoxycholic acid (13-15 mg/kg/day); fat-soluble vitamins; cholestyramine for pruritus; transplantation; colchicine, methotrexate in selected cases

Primary sclerosing cholangitis (PSC) (*NEJM* 1995;332:924)
- Definition: idiopathic cholestasis with fibrosis, structuring and dilatation of *intra- and extrahepatic* bile ducts
- Epidemiology: young *men* (age 20-50), associated with IBD in 70% of cases (UC >> CD)
- Clinical manifestations: pruritus, jaundice, fevers, RUQ pain, cholangiocarcinoma
- Diagnostic studies: ↑ bilirubin, ↑ Aϕ, ⊕ p-ANCA in 70%, MRCP/ERCP → *multifocal beaded bile duct strictures*; "onion-skin" lesions around bile ducts on liver bx
- Treatment
  high dose ursodeoxycholic acid (20-30 mg/kg/day), ? cholestyramine, fat-soluble vitamins
  endoscopic dilation and short-term stenting of dominant bile duct strictures
  liver transplantation (↑ risk of post-transplant duct strictures)

Budd-Chiari syndrome (*NEJM* 2004;350:578)
- Definition: occlusion of the hepatic veins or IVC
- Etiologies: hypercoagulable states (typically MPD, PNH, OCP), tumor invasion (HCC, renal, adrenal), membranous web, trauma, idiopathic
- Clinical manifestations: hepatomegaly, RUQ pain, ascites
- Diagnostic studies: ± ↑ transaminases & Aϕ; Doppler U/S of hepatic veins (85% sens. & spec.; CT (I+) or MRI/MRA; "spiderweb" pattern on hepatic venography; liver bx showing congestion (in Pt w/o evidence of right-sided CHF)
- Treatment: anticoagulation (heparin → warfarin), thrombolysis if acute thrombosis; TIPS (portocaval gradient <10) or surgical shunt (gradient >10); liver transplantation

Veno-occlusive disease (VOD) (*Mayo* 2003;78:589)
- Definition: occlusion of hepatic venules
- Etiology: stem cell transplant, chemotherapy, XRT, Jamaican bush tea
- Clinical manifestations: hepatomegaly, RUQ pain, ascites, weight gain, ↑ bilirubin
- Diagnostic studies: U/S usually not helpful, dx made clinically or, if necessary, by liver bx
- Treatment: mainly supportive

• ASCITES •

Etiologies	
Portal hypertension related SAAG ≥1.1	**Non-portal hypertension related SAAG <1.1**
Sinusoidal **cirrhosis** (81%), including SBP acute hepatitis extensive malignancy (HCC or mets) *Post-sinusoidal* right-sided CHF incl. constriction & TR Budd-Chiari syndrome, VOD *Pre-sinusoidal* portal or splenic vein thrombosis schistosomiasis	**Peritonitis**: TB, ruptured viscus (↑ amy) **Peritoneal carcinomatosis** **Pancreatitis** Vasculitis Hypoalbuminemic states: nephrotic syndrome, protein-losing enteropathy Meigs' syndrome

Pathophysiology
- "Underfill" theory: portal hypertension → transudation of fluid into peritoneum → ↓ plasma volume → renal Na retention
- "Overflow" theory: hepatorenal reflex → Na retention
- Peripheral vasodilatation theory (favored): portal hypertension → systemic vasodilatation (? due to release of nitric oxide) → ↓ effective arterial volume → renal Na retention
- Hypoalbuminemia → ↓ serum oncotic pressure
- ↑ hepatic lymph production

Workup
- Detection: shifting dullness, fluid wave has 60% sens.; U/S detects if >100 cc
- **Serum-ascites albumin gradient (SAAG)**; >95% accuracy (*Annals* 1992;117:215)
  ≥1.1 g/dL → portal hypertension related; <1.1 g/dL → non-portal hypertension related
- Ascites fluid total protein (AFTP): useful when SAAG ≥1.1 to distinguish cirrhosis (↓ AFTP <2.5 g/dL) from cardiac ascites (AFTP >2.5 g/dL)
- If portal hypertensive etiology, consider standard cirrhosis w/u (see "Cirrhosis")
- Rule-out infection: cell count with differential, gram stain & culture (± AFB) + *bedside inoculation* of blood culture bottles (yield 90%) (*Gastroenterology* 1988;95:1351)
- Other tests as indicated (e.g., amylase, triglycerides, adenosine deaminase, cytology)

Treatment (*NEJM* 1994;330:337; *Hepatology* 1998;27:264)
- ↓ **Na intake** (1-2 g/d); free H_2O restriction *if* hyponatremic
- **Diuretics** (effective in 80% of cases)
  spironolactone (start 100 mg po qd) ± furosemide (start 40 mg po qd); ↑ in proportion
  goals: diurese ~1L/day, steady wt loss, urinary Na/K ratio >1 (indicating effective blockade of endogenous aldosterone)
- Options for refractory ascites (ensure diet & medicine compliance)
  Large volume paracentesis: remove 4-6 L; ± albumin replacement (fewer asymptomatic chemical abnormalities; no Δ in mortality)
  TIPS: ↓↓ ascites in 75%, ↑ CrCl, ↑ transplantation-free survival (*NEJM* 2000;342:1701) but ? ↑ encephalopathy, 40% need TIPS revision, no Δ quality of life (*Gastro* 2003;124:634) consider if refractory ascites, Child's class A or B, minimal encephalopathy
  Liver transplantation, if patient is a candidate

Complications
- Spontaneous bacterial peritonitis (see next page)
- Hepatorenal syndrome (see "Cirrhosis")
- Pleural effusions

Bacterial peritonitis

- Definitions and diagnosis

Type	Ascites cell count/mm³	Ascites culture
Sterile	<250 polys	⊖
Spontaneous bacterial peritonitis (SBP)	>250 polys	⊕ (one organism)
Culture-negative neutrocytic ascites (CNNA)	>250 polys	⊖
Non-neutrocytic bacterascites (NNBA)	<250 polys	⊕ (one organism)
Secondary	>250 polys	⊕ (polymicrobial)
Peritoneal dialysis-associated	>100 with poly predom.	⊕

- **SBP**
  - epidemiology: occurs in 19% of cirrhotics; risk factors = AFTP <1.0 g/dl, serum bilirubin >2.5 mg/dl, prior SBP
  - clinical manifestations: fever, abdominal pain, rebound tenderness, Δ MS
    - clinical signs may be unreliable; ∴ have a low threshold for diagnostic paracentesis
  - pathogens: 70% GNR (***E. coli*, *Klebsiella***), 30% GPC (***S. pneumococcus***, other streptococci, *Enterococcus*)
  - treatment: cefotaxime 2 gm IV q 8hrs × 5 d; IV albumin 1.5 g/kg at dx and 1 g/kg on day 3 results in survival benefit (*NEJM* 1999;341:403)
  - prophylaxis (if h/o SBP, current GIB, or ? AFTP <1.0 g/dL): norfloxacin 400 mg PO qd or bactrim DS qd
- **CNNA**: variant of SBP with similar clinical course; also treated with antibiotics
- **NNBA**: often resolves without treatment; follow patient closely
- **Secondary** (intraabdominal abscess or perforated viscus)
  - polymicrobial
  - usually AFTP >1.0 g/dl, ascitic fluid glucose <50 mg/dl, or ascitic fluid LDH >225 U/L
  - treatment: 3rd gen. cephalosporin + metronidazole
    - CT scan and likely exploratory laparotomy for definitive diagnosis and treatment
- **Peritoneal dialysis-associated**
  - pathogens: 70% GPC, 30% GNR
  - treatment: vancomycin + gentamicin (IV load then administer in PD)

Portal vein thrombosis (PVT)

- Etiologies: cirrhosis, neoplasm (pancreas, HCC), intraabdominal inflammation/infection, hypercoagulable state (including MPS), surgery, trauma
- Clinical manifestations: pain (with acute thrombosis), variceal bleeding, splenomegaly, ascites
- Diagnostic studies: LFTs usually normal; U/S with Doppler, CT (I+), MRA, angiography
- Treatment: as for portal hypertension; ? anticoagulation, ? surgery

• BILIARY TRACT DISEASE •

CHOLELITHIASIS ("GALLSTONES")

Epidemiology
- >10% adults in the U.S. have gallstones; ↑ prevalence in women, Native Americans, and with increasing age, obesity, and pregnancy

Pathogenesis
- Bile = bile salts, phospholipids, cholesterol. ↑ cholesterol saturation in bile → gallstones.

Types of gallstones
- Mixed (80%): multiple stones, mostly cholesterol, may calcify (15-20%)
- Cholesterol (10%): usually single stone, large, uncalcified
- Pigment (10%): unconjugated bilirubin (hence seen in chronic hemolysis) and calcium

Clinical manifestations
- History: May be asymptomatic (symptoms develop in ~2%/yr)
  biliary "colic" = episodic RUQ or epigastric abdominal pain that begins abruptly, is continuous, resolves slowly, and lasts for 30 min to 3 hr
  associated **nausea**; may be precipitated by **fatty foods**
- Physical exam: afebrile, ± RUQ tenderness

Diagnostic studies
- RUQ U/S: sensitivity and specificity >90-95%, can show complications (cholecystitis and cholangitis)

Treatment
- Cholecystectomy (usually laparoscopic) if symptomatic
- ? Oral dissolution therapy (ursodeoxycholic acid) in patients who refuse or who are not surgical candidates

Complications
- Cholecystitis (30% of symptomatic biliary colic → cholecystitis within 2 years)
- Cholangitis
- Pancreatitis
- Gallbladder carcinoma (~1%)

CHOLECYSTITIS

Definition
- Inflammation of the gallbladder

Pathogenesis
- Obstruction of the cystic duct by a gallstone
- Acalculous (? ischemic)

Clinical manifestations
- History: nausea & vomiting (>50% of Pts), fever, steady severe epigastric and RUQ pain
- Physical examination: **RUQ tenderness, Murphy's sign** = ↑ RUQ pain on inspiration, ± palpable gallbladder
- Laboratory evaluation: ↑ WBC, ± ↑ bilirubin and Aϕ, and ± ↑ amylase (even in absence of pancreatitis); transaminases >500 U or bilirubin >4 mg/dL → choledocholithiasis

Diagnostic studies (*JAMA* 2003;289:80)
- **RUQ U/S**: high sens. and spec. for gallstones; specific signs of cholecystitis include pericholecystic fluid, edema of the gallbladder wall, and a sonographic Murphy's sign
- Cholescintigraphy (**HIDA scan**): most sensitive test for acute cholecystitis. Procedure involves IV injection of radiolabeled HIDA, which is selectively secreted into biliary tree. In acute cholecystitis, HIDA enters the common bile duct (CBD) but not the gallbladder.

Treatment
- NPO, IV fluids, antibiotics (*E. coli*, *Klebsiella*, enterococcus, and *Enterobacter* are the usual pathogens)
- Semiurgent cholecystectomy (usually within 72 hrs)
- Cholecystostomy and percutaneous drainage in patients too sick for surgery
- ERCP or CBD exploration to r/o choledocholithiasis in patients with jaundice, cholangitis or stone in CBD on U/S

Complications
- Perforation
- Empyema
- Emphysematous gallbladder due to infection by gas-forming organisms
- Cholecystenteric fistula (to duodenum, colon, or stomach): can see air in biliary tree
- Gallstone ileus: bowel obstruction (usually at terminal ileum) due to stone in intestine that passed through a fistula

CHOLEDOCHOLITHIASIS

Definition
- Gallstone lodged in the common bile duct (CBD)

Epidemiology
- Occurs in 15% of patients with gallstones

Clinical manifestations
- Asymptomatic (50%)
- Biliary colic
- Jaundice

Diagnostic studies
- RUQ U/S: dilated ducts (but sensitivity only 33% for detecting CBD stones)
- Cholangiogram (ERCP, percutaneous, or operative), endoscopic ultrasound

Treatment
- ERCP and papillotomy with stone extraction

Complications
- Cholangitis
- Pancreatitis
- Cholecystitis
- Stricture

CHOLANGITIS

Definition
- Common bile duct (CBD) obstruction → infection proximal to the obstruction

Etiologies
- CBD stone
- Stricture
- Neoplasm (biliary or pancreatic)
- Infiltration with flukes (*Clonorchis sinensis, Opisthorchis viverrini*)

Clinical manifestations
- Charcot's triad: RUQ pain, jaundice, fever/chills
- Reynold's pentad: Charcot's triad + shock and Δ MS

Diagnostic studies
- ERCP

Treatment
- Antibiotics
- Decompression of the biliary tree via ERCP

• ACID-BASE DISTURBANCES •

GENERAL

Definitions
- **Acidemia** → pH < 7.36, **alkalemia** → pH > 7.44
- **Acidosis** → process that raises $[H^+]$; **alkalosis** → process that decreases $[H^+]$
- Primary disorders: metabolic acidosis or alkalosis, respiratory acidosis or alkalosis
- Compensation
  - respiratory: hyper- or hypoventilation alters P_aCO_2 to counteract 1° metabolic process
  - renal: excretion/retention of H^+/HCO_3 by kidneys to counteract 1° respiratory process
  - respiratory compensation occurs in mins; renal compensation takes hrs to days
  - *compensation never fully corrects pH;* if pH normal, consider mixed disorder

Workup
- Determine **primary disorder:** ✓ pH, P_aCO_2, HCO_3
- Determine if **degree of compensation** is appropriate

Primary Disorders				
Primary disorder	**Problem**	**pH**	**HCO_3**	**P_aCO_2**
Metabolic acidosis	gain of H^+ or loss of HCO_3	↓	⇓	↓
Metabolic alkalosis	gain of HCO_3 or loss of H^+	↑	⇑	↑
Respiratory acidosis	hypoventilation	↓	↑	⇑
Respiratory alkalosis	hyperventilation	↑	↓	⇓

Compensation for Acid/Base Disorders	
Primary disorder	**Expected compensation**
Metabolic acidosis	↓ $P_aCO_2 = 1.25 \times \Delta HCO_3$ (also, $PaCO_2$ = last two digits of pH)
Metabolic alkalosis	↑ $P_aCO_2 = 0.75 \times \Delta HCO_3$
Acute respiratory acidosis	↑ $HCO_3 = 0.1 \times \Delta P_aCO_2$ (also, ↓ pH = $.008 \times \Delta P_aCO_2$)
Chronic respiratory acidosis	↑ $HCO_3 = 0.4 \times \Delta P_aCO_2$ (also, ↓ pH = $.003 \times \Delta P_aCO_2$)
Acute respiratory alkalosis	↓ $HCO_3 = 0.2 \times \Delta P_aCO_2$
Chronic respiratory alkalosis	↓ $HCO_3 = 0.4 \times \Delta P_aCO_2$

Mixed disorders (more than one primary disorder at the same time)
- If compensation is less than or greater than predicted then there may be 2 disorders:
  - P_aCO_2 too low → concomitant 1° resp. alk.; P_aCO_2 too high → concomitant 1° resp. acid.
  - HCO_3 too low → concomitant 1° met. acid.; HCO_3 too high → concomitant 1° met. alk.
- Normal pH *but*...
  - ↑ P_aCO_2 + ↑ HCO_3 → resp. acid. + met. alk.
  - ↓ P_aCO_2 + ↓ HCO_3 → resp. alk. + met. acid.
  - normal P_aCO_2 & HCO_3, *but* ↑ AG → AG met. acid. + met. alk.
  - normal P_aCO_2, HCO_3, & AG → no disturbance *or* non-AG met. acid. + met. alk.
- *Cannot* have resp. acid. and resp. alk. simultaneously (one either hypo- or hyperventilates)

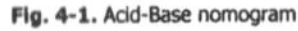

Fig. 4-1. Acid-Base nomogram

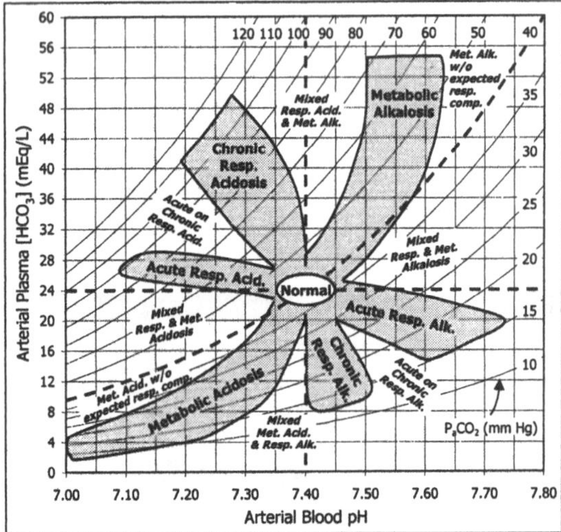

N.B., If ABG not available, can use VBG, but note that pH ~0.04 ↓, $PaCO_2$ ~8 mm Hg ↑, and HCO_3 ~2 mEq ↑. (Adapted from Brenner BM, ed. *Brenner & Rector's The Kidney*, 5th ed., 1996 and Ferri F, ed. *Practical Guide to The Care of the Medical Patient*, 5th ed., 2001)

METABOLIC ACIDOSIS

Workup

- ✓ **anion gap** (AG) = Na - (Cl + HCO_3) = unmeasured anions - unmeasured cations
  most unmeasured anions come from albumin; ∴ expected AG is [albumin] x 2.5 = 10
  (given normal albumin of 4; if albumin = 3 g/dl, expected AG would be 7.5)
  low AG → ↓ alb or ↑ cations (Ca, Mg, K, Ig, Li); if ↑ glc, use measured *not* corrected Na
  AG normal → non-AG metabolic acidosis (see below)
  ↑ AG → AG metabolic acidosis (see below)
- If ↑ AG, ✓ **delta-delta** (ΔΔ): way to assess if more than just AG met. acid. affecting HCO_3
  ΔHCO_3 = (24 - HCO_3); ΔAG = (calculated AG – expected AG)
  $\Delta HCO_3 \approx \Delta AG$ → pure AG metabolic acidosis
  $\Delta HCO_3 > \Delta AG$ → simultaneous non-AG acidosis
  $\Delta HCO_3 < \Delta AG$ → simultaneous metabolic alkalosis [esp. if $\Delta HCO_3 < (\Delta AG \div 2)$; if ΔHCO_3 only slightly less than ΔAG, may be due to non-HCO_3 buffering of acid]

Etiologies of AG Metabolic Acidosis	
Category	**Etiologies**
Ketoacidosis	**Diabetes mellitus**, alcoholism, starvation
Lactic acidosis	**Circulatory or respiratory failure**, sepsis **Ischemic bowel or limb**, seizures, malignancy, hepatic failure Carbon monoxide or cyanide poisoning, metformin
Renal failure	Accumulation of organic anions such as phosphates, sulfates, etc.
Ingestions	**Methanol**: manifestations include blurred vision **Ethylene glycol**: manifestation include ΔMS, cardiopulmonary failure, calcium oxalate crystals and renal failure **Paraldehyde** **Salicylates**: metabolic acidosis (from lactate, ketones) + respiratory alkalosis due to stimulation of CNS respiratory center

Workup for AG metabolic acidosis

- ✓ for **ketonuria** (dipstick acetoacetate) or plasma β-hydroxybutyrate (βOHB)
  Note that urine acetoacetate is often not present in early ketoacidosis due to shunting to βOHB; ∴ acetoacetate may later turn ⊕, but this does not signify worsening disease
- If ⊖ ketones, ✓ **renal function, lactate, toxin screen**, and **osmolal gap**
- **Osmolal gap** (OG) = measured osmoles - calculated osmoles
  calculated osmoles = (2 × Na) + (glucose/18) + (BUN/2.8)
  correct OG for ethanol; ethanol (mg/dl) contribution to OG = EtOH/4.6
  corrected OG >10 → suggests ingestion (methanol, ethylene glycol)

Etiologies of Non-AG Metabolic Acidosis	
Category	**Etiologies**
GI losses of HCO_3	Diarrhea, intestinal or pancreatic fistulas or drainage
Renal tubular acidoses (RTAs)	*See section on RTAs below*
Ureteral diversion	Colonic Cl^-/HCO_3^- exchange, ammonium reabsorption
Early renal failure	Impaired generation of ammonia
Dilutional	Due to rapid infusion of bicarbonate-free intravenous fluids
Post-hypocapnia	Respiratory alkalosis → renal wasting of HCO_3; rapid correction of resp. alk. → transient acidosis until HCO_3 regenerated

Workup for non-AG metabolic acidosis

- Evaluate history for causes (e.g. diarrhea, medications, saline administration)
- ✓ **urine anion gap** (UAG) = (U_{Na} + U_K) - U_{Cl}
  UAG = unmeasured anions - unmeasured cations; as NH_4^+ is primary unmeasured cation, UAG is an indirect assay for renal NH_4^+ excretion (*NEJM* 1988;318:594)
- ⊖ UAG → ↑ renal NH_4^+ excretion → appropriate renal response to acidemia
  GI causes, type II RTA, exogenous acid or dilutional
  urine pH will become elevated (>5.3) after IV bicarbonate load (0.5-1 mEq/kg/hr) in type II RTA but not in non-renal causes (diarrhea, dilution, exogenous acid)
- ⊕ UAG → failure of kidneys to secrete NH_4^+
  type I or IV RTA, early renal failure; plasma K usually low in type I and high in type IV
- Interpretation of UAG assumes Pt is not volume deplete or ketotic → ⊕ UAG

Renal tubular acidoses (RTAs)

- **Type I (distal)**
  pathophysiology: defective distal H^+ secretion
  etiologies: Sjögren's, SLE, hepatitis, nephrocalcinosis, amphotericin, multiple myeloma
- **Type II (proximal)**
  pathophysiology: ↓ proximal reabsorption of HCO_3
  etiologies: Fanconi's, amyloidosis, multiple myeloma, acetazolamide
- **Type IV (hypoaldosteronism)**
  pathophysiology: ↓ aldo → ↑ K → ↓ NH_3 synthesis → ↓ urine acid carrying capacity
  etiologies
    ↓ renin: diabetic nephropathy, NSAIDs, chronic interstitial nephritis
    normal renin, ↓ aldo synthesis: ACEI, ARBs, heparin, 1° adrenal disorders
    ↓ response to aldosterone
      medications: K-sparing diuretics, TMP-SMX, pentamidine, CsA, tacrolimus
      tubulointerstitial disease: sickle cell, SLE, amyloid, diabetes

Renal Tubular Acidosis						
Type	Location	Acidosis	UAG	U pH	$FeHCO_3$†	Serum K
I	Distal	severe	⊕	>5.3	<3%	↓
II	Proximal	moderate	±	<5.3*	>15%	↓
IV	Hypoaldo	mild	⊕	<5.3	<3%	↑

* In type II RTA, urine pH will rise above 5.3 in the setting of an HCO_3 load
† $FeHCO_3$ should be checked after an HCO_3 load

Fig. 4-2. Approach to metabolic acidosis

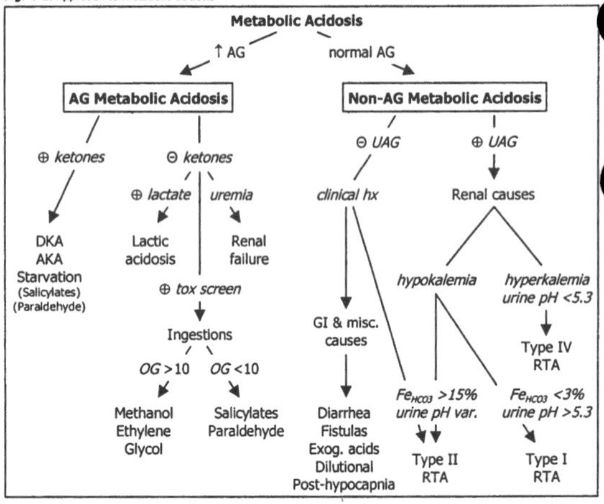

METABOLIC ALKALOSIS

Pathophysiology

- Requires *initiating event* and *maintenance factors*
- *Initiating event*
  - **loss of H^+** from GI tract or kidneys
  - **exogenous alkali**
  - **contraction alkalosis**: diuresis → excretion of HCO_3-poor fluid → extracellular fluid "contracts" around fixed amount of HCO_3 → ↑ HCO_3 concentration. Also, volume depletion → ↑ aldo → H^+ excretion & HCO_3^- retention (see below).
  - **post-hypercapnia**: respiratory acidosis → renal compensation with HCO_3 retention; rapid correction of respiratory disorder (i.e., with intubation) → transient excess HCO_3 until kidneys excrete it
- *Maintenance factors*
  - **volume depletion** → ↑ proximal reabsorption of $NaHCO_3$ and ↑ aldosterone (see next)
  - **hyperaldosteronism** (either 1° or 2°) → distal Na reabsorption in exchange for K^+ and H^+ excretion (and consequent HCO_3 retention)
  - **hypokalemia** → transcellular K^+/H^+ exchange

Etiologies of Metabolic Alkalosis	
Category	**Etiologies**
Saline-responsive	**GI loss of H^+**: vomiting, NGT drainage, villous adenoma **Diuretic use** **Volume depletion** post-hypercapnia
Saline-resistant	*Hypertensive* **(mineralocorticoid excess)** 1° hyperaldosteronism (e.g., Conn's syndrome) 2° hyperaldosteronism non-aldo (e.g., Cushing's, Liddle's, exogenous mineralocorticoids) *Normotensive* severe hypokalemia exogenous alkali load Bartter's syndrome, Gitelman's syndrome

Workup

- Check **volume status** and **U_{Cl}**
  - U_{Cl} <20 mEq/L → saline-responsive
  - U_{Cl} >20 mEq/L → saline-resistant (unless diuretics actively in use)
  - (n.b., U_{Na} unreliable determinant of volume status as alkalemia → ↑ HCO_3 excretion → ↑ Na excretion; negatively charged HCO_3 "drags" Na^+ along)
  - If U_{Cl} >20 and volume replete, ✓ **blood pressure**

Fig. 4-3. Approach to metabolic alkalosis

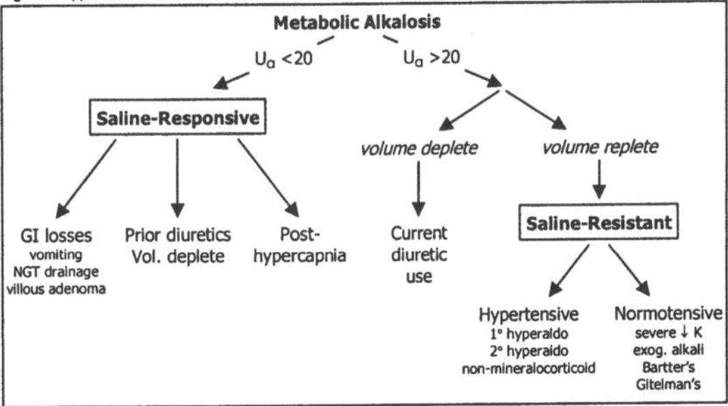

RESPIRATORY ACIDOSIS

Etiologies

- **CNS depression**: sedatives, CNS trauma
- **Neuromuscular disorders**: myasthenia gravis, Guillain-Barré, poliomyelitis, ALS, muscular dystrophy, severe hypophosphatemia
- **Upper airway abnormalities**: acute airway obstruction, laryngospasm, obstructive sleep apnea, esophageal intubation
- **Lower airway abnormalities**: asthma, COPD
- Lung parenchyma abnormalities (often cause hypoxia → ↑ RR → resp. alk., but eventual muscle fatigue → resp. acid.): pneumonia, pulmonary edema, restrictive lung disease
- Thoracic cage abnormalities: pneumothorax, flail chest, kyphoscoliosis

RESPIRATORY ALKALOSIS

Etiologies

- **Hypoxia → hyperventilation**: pneumonia, pulmonary edema, PE, restrictive lung disease
- ***Primary hyperventilation***

  CNS disorders, pain, anxiety
  drugs: salicylates, progesterone
  pregnancy
  sepsis
  hepatic failure

• SODIUM AND WATER HOMEOSTASIS •

Overview

General

- Disorders of serum sodium are generally due to Δs in *total body water*, not sodium
- Hyper- or hypoosmolality → water shifts → Δs in brain cell volume → Δ MS, seizures

Key hormones

- **Antidiuretic hormone (ADH)**: primary hormone that regulates *sodium concentration*
  stimuli for secretion: hyperosmolality, ↓↓ effective arterial volume (EAV)
  action: open water channels in collecting ducts → passive water reabsorption
  urine osmolality is an indirect functional assay of the ADH-renal axis
  U_{osm} range: 60 mOsm/L (no ADH activity) to 1200 mOsm/L (maximal ADH activity)
- **Aldosterone**: primary hormone that regulates *total body sodium* (and ∴ volume)
  stimuli for secretion: hypovolemia (via renin and angiotensin II), hyperkalemia
  action: isoosmotic reabsorption of sodium in exchange for potassium or H^+
  aldosterone excess → hypertension, hypokalemia, metabolic alkalosis
  reduced aldosterone activity → hypovolemia, hyperkalemia, metabolic acidosis

Hyponatremia

Pathophysiology

- **Excess of water relative to sodium**; almost always due to ↑ **ADH**
- ↑ ADH may be *appropriate* (e.g., hypovolemia or hypervolemia but with ↓ EAV)
- ↑ ADH may be *inappropriate* (SIADH)
- Rarely, ↓ ADH (appropriately suppressed), but kidney unable to maintain normal $[Na]_{serum}$:
  net free H_2O retention = free H_2O intake – (solute load/U_{osm})
  primary polydipsia: ingestion of massive quantities (usually >12 L/d) of free H_2O
  overwhelms diluting ability of kidney (normal solute load ~750 mOsm/d, minimum U_{osm} = 60 mOsm/L → excrete in ~12 L; if H_2O ingestion exceeds this, ⊕ H_2O retention)
  "tea & toast" and *"beer potomania"*: ↓↓ daily solute load, ↑ free H_2O
  insufficient solute load to excrete free H_2O (250 mOsm/d, minimum U_{osm} = 60 mOsm/L → excrete in ~4 L; if H_2O ingestion exceeds this, ⊕ H_2O retention)

Workup (*NEJM* 2000;342:1581)

- Measure **plasma osmolality**
  Hypotonic hyponatremia most common scenario; true excess of free H_2O relative to Na
  Hypertonic hyponatremia: excess of another effective osmole (e.g., glc, mannitol) that draws H_2O intravascularly; each 100 mg/dL ↑ glc >100 mg/dL → ↓ [Na] by 2.4 mEq/L
  Isotonic hyponatremia: lab artifact from hyperlipidemia or hyperproteinemia (if using ion-sens. electrodes); absorption of glycine or sorbitol bladder irrigation during uro proced.
- For hypotonic hyponatremia, ✓ **volume status** (vital signs, orthostatics, JVP, skin turgor, mucous membranes, peripheral edema, BUN, Cr, uric acid)
- **U_{osm}** usually *not* helpful diagnostically, because almost always >300
  (exceptions: U_{osm} <100 in 1° polydipsia & ↓ solute intake, but usually obvious on hx)
  moreover, U_{osm} >300 = ADH ≠ SIADH; must clinically determine if approp. or inapprop.
  however, U_{osm} very important when deciding on *treatment* (see below)
- If euvolemic and ↑ U_{osm}, evaluate for adrenal insufficiency and hypothyroidism

Fig. 4-4. Approach to hyponatremia

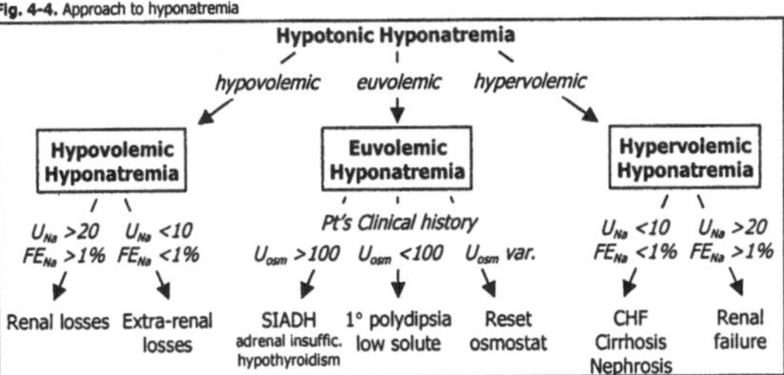

Hypovolemic hypotonic hyponatremia

- **Renal losses** (U_{Na} >20 mEq/L, FE_{Na} >1%): diuretics (espec. thiazides), salt-wasting nephropathy, adrenal insufficiency
- **Extra-renal losses** (U_{Na} <10 mEq/L, FE_{Na} <1%): GI losses (e.g., diarrhea), third-spacing (e.g., pancreatitis), inadequate intake, insensible losses

Euvolemic hypotonic hyponatremia

- **SIADH** (eu- or mildly hypervolemic, inappropriately ↑ U_{Osm}, normal U_{Na}, low BUN & UA)
  pulmonary pathology: pneumonia, asthma, COPD, SCLC, PTX, ⊕ pressure ventilation
  intracranial pathology: trauma, stroke, hemorrhage, tumors, infection, hydrocephalus
  drugs: antipsychotics, antidepressants, thiazides
  miscellaneous: pain, nausea, post-operative state
- **Endocrinopathies**: ↑ ADH activity seen in *adrenal insufficiency* (volume depletion + co-secretion of ADH & CRH) and *hypothyroidism* (↓ CO & ↓ GFR)
- **Psychogenic polydipsia** (U_{osm} <100, low UA): usually requires intake >12 L/d
- **Low solute**: "tea & toast"; "beer potomania"
- Reset osmostat (ADH physiology reset to regulate a lower $[Na]_{serum}$)

Hypervolemic hypotonic hyponatremia

- **CHF** (↓ CO → ↓ EAV; U_{Na} <10 mEq/L, FE_{Na} <1%)
- **Cirrhosis** (ascites → ↓ EAV; U_{Na} <10 mEq/L, FE_{Na} <1%)
- **Nephrotic syndrome** (hypoalbuminemia → edema → ↓ EAV; U_{Na} <10 mEq/L, FE_{Na} <1%)
- **Advanced renal failure** (U_{Na} >20 mEq/L)

Treatment

- **Goals of treatment**
  Asymptomatic hyponatremia: correct $[Na]_{serum}$ at rate of ≤0.5 mEq/L/hr
  Symptomatic hyponatremia: *initial* rapid correction of Na (2 mEq/L/hr) until sx resolve
  Rate of ↑ of Na *should not exceed 12 mEq/L/day* to avoid central pontine myelinolysis
  (CNS demyelinization → Δ MS, spastic paralysis, pseudobulbar palsy)
- **Methods of treating hyponatremia**
  Free water restrict
  Remove stimulus for ADH: volume replete, ↑ EAV, treat pulmonary pathology, etc.
  Demeclocycline (ADH antagonist)
  Normal saline: useful *only* to Rx volume depletion
  in SIADH can *worsen* hyponatremia if U_{osm} > $infusate_{osm}$ (=308)
  e.g., if infuse 1 L NS (=154 mEq of Na or 308 mOsm of solute in 1 L free of H_2O) in Pt with SIADH

  initially ↑ serum Na: $\Delta[Na]_{serum}$ per L infusate $= \dfrac{[Na]_{infusate} - [Na]_{serum}}{TBW + 1}$ {Eq 1}

  where TBW = 0.60 × ideal body weight (IBW) (× 0.85 if female and × 0.85 if elderly)
  however, above assumes entire infusate retained *without any output of Na or H_2O*
  if Pt euvolemic, as in SIADH, then infused Na will be excreted
  amount of free H_2O the osmoles in 1 L of an infusate is excreted in depends on U_{osm}:

  $$\left[\frac{osm_{infusate}}{U_{osm}} - 1\right] = \Delta TBW$$ (⊕ → net excretion; ⊖ → net retention) {Eq 2}

  e.g., U_{osm}=616, 308 mOsm solute excreted in 0.5 L H_2O → net gain 0.5 L H_2O → ↓ [Na]
  Hypertonic saline (=513 mEq of Na or 1026 mOsm of solute per L) used in severe cases of SIADH
  ± loop diuretic to prevent hypervolemia
  as excretion of Na and H_2O takes time, use {Eq 1} to guide initial rate of infusion
  N.B.: these formulae are only estimates; ∴ one must recheck serum Na frequently
- **Hypovolemic hyponatremia**: *normal saline*
  titrate infusion to replete volume status and ∴ remove stimulus for ADH
  once ADH off, U_{osm} will ↓, kidneys will excrete free H_2O, and serum Na will correct rapidly
- **Hypervolemic hyponatremia**: *free water restrict ± diuresis ± ↑ EAV*
  (e.g., vasodilators in CHF, colloid infusion in cirrhosis or nephrotic syndrome)
- **SIADH**: *free water restrict + Rx underlying cause, if possible*
  if ⊕ sx or Na fails to ↑ → hypertonic saline + loop diuretic ± demeclocycline

HYPERNATREMIA

Pathophysiology (*NEJM* 2000;342:1493)

- Deficit of water relative to sodium
- Usually **loss of hypotonic fluid**; occasionally infusion of hypertonic fluid
- ***And*** **impaired access to free water** (e.g. intubation, Δ MS): hypernatremia powerful thirst stimulus; ∴ usually only develops in Pts w/o access to H_2O
- By definition, all Pts are hypertonic; Pts can be either hypo-, eu-, or hypervolemic

Hypovolemic hypernatremia

- **Renal H_2O losses**: osmotic diuresis from glc (uncontrolled DM), mannitol, or urea
- **Extra-renal H_2O losses**: diarrhea (infectious, lactulose); insensible (fever, exercise)

Euvolemic hypernatremia

- **Diabetes insipitus (DI)**: ADH deficiency (central) or renal ADH resistance (nephrogenic)
  - **Central**: trauma, surgery, hemorrhage, infection, granulomas, tumor, hypoxia, anorexia
  - **Nephrogenic**
    - drugs: **Li**, amphotericin, demeclocycline, foscarnet, cidofovir
    - metabolic: **hypercalcemia**, severe hypokalemia
    - tubulointerstitial: polycystic, sickle cell, Sjögren's, sarcoid, amyloidosis, pregnancy
  - DI usually presents as *severe polyuria* and *mild hypernatremia*; see "Polyuria" for details
- Seizures, exercise: intracellular osmole generation → water shifts → transient ↑ $[Na]_{serum}$
- Reset osmostat

Hypervolemic hypernatremia

- Hypertonic saline administration: can be seen in code resuscitation with aggressive $NaHCO_3$
- Mineralocorticoid excess: usually mild hypernatremia caused by ADH suppression

Workup

- ✓ **volume status** (vital signs, orthostatics, JVP, skin turgor, mucous membranes, peripheral edema, BUN, Cr, uric acid)
- If hypovolemic, ✓ U_{osm} & U_{Na} to determine whether **renal** (U_{osm} 300-600; U_{Na} >20 mEq/L) or **extra-renal** (U_{osm} >600; U_{Na} <20 mEq/L) source of **free water loss**
- If euvolemic, ✓ U_{osm} to evaluate for complete (U_{osm} <300) or partial (U_{osm} 300-600) **DI** see "Polyuria" below for full details of DI workup

Fig. 4-5. Approach to hypernatremia

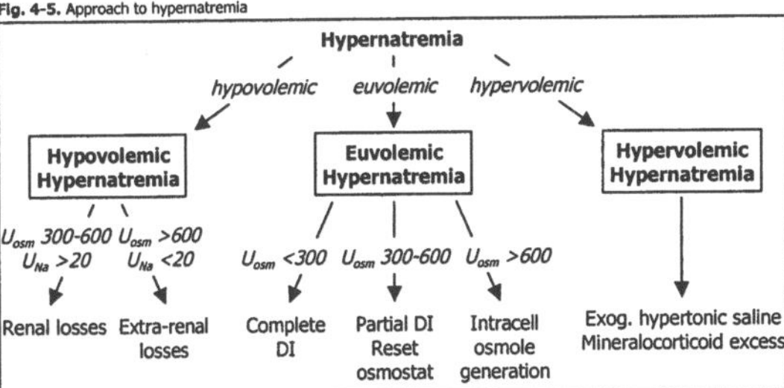

Treatment

- **Replete free H_2O deficit** via IVF or enteral feeds

$$\textbf{Free } \mathbf{H_2O} \textbf{ deficit} = \text{TBW} \times \left(\frac{[\text{Na}]_{\text{serum}} - 140}{140} \right)$$

where TBW = 0.60 × ideal body weight (IBW) (× 0.85 if female and × 0.85 if elderly)

$$\Delta[\text{Na}]_{\text{serum}} \text{ per L infusate} = \frac{[\text{Na}]_{\text{serum}} - [\text{Na}]_{\text{infusate}}}{\text{TBW} + 1}$$

To avoid cerebral edema, correct $[Na]_{serum}$ at rate of ≤0.5 mEq/L/hr
Need to **recheck sodium frequently** as formulae are only estimates

- **Restore access to H_2O** or supply daily requirement of H_2O (≥1 L/d)
- **Correct volume status**
  hypovolemia hypernatremia: ¼ or ½ NS
  hypervolemic hypernatremia: D_5W + loop diuretic
- **DI**
  central DI: desmopressin (dDAVP)
  nephrogenic DI: treat underlying cause if possible; salt restriction + thiazide diuretics (reduces delivery of filtrate to diluting segment of kidney)

POLYURIA

Definition and pathophysiology
- **Polyuria** defined as >3L UOP per day
- Can be due to an *osmotic* or a *water* diuresis
- In inpatients almost always due to osmotic diuresis, whereas both water diuresis (DI) and osmotic diuresis (e.g., uncontrolled diabetes mellitus) can be seen in outpatients

Workup
- Perform a timed urine collection (6 hrs sufficient) and measure U_{osm}
- 24-hr osmole excretion rate = 24-hr UOP (actual or estimate) × U_{osm}
- >1000 mOsm/day → osmotic diuresis
- <800 mOsm/day → water diuresis

Osmotic diuresis
- Etiologies
  Glucose (uncontrolled diabetes mellitus)
  Mannitol
  Urea: recovering ARF, high protein feeds (TPN, tube feeds), hypercatabolism (e.g., burn patients), GI bleed, corticosteroids
  NaCl administration
- Treatment: address underlying cause, replace free water deficit if present (see section on hypernatremia), and address ongoing water losses as a result of the diuresis

Water diuresis
- Etiologies: DI (Na_{serum} >140) or 1° polydipsia (Na_{serum} <140)
  see "Hypernatremia" above for list of causes of central and nephrogenic DI
- Workup of DI: U_{osm} <300 (complete) or 300-600 (partial)
  water deprivation test: deprive until P_{osm} >295 and U_{osm} <300, then administer vasopressin (5U SC) or dDAVP (10 μg intranasal):
    U_{osm} ↑ by >50% = central DI
    U_{osm} unΔ'd = nephrogenic DI
- Treatment of DI
  Central: desmopressin (dDAVP)
  Nephrogenic: treat underlying cause if possible; salt restriction + thiazide diuretics

• POTASSIUM HOMEOSTASIS •

OVERVIEW

Renal handling (*Lancet* 1998;352:135)
- Potassium excretion regulated at distal nephron
- ↑ renal excretion triggered by: hyperkalemia, ↑ distal Na delivery, ↑ urine flow rate, metabolic alkalosis, ↑ aldosterone
- Transcellular shifts: most common cause of acute change in serum potassium
  Acid-base disturbance: K^+/H^+ exchange across cell membranes
  Insulin → stimulates Na-K ATPase → hypokalemia
  Catecholamines → stimulate Na-K ATPase → hypokalemia; reversed by β-blockers
  Digoxin → blocks Na-K ATPase → hyperkalemia
  Massive necrosis (e.g., tumor lysis, rhabdo, ischemic bowel) → release of intracellular K
  Hypo- or hyperkalemic periodic paralysis: rare disorders due to channel mutations

HYPOKALEMIA

Transcellular shifts
- Alkalemia, insulin, catecholamines, hypokalemic periodic paralysis (Ca channelopathy)

Renal potassium losses
- Hypo- or normotensive
  acidosis: DKA, RTA (predominantly type I, also type II)
  alkalosis
    diuretics, vomiting/NGT drainage (via 2° hyperaldosteronism)
    Bartter's syndrome (loop of Henle dysfxn → furosemide-like effect; *NEJM* 1999;340:1177)
    Gitelman's syndrome (distal convoluted tubule dysfxn → thiazide-like effect)
  Mg depletion: mechanism unclear, variable acid-base
- Hypertensive: mineralocorticoid excess → hypertension, hypokalemia, metabolic alkalosis
  1° hyperaldosteronism (e.g., Conn's syndrome)
  2° hyperaldosteronism (e.g., renovascular disease, renin-secreting tumor)
  non-aldosterone mineralocorticoid (e.g., Cushing's, Liddle's, exogenous mineralocort.)

GI potassium losses
- GI losses *plus* acidosis: diarrhea, laxative abuse, villous adenoma
- Vomiting & NGT drainage usually manifest as *renal losses* due to 2° hyperaldo & met. alk.

Clinical manifestations
- Nausea, vomiting, weakness, muscle cramps
- ECG: U waves, ± ↑ QT interval, ventricular ectopy (PVCs, VT, VF)

Workup (*NEJM* 1998;339:451)
- Rule-out transcellular shifts: alkalemia, insulin, catecholamines
- ✓ 24-hr $\mathbf{U_K}$ and **trans-tubular potassium gradient** (TTKG) = $(U_K/P_K) / (U_{osm}/P_{osm})$
  U_K >30 mEq/d or >15 mEq/L or TTKG >7 → renal loss
  U_K <25 mEq/d or <15 mEq/L or TTKG <3 → extrarenal loss
- If renal losses, ✓ **BP** and **acid-base status**

Fig. 4-6. Approach to hypokalemia

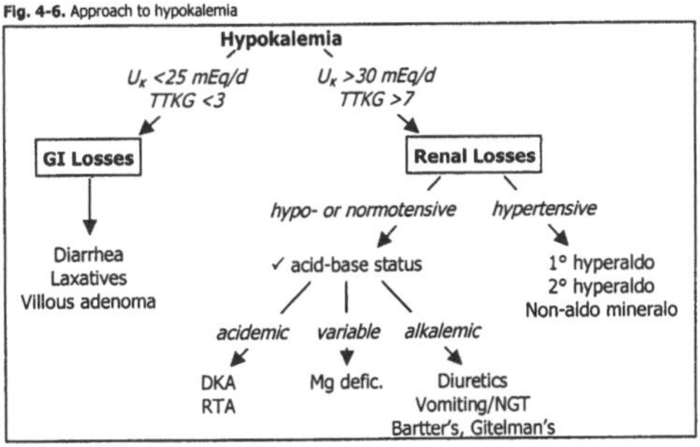

Treatment

- *If true potassium deficit:* **potassium repletion** (↓ 1 mEq/L ≈ 200 mEq total body loss) KCl 40 mEq PO q 4-6 hrs if non-urgent, KCl 10 mEq/hr IV if urgent, recheck K frequently
- Beware of excessive potassium repletion if transcellular shift cause of hypokalemia
- Treat underlying cause (if hydration needed, avoid dextrose-containing solutions as dextrose → ↑ insulin → intracellular potassium shifts)
- Replete Mg as necessary

HYPERKALEMIA

Transcellular shifts

- Acidosis, β-blockers, insulin defic. (untreated DM), dig intoxication, massive cellular necrosis, hyperkalemic periodic paralysis (Na channelopathy; weakness *precipitated* by K, serum K levels may be only modestly elevated during an attack)

↓ renal excretion of potassium

- ↓ **GFR** (including urinary tract obstruction)
- Normal GFR but **hypoaldosteronism**

Hyperkalemia with normal GFR (↓ effective aldosterone function)	
Mechanism	**Etiologies**
↓ renin	**Diabetic nephropathy**, **NSAIDs**, acute GN, HIV, chronic interstitial nephritis
↓ aldosterone production (normal renin)	**ACEI**, **ARBs**, heparin, 1° adrenal disorders
↓ tubular response to aldosterone	Medications: **K-sparing diuretics**, **TMP-SMX**, pentamidine, CsA, tacrolimus Tubulointerstitial disease: sickle cell, SLE, amyloid, diabetes

Clinical manifestations

- Weakness, nausea, paresthesias, palpitations
- ECG: peaked T waves, ↑ PR interval, ↑ QRS width, sine wave pattern, PEA

Workup

- r/o pseudohyperkalemia (IVF containing K, hemolysis during venipuncture, ↑ plt or WBC)
- Rule-out transcellular shift: acidosis, β-blockers, insulin defic., dig, massive cellular necrosis
- Assess GFR (estimated CrCl)
- If normal GFR, calculate **trans-tubular potassium gradient** (TTKG) = $(U_K/P_K)/(U_{osm}/P_{osm})$ TTKG <7 → ↓ effective aldosterone function; TTKG >7 → normal aldosterone function

Treatment of Hyperkalemia			
Intervention	**Dose**	**Onset**	**Comment**
Calcium gluconate **Calcium chloride***	1-2 amps IV	few min	transient effect stabilizes cell membrane
Insulin	reg. insulin 10 U IV + 1-2 amps $D_{50}W$	15-30 min	transient effect drives K into cells
Bicarbonate	1-3 amps IV	15-30 min	transient effect drives K into cells in exchange for H
β2 agonists	albuterol 10-20 mg inh. or 0.5 mg IV	30-90 min	transient effect drives K into cells
Kayexalate	30-90 g PO/PR	1-2 hrs	↓ total body K exchanges Na for K in gut
Diuretics	furosemide ≥ 40 mg IV	30 min	↓ total body K
Hemodialysis			↓ total body K

*calcium chloride contains more calcium and is typically reserved for use in codes

- *Rate of onset* important to note when establishing a treatment plan
- Calcium helps prevent cardiac complications; ∴ should be initial Rx, esp. if ECG Δs present
- Insulin, bicarbonate, and β2 agonists should follow to ↓ plasma K
- Treatments that eliminate total body K essential as other Rxs will wear off with time; kayexalate ± diuretics may be effective in many cases, but emergent hemodialysis should be considered in life-threatening situations

• URINALYSIS •

Urine dipstick	
Measurement	**Significance and uses**
Specific gravity	estimates U_{osm}: each thousandth of SG above 1 ≈ 30 points of osmoles (e.g. SG = 1.010 → U_{osm} ≈ 300) note that heavy substances (protein, glucose, contrast) can elevate SG more than U_{osm}
pH	range: 4.5-8.5; useful in w/u of stones and RTAs
Protein	measures albumin; marker for glomerular dysfunction
RBC	seen in glomerulonephritis, nephrolithiasis, urinary tract malignancy, and traumatic injury; also ⊕ with myoglobinuria (seen in rhabdomyolysis)
WBC (leukocyte esterase)	suggests inflammation (UTI, interstitial nephritis, GN)
Ketones	detects acetoacetate (seen in ketoacidosis); does *not* detect β-hydroxybutyrate
Nitrite	suggests presence of Enterobacteriaceae
Bilirubin	↑ in biliary or hepatic disease
Glucose	⊕ in hyperglycemia, pregnancy, Fanconi's syndrome

Urine Sediment (microscopic examination)	
Method: centrifuge test tube × 3-5 minutes at 1500-3000 RPM; pour off supernatant in one motion; allow residual urine to drip to bottom; resuspend pellet by agitating base of tube; pour suspension onto slide, place coverslip; view under "high - dry" power; phase contrast for RBC morphology.	
Cells	RBCs: assess amount & morphology (many dysmorphic → glomerular) WBCs: PMNs (UTI) *vs.* eosinophils (AIN; may require special stain) Epithelial cells: tubular cells (ATN), transitional cells (from bladder or ureters), squamous cells
Casts	*Proteins molded in lumen of renal tubule ± entrapped cellular elements* RBC → glomerulonephritis WBC → AIN, pyelonephritis, GN Tubular cell → ATN Granular: degenerating cellular casts → any tubular injury; ("muddy brown" = pigmented, coarse granular casts → ATN) Hyaline: Tamm-Horsfall protein (non-specific) Waxy and broad → advanced renal failure
Crystals	*Differentiated on basis of shape and pH of urine* Calcium oxalate monohydrate: spindle, oval or dumbbell shaped Calcium oxalate dihydrate: envelope shaped or octahedral Uric acid: variable shape; polychromatic under polarized light Cystine: hexagon shaped Struvite: coffin-lid shaped; seen at a high pH in association with chronic upper UTI with urea-splitting organisms (e.g., *Proteus*)

PROTEINURIA

Etiologies of Proteinuria		
Category	**Description**	**Etiologies**
Glomerular (usually >2-3 g/d)	Disruption of filtration barrier → lose albumin	Nephritic or nephrotic glomerular disease
Tubulointerstitial (usually <2 g/d)	↓ reabsorption of freely filtered proteins → lose globulins	Acute tubular necrosis Acute interstitial nephritis Fanconi's syndrome
Overflow	↑ production of freely filtered proteins	Multiple myeloma Myoglobinuria Myelogenous leukemia
Isolated	By def'n: asx, normal renal fxn, sed, & imaging, no h/o renal disease	Functional (fever, exercise, CHF) Orthostatic (only when upright) Idiopathic (transient or persistent)

Workup

- **Urine dipstick**
  approximate concen.: 1+ ≈30 mg/dL, 2+ ≈100 mg/dL, 3+ ≈300 mg/dL, 4+ >2000 mg/dL
  insensitive for microalbuminuria and myeloma light chains
- **Spot urine**: protein (mg/dl)/creatinine (mg/dl) ≈ g/day of proteinuria (*NEJM* 1983;309:1543)
  unlike urine dipstick, will detect myeloma light chains
- **24° urine protein** for definitive quantification
  Cr ≥20 mg/kg in males or ≥15 mg/kg in females suggests adequate 24-hr urine collection
- **Urine protein electrophoresis (UPEP)**
- Urine sediment
  hematuria, dysmorphic RBCs, RBC casts → glomerulonephritis
  oval fat bodies, fatty casts, free fat droplets → nephrotic syndrome
  WBCs, WBC casts, tubular casts, granular casts → tubulointerstitial process
- Serum: electrolytes, BUN, Cr, SPEP, triglycerides, cholesterol
- Renal imaging and/or biopsy

Treatment

- Disease specific
- **ACEIs** and **ARBs** ↓ proteinuria and disease progression in proteinuric renal disease (*NEJM* 1993;329:1462 & 1996; 334:939, RENAAL, *NEJM* 2001; 345:861)

HEMATURIA

Etiologies of Hematuria	
Extrarenal (far more common)	**Intrarenal**
Nephrolithiasis Neoplasm: transitional cell, prostate Infection: cystitis, urethritis, prostatitis Foley trauma	Nephrolithiasis or crystalluria Neoplasm Infection Trauma Vascular: renal infarcts, renal vein thrombosis Glomerulonephritis

Workup (*NEJM* 2003;348:2330)

- **Urine dipstick**: ⊕ if >3 RBCs; ⊕ dipstick and ⊖ sediment → myo- or hemoglobinuria
- **Urine sediment**: dysmorphic RBCs or RBC casts → glomerulonephritis → renal bx
- If no evidence of glomerulonephritis:
  r/o UTI
  ✓ urine cytology
  renal imaging: helical CT (r/o neoplasia of upper tract), cystoscopy (r/o bladder neoplasia), ? U/S (r/o obstruction or parenchymal disease)

• RENAL FAILURE •

ACUTE RENAL FAILURE (ARF)

Definitions (*NEJM* 1996;334:1448 & 1998;338:671, *JAMA* 2003;289:747)

- Acute deterioration in renal function manifested by ↑ Cr
  research def'ns: ↑ Cr ≥0.5 mg/dL in ≤2 wks or ↑ Cr ≥20% if baseline Cr >2.5 mg/dL
- Oliguria: UOP = 100-400 ml/24 hrs; anuria: UOP <100 ml/24 hrs

Workup

- **History and physical**: special attention to recent procedures and medications, vital signs, volume status, signs and symptoms of obstruction, vascular disease or systemic disease
- **Urine evaluation**: output, urinalysis, sediment, electrolytes and osmolality
- **Fractional excretion of sodium (FE_{Na})** = $(U_{Na}/P_{Na})/(U_{Cr}/P_{Cr})$
  <1% → prerenal, contrast, or glomerulonephritis; >2% → ATN
  in setting of diuretics, ✓ $FE_{UN} = (U_{UN}/P_{UN})/(U_{Cr}/P_{Cr})$; <35% → prerenal etiology
- Renal U/S: useful to r/o obstruction and evaluate kidney size to estimate chronicity of RF
- Renal biopsy: consider if suspect AGN
- Serologies (if indicated): see "Glomerular Disease"

Etiologies & Diagnosis of Acute Renal Failure		
Etiologies		**U/A, Sediment, Indices**
Prerenal	**Hypovolemia** **↓ CO** **Systemic vasodilatation** **Renal vasoconstriction** ACEI, ARBs, NSAIDs, contrast dye, CsA, tacrolimus cirrhosis (hepatorenal syndrome) **Large vessel**: RAS (bilateral + ACEI), thrombosis, embolism, dissection, vasculitis	Bland Transparent hyaline casts FE_{Na} <1% BUN/Cr >20
Intrinsic	**Acute tubular necrosis (ATN)** *Ischemia:* progression of prerenal disease *Toxins* Drugs: AG, amphotericin, cisplatin Pigments: myoglobin, hemoglobin Proteins: Ig light chains *Contrast Induced ARF (CIARF):* ↓ RBF + toxin	Pigmented granular "muddy brown" casts in ~75% (± in CIARF) ± RBCs & protein from tubular damage FE_{Na} >2% (except pigment & CIARF)
	Acute interstitial nephritis (AIN) *Allergic:* β-lactams, sulfa-based drugs, NSAIDs *Infection:* pyelonephritis *Infiltrative:* sarcoid, lymphoma, leukemia	WBCs, WBC casts, ± RBCs ⊕ eos in abx (~90%) ⊕ lymphs in NSAIDs
	Renovascular (small vessel) HUS/TTP, DIC, preeclampsia cholesterol emboli, endocarditis hypertensive crisis, scleroderma renal crisis	± RBCs ⊕ eos in cholesterol emboli
	Glomerulonephritis (see "Glomerular Disease")	Dysmorphic RBCs & RBC casts
Postrenal	**Bladder neck**: BPH, prostate cancer, neurogenic bladder, anticholinergic meds **Ureteral**: malignancy, lymphadenopathy, retroperitoneal fibrosis, nephrolithiasis (bilateral or if solitary kidney) **Tubular**: precipitation of crystals	Bland ± RBCs if nephrolithiasis

Contrast-induced acute renal failure (CIARF)

- Incidence: usually in Pts w/ underlying renal disease (especially diabetes) or dehydration
- Dye: non-ionic (*Kidney Int* 1994;47:259) & iso-osmolar contrast (*NEJM* 2003;348:491) safer
- Clinical: Cr ↑ w/in 24 hrs, peaks in 3-5 d, resolves in 7-10 d
- Prevention
  pre- and post-hydration (*NEJM* 1994;331:1416)
  use non-ionic & low- or iso-osmolar contrast & minimize dye load
  hold ACEI, NSAIDs, no benefit to fenoldopam (*JAMA* 2003;290:2284)
  N-acetylcysteine 600 mg PO bid on day prior to and day of contrast (*NEJM* 2000;343:180; *JAMA* 2003;289:553; *Lancet* 2003;362:598)
  ? hemofiltration (before & for 24 hrs after) if high-risk (Cr >2.0; *NEJM* 2003;349:1333)

Complications

- Volume overload (CHF)
- Hyperkalemia, hyperphosphatemia
- Metabolic acidosis
- Uremia (nausea, vomiting, encephalopathy, pericarditis)
- After relief of obstruction
  hypotonic diuresis (2° buildup of BUN, tubular damage); Rx with IVF (½ NS)
  hemorrhagic cystitis (rapid Δ in size of bladder vessels); avoid by decompressing slowly

Treatment

- Treat underlying disorder; avoid nephrotoxic insults; review dosing of renally cleared drugs
- Optimize hemodynamics (both MAP & CO)
- *No* benefit to dopamine (*Lancet* 2000;356:2139), diuretics (although Pts who fail to ↑ UOP to diuretics have worse outcome, *JAMA* 2002;288:2547), mannitol, or ANP (*NEJM* 1997;336:828)
- Indications for urgent dialysis (when condition refractory to conventional therapy)
  Acid-base disturbance: acidemia
  Electrolyte disorder: hyperkalemia
  Intoxication: methanol, ethylene glycol
  Overload of volume
  Uremia: pericarditis, encephalopathy, bleeding

CHRONIC KIDNEY DISEASE (CKD)

Definition and etiologies

- ≥3 mos of **reduced GFR** (<60 ml/min/1.73 m^2) *and/or* **kidney damage** (abnormal pathology, blood/urine markers, or imaging)
- Prevalence 11% in US; serum Cr poor estimate of GFR and may underdiagnose CKD
- Etiologies include diabetes mellitus, hypertension, polycystic kidney disease, glomerulonephritis, drug-induced, myeloma, progression of ARF

Stages of CKD

Stage	GFR	Goals
1 (nl or ↑ GFR)	>90	Dx/Rx of underlying condition & comorbidities, slow progression. Cardiovascular risk reduction
2 (mild)	60-89	Estimate progression
3 (moderate)	30-59	Evaluate and treat complications
4 (severe)	15-29	Prepare for renal replacement therapy (RRT)
5 (kidney failure)	<15 or dialysis	Dialysis if uremic

(Adapted from *Am J Kidney Dis* 2002;39:S1)

Signs and Symptoms of Uremia

System	Manifestations
General	Nausea, anorexia, malaise, fetor uremicus, metallic taste, pruritis, uremic frost (white crystals in & on skin), susceptibility to drug O/D
Neurologic	Encephalopathy (Δ MS, ↓ memory & attention), seizures, myoclonus, neuropathy
Cardiovascular	Pericarditis, accelerated atherosclerosis, hypertension, hyperlipidemia, volume overload, CHF, cardiomyopathy
Hematologic	Anemia, bleeding (due to platelet dysfunction)
Metabolic	↑ K, ↑ PO_4, acidosis, ↓ Ca, 2° hyperparathyroidism, osteodystrophy

Calcium/Phosphate Balance in CKD

Ca	PO_4	PTH	Process	Treatment
↓	↓	↑	Vitamin D deficiency	Daily 1,25-OH vit D PO
↓	↑	↑	2° hyperparathyroidism	Phosphate binders
↓	↑	↑↑↑	Severe 2° hyperparathyroidism	Phosphate binders IV pulse vit D with HD
↑	var	↓	Excessive Ca/vitamin D replacement	stop treatment

Treatment

- **General**: early nephrology referral & consideration of dialysis & transplant
  avoid subclavian lines to maintain site for future access
  preserve one arm (avoid blood draws) for future HD access
- **Dietary restrictions**: sodium (if hypertensive), potassium (usually if oliguric), PO_4, Mg
- **ACEI**: slow progression of diabetic and non-diabetic nephropathy (*NEJM* 1993;329:1456 & 1996;334:939); need to *follow K very closely*: if ↑ → low K diet ± kayexalate ± diuretic
- **ARBs**: slow progression of diabetic renal disease (*NEJM* 2001;345:851, 861, 870); combination of ACEI + ARB ? superior to either alone (COOPERATE, *Lancet* 2003;361:117)
- **Hematologic**
  anemia: erythropoietin (start 80-120 U/kg SC, divided 3x/wk); iron supplementation
  uremic bleeding: desmopressin (dDAVP) 0.3 µg/kg IV or 3 µg/kg intranasally
- **Metabolic**
  hyperkalemia: kayexalate as needed; see "Hyperkalemia"
  metabolic acidosis: can treat with bicarbonate or sodium citrate if HCO_3 <22
  vitamin D deficiency: daily 1,25-OH vitamin D PO
  severe 2° hyperparathyroidism: calcitriol or paricalcitol (? ↑ survival, *NEJM* 2003;349:446)
  hyperphosphatemia: phosphate binders
    if ↑ PO_4 & ↓ Ca → calcium acetate (PhosLo) or calcium carbonate
    if refractory ↑ PO_4 or in setting of ↑ Ca → sevelamer (Renagel)
    if severe ↑ PO_4 → aluminum hydroxide (Amphojel), *short-term use only*

DIALYSIS

Hemodialysis (HD) (*NEJM* 1998;338:1428 & 339:1054)

- Physiology: blood flows along one side of semipermeable membrane, dialysate along other. Fluid removal (i.e., salt + H_2O) via transmembrane pressure (TMP) gradient. Solute removal via transmembrane concentration gradient and inversely proportional to size (∴ effective removal of K, urea, and creatinine, but not PO_4).
- Access: temporary or tunneled double-lumen central catheter, AV fistula, AV graft
- Typical orders: volume removal goals, K in dialysate bath, anticoagulation
- Complications: hypotension, arrhythmia, HIT, vascular access complications

Continuous Veno-Venous Hemofiltration (CVVH) (*NEJM* 1997;336:1303)

- Physiology: based on *ultrafiltration* rather than dialysis. Blood under pressure passes down one side of a highly permeable membrane allowing both water and solutes (K, urea, creatinine, and PO_4) to pass across the membrane via TMP gradient. Filtrate is discarded; replacement fluid (solute concentrations similar to plasma) infused. Fluid balance precisely controlled by adjusting amount of effluent and replacement fluid.
- Access: double-lumen central venous catheter
- Typical orders: type of replacement fluid (HCO_3- or citrate-based), ± K and Ca
- Complications: hypotension, ↓ Ca, ↓ PO_4, vascular access complications

Peritoneal Dialysis (PD) (*Perit Dial Int* 2001;21:25)

- Physiology: gravity assisted infusion into peritoneum which acts as membrane; control water and NaCl balance by choosing appropriate glucose concentrations; very long dwell times pull out less fluid as glucose equilibrates.
- Access: temporary catheter inserted midline, permanent catheter inserted in OR
- Typical orders for CAPD (continuous ambulatory peritoneal dialysis):
  PD fluid = 1.5% dextrose, 2.5% dextrose, or 4.25% dextrose
  buffer (lactate, acetate, bicarbonate), Na^+, K^+, Ca^{2+}, Mg^{2+}
  optional additives: insulin; K; heparin (no systemic absorption)
  infuse 10 min, dwell 30 min – 5.5 hrs, drain 20 min
- Can use overnight cycler device that infuses & drains more rapidly, with shorter dwells, while Pts sleep. Called automated or continuous cycling peritoneal dialysis (APD, CCPD).
- Complications
  peritonitis (abdominal pain, tenderness, cloudy drainage)
    diagnosis: WBC >100 and >50% PMNs
    spectrum: 60-70% GPC, 15-20% GNR, remainder no bugs or fungal
    treatment: antibiotics IV or in PD, catheter removal if fungal peritonitis
  hyperglycemia: exacerbated by inflammation, long dwell times, and higher glc

• GLOMERULAR DISEASE •

Overview

Definitions

- **Nephritic syndrome**: hypertension, edema, renal failure, hematuria, RBC casts, ± proteinuria (*NEJM* 1998; 339:888)
  - acute glomerulonephritis (AGN) = develops rapidly
  - rapidly progressive glomerulonephritis (RPGN) = develops over wks with 50% loss of GFR in ≤3 mos and with biopsy revealing crescents in >50% of glomeruli
- **Nephrotic syndrome**: proteinuria >3.5 g/day, hypoalbuminemia <3.5 mg/dL, edema, hypercholesterolemia (*NEJM* 1998;338:1202)
- Some diseases can present with components of *both* syndromes

Nephritic Syndrome

ANCA ⊕ Vasculitis (pauci-immune or minimal staining)						
Disease	**Gran.**	**Renal**	**Pulm.**	**Asthma**	**ANCA Type***	**ANCA ⊕**
Wegener's granulomatosis	⊕	80%	90%	–	c-ANCA (anti-PR3)	90%
Microscopic polyangiitis	–	90%	50%	–	p-ANCA (anti-MPO)	70%
Churg-Strauss syndrome	⊕	45%	70%	⊕	p-ANCA (anti-MPO)	50%

*Predominant ANCA type; either p- or c-ANCA can be seen in all three disease. (*NEJM* 1997;337:1512)

Anti-GBM disease (linear staining)			
Disease	**Glomerulonephritis**	**Pulm hemorrhage**	**Anti-GBM**
Goodpasture's	⊕	⊕	⊕
Anti-GBM disease	⊕	–	⊕

Immune Complex (IC) disease (granular staining)	
Renal-limited diseases	**Systemic diseases**
Post-streptococcal GN (PSGN, ⊕ ASLO, ↓ C3)	**SLE** (⊕ ANA, anti-dsDNA, ↓ C3)
Membranoproliferative GN (MPGN, ↓ C3)	**Endocarditis** (fever, ⊕ BCx, valvular disease, ↓ C3)
Fibrillary glomerulonephritis (normal C3)	**Cryoglobulinemia** (⊕ cryoprecipitate, ↓ C3, HCV Ab)
IgA nephropathy (normal C3)	**Henoch-Schönlein purpura** (IgA nephropathy + systemic vasculitis, normal C3)

Workup (*Archives* 2001;161:25)

- ANCA, anti-GBM, complement levels (C3)
- Depending on clinical hx ✓: ANA, ASLO, blood cultures, cryocrit, hepatitis serologies
- Renal biopsy with immunofluorescence (IF)

Fig. 4-7. Approach to nephritic syndrome

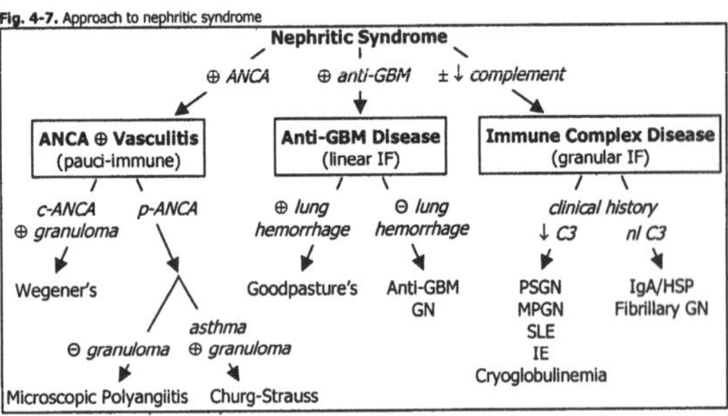

Treatment

- ANCA ⊕ disease: *immediate* steroids + cyclophosphamide (*Annals* 1992;116:488)
- Anti-GBM dis.: *immediate* steroids + cytotoxic agent ± plasmapheresis (*Medicine* 1985;64:219)
- IC disease: ? steroids ± alkylating agents for renal diseases; treat underlying diseases
  proliferative lupus nephritis: ? short-term IV cyclophosphamide → mycophenolate mofetil or azathioprine (*NEJM* 2004;350:971)

Nephrotic Syndrome

Primary glomerular diseases

(Grouped by pathology; all can be idiopathic or associated with systemic diseases which are listed below.)

- **Focal segmental glomerulosclerosis** (FSGS, 40%)
  sustained glomerular hyperfiltration, diabetes
  HIV ("collapsing variant"), heroin
- **Membranous nephropathy** (MN, 30%)
  infection (HBV, HCV, syphilis)
  autoimmune (SLE, RA, Sjögren's)
  carcinomas (breast, lung, colon)
  drugs (gold, penicillamine, ACEI, NSAIDs)
- **Minimal change disease** (MCD, 20%)
  NSAIDs, Hodgkin's disease & other lymphoproliferative disorders, HIV
- **Membranoproliferative glomerulonephritis** (MPGN, 5%)
  Type I (subepithelial C3 & Ig deposits)
    infection (endocarditis, HIV, HBV, HCV)
    IC diseases (SLE, cryoglobulinemia, Sjögren's)
    lymphoproliferative disorders (leukemia, lymphoma)
  Type II ("dense deposit disease" w/ C3 only; due to IgG autoAb = *C3 nephritic factor*)
- **Fibrillary-immunotactoid glomerulopathy** (1%)
- **Mesangial proliferative GN** (likely atypical forms of MCD or FSGS, 5%)
- **IgA nephropathy** (usually asx hematuria)

Systemic diseases

- **Diabetes mellitus**: nodular glomerulosclerosis (Kimmelsteil-Wilson lesion); large kidneys
  hyperfiltration → microalbuminuria → dipstick ⊕ → nephrotic range (10-15 yrs)
  concomitant proliferative retinopathy seen in 90% of type 1 and 60% of type 2
- **Amyloidosis:** large kidneys
- **SLE**: typically with MN (WHO type V)
- **Cryoglobulinemia**: typically with MPGN

Workup (*Archives* 2001;161:25)

- Urine sediment: usually benign w/o concurrent nephritis; ± oval fat bodies
- r/o secondary causes
  ↑ Hb_{A1C} + retinopathy → presumpt. dx of diabetic nephropathy unless another suggested
  ANA, anti-dsDNA, complement (C3, C4, CH50), SPEP, fat pad biopsy, cryocrit
  HBV, HCV, HIV, RPR
- Renal biopsy

Treatment

- **General management**: protein supplementation; Na restriction and diuretics for edema; diet and pharmacologic therapy for hyperlipidemia
- **ACEI/ARB**: ↓ proteinuria and progression to ESRD (*NEJM* 1993;329:145 & 2001;345:861; *Lancet* 1997;349:1857 & 1999;354:359)
- Primary glomerular disease: steroids ± cytotoxic therapy (e.g., cyclophosphamide, chlorambucil) (*NEJM* 1989;320:8 & 1992;327:599)
- Secondary causes: treat underlying disease

Complications

- Malnutrition (protein loss)
- Thrombosis (especially renal vein, because loss of ATIII, other endogenous anticoagulants)
- Infection (especially encapsulated organisms, because loss of immunoglobulin)
- Accelerated atherosclerosis (hypercholesterolemia)

• NEPHROLITHIASIS •

Pathogenesis
- ↑ excretion of solutes (e.g., hypercalciuria, hyperoxaluria, hyperuricosuria)
- ↓ urine volume
- Abnormal urine pH
  alkaline → precipitation of calcium phosphate and struvite stones
  acidic → precipitation of uric acid, cystine, and calcium oxalate stones
- Absence of inhibitors (e.g., citrate)

Stone types
- Calcium oxalate
- Calcium phosphate
- Uric acid
- Magnesium ammonium phosphate ("struvite" or "triple phosphate")
- Cystine

Etiologies
- **Idiopathic**: hypercalciuria, hyperoxaluria, hyperuricosuria, hypocitraturia
- Secondary
  hypercalciuria: primary hyperparathyroidism, type 1 RTA, sarcoidosis
  hyperoxaluria: Crohn's disease or other ileal disease with intact colon
  hyperuricosuria: myelo- and lymphoproliferative disorders
- **Structural renal disease**: polycystic kidney disease, medullary sponge disease, horseshoe kidney
- **Infection**: urea-splitting organisms (e.g., *Proteus*) → ↑ NH_3 and alkali urine

Clinical manifestations
- **Hematuria**
- **Renal colic**: flank pain → groin
- **Ureteral obstruction** (stones >5-7 mm are unlikely to pass spontaneously)
- **Acute renal failure** if bilateral obstruction or unilateral obstruction of solitary kidney
- **UTI**: ↑ risk of infection proximal to stone; urinalysis of distal urine may be normal

Workup
- Spiral CT scan is first choice for imaging (*J Urol* 1998;159:735)
- Urinalysis, urine sediment, urine culture, electrolytes, BUN, Cr, Ca, PO_4, PTH, uric acid
- 24 hour urine for Ca, PO_4, uric acid, oxalate, citrate, Na, Cr, pH (should be done outside of acute setting)

Acute treatment
- Narcotic analgesia and aggressive PO/IV hydration
- **Strain urine** for gravel/stones for stone analysis
- Antibiotics as needed for UTI
- Hospitalization indications: obstruction, infection, intractable pain, not taking POs
- Indications for **immediate urologic evaluation**: obstruction, infection
- Urologic interventions: lithotripsy, cystoscopic stenting, percutaneous nephrostomy, stone removal

Chronic treatment
- Identify and treat underlying disease
- ↑ fluid intake (>2 L/day)
- Calcium stones: (*NEJM* 2002;346:77)
  ↓ Na & meat intake (both → calciuria); **thiazides** → ↓ urinary calcium excretion
  avoid limiting calcium intake as causes hyperoxaluria and ↑ risk of osteoporosis
- Uric acid: urine alkalinization (with potassium citrate), allopurinol
- Hypocitraturia: K-citrate replacement
- Magnesium ammonium phosphate: antibiotics to treat UTI

• ANEMIA •

GENERAL

Definition
- ↓ in RBC mass: Hct <41% or Hb <13.5 g/dl (men) or Hct <36% or Hb <12 g/dl (women)

Clinical manifestations
- Symptoms: ↓ O_2 delivery → fatigue, exertional dyspnea, angina (in pt w/ CAD)
- Signs: pallor (mucous membranes, palmar creases), tachycardia, orthostatic hypotension
- Other findings: **jaundice** (hemolysis), **splenomegaly** (thalassemia, neoplasm, chronic hemolysis), **petechiae/purpura** (bleeding disorder), **glossitis** (iron, folate, vitamin B_{12} deficiency), **koilonychia** (iron deficiency), **neurologic abnormalities** (B_{12} deficiency)

Diagnostic evaluation
- History: bleeding, systemic illness, drugs, exposures, alcohol, diet (including **pica**), FHx
- CBC with differential; RBC parameters including reticulocyte count, MCV, RDW
- **Reticulocyte index** (RI) = [reticulocyte count × (Pt's Hct/normal Hct)]/maturation factor
  maturation factors for a given Hct: 45% = 1.0, 35% = 1.5, 25% = 2.0, 20% = 2.5
  RI >2% → adequate marrow response; RI <2% → hypoproliferation
- **Peripheral smear**: select area where RBCs evenly spaced and very few touch each other

Peripheral Smear Findings	
Feature	**Abnormalities and diagnoses**
Size	normocytic vs. microcytic vs. macrocytic → see below
Shape	**anisocytosis** → unequal RBC size; **poikilocytosis** → irregular RBC shape **spherocytes** → HS, AIHA; **sickle** cells → sickle cell anemia **tear drop** cells → myelophthisic anemia, megaloblastic anemia, thalassemia **schistocytes**, helmet cells → MAHA (e.g., DIC, TTP/HUS), mechanical valve echinocytes = **burr** cells (even, regular projections) → uremia acanthocytes = **spur** cells (irregular projections) → liver disease **target** cells→ liver disease, hemoglobinopathies, splenectomy **bite** cells (removal of Heinz bodies by phagocytes) → G6PD deficiency **rouleaux** → hyperglobulinemia (e.g., multiple myeloma)
Intra-RBC findings	**basophilic stippling** (ribosomes) → abnl Hb, sideroblastic, megaloblastic **Heinz bodies** (denatured Hb) → G6PD deficiency, thalassemia **Howell-Jolly bodies** (nuclear fragments) → splenectomy, sickle cell **nucleated** RBCs → hemolysis, extramedullary hematopoiesis
WBC findings	**hypersegmented** (>5 lobes) PMNs: megaloblastic anemia **toxic granules** (coarse, dark blue) and **Döhle bodies** (blue patches of dilated endoplasmic reticulum) → sepsis, severe inflammation **pseudo-Pelger-Huët anomaly** (bilobed nucleus, "pince-nez") → MDS **blasts** → leukemia, lymphoma; **Auer rods** → acute leukemia

- Additional laboratory evaluations as indicated: hemolysis labs (if RI >2%), iron, folate, B_{12}, LFTs, BUN and Cr, TFTs, Hb electrophoresis, enzyme analyses, gene mutation screens
- **Bone marrow (BM) aspirate and biopsy (bx)** with cytogenetics as indicated

Fig. 5-1. Approach to anemia

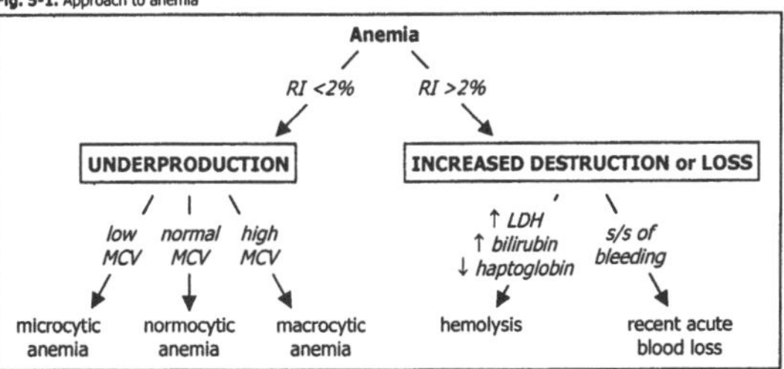

MICROCYTIC ANEMIAS

Iron deficiency
- ↓ marrow iron → ↓ ferritin → ↓ Fe & ↑ TIBC → ↓ heme synthesis → anemia & microcytosis
- Special clinical manifestations: angular cheilosis, atrophic glossitis, pica (consumption of non-nutritive substances such as ice, inorganic materials), koilonychia (nail spooning) Plummer-Vinson syndrome (iron deficiency anemia, esophageal web & atrophic glossitis)
- Etiologies: **chronic bleeding** (GI, menstrual, etc.), ↓ **supply** (malnutrition; ↓ absorption due to celiac sprue, Crohn's, subtotal gastrectomy), or ↑ **demand** (pregnancy)
- Diagnosis: ↓ **Fe**, ↑ **TIBC**, ↓ **ferritin** (<12 *very* suggestive), **Fe/TIBC <18%**, ↑ RDW, ↓ marrow iron; unless history points to a different etiology, *initiate workup for GI bleeding*
- Treatment: Fe supplementation (~6 wks to correct anemia; ~6 mos to replete Fe stores)

Thalassemias
- Pathophysiology: ↓ synthesis of α- or β-globin chains of Hb → ≠ subunits → destruction of RBCs and erythroid precursors; ∴ anemia from hemolysis *and* ineffective erythropoiesis
- **α-thalassemia**: deletions in the α-globin gene complex on chromosome 16
  4 α genes → normal; 3 α genes → α-thalassemia-2 trait = silent carrier
  2 α genes → α-thalassemia-1 trait or α-thalassemia minor = mild microcytic anemia
  1 α gene → HbH (β4) disease = severe anemia, hemolysis, and splenomegaly
  0 α genes → Hb Barts (γ_4) = intrauterine hypoxia and hydrops fetalis
- **β-thalassemia**: mutations in the β-globin gene on chr. 11 → absent or ↓ gene product
  1 mutated β gene → thalassemia minor = mild microcytic anemia (no transfusions)
  2 mutated β genes → thalassemia intermedia (occasional transfusions) or thalassemia major (= Cooley's anemia; transfusion-dependent) depending on severity of mutations
- Special clinical manifestations (in severe cases): chipmunk facies, pathologic fractures, hepatosplenomegaly, high-output CHF, bilirubin gallstones, iron overload syndromes
- Diagnosis: MCV very low (<70), **normal Fe, MCV/RBC count <13**, ± ↑ retics, basophilic stippling; **Hb electrophoresis**: ↑ HbA_2 ($\alpha_2\delta_2$) in β-thal; *normal* pattern in α-thal trait
- Treatment: folic acid; transfusions + deferoxamine; splenectomy if ≥50% ↑ in transfusion requirement; consider allogeneic HSCT in children with severe β–thalassemia major

Anemia of chronic disease (ACD)
- Pathophysiology: impaired iron utilization & ↓ epo-responsiveness due to cytokines in the setting of autoimmune disorders, chronic infection/inflammation, and malignancy
- Diagnosis: ↓ **Fe**, ↓ **TIBC**, ± ↑ **ferritin**; usually normocytic but can by microcytic if severe
- Treatment: treat underlying disease ± erythropoietin; *iron supplementation without benefit*

Sideroblastic anemia
- Pathophysiology: defective heme biosynthesis within RBC precursors
- Etiologies: **hereditary**, **idiopathic** (**MDS**), **reversible** (alcohol, lead, isoniazid, chloramphenicol, copper deficiency, hypothermia)
- Special clinical manifestations: hepatosplenomegaly, iron overload syndromes
- Diagnosis: can be micro-, normo-, or macrocytic; variable population of hypochromic RBCs; ↑ Fe, normal TIBC, ↑ ferritin, basophilic stippling, RBC **Pappenheimer bodies** (iron-containing inclusions), **ringed sideroblasts** (with iron-laden mitochondria) in BM
- Treatment: treat reversible causes; supportive transfusions for severe anemia; high-dose pyridoxine for some hereditary cases

Fig. 5-2. Approach to microcytic anemias

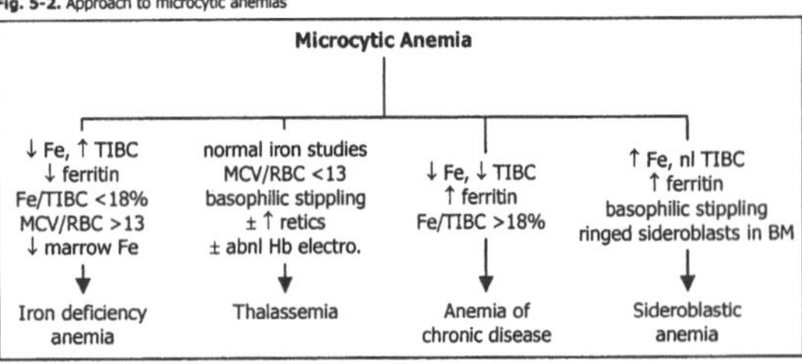

Normocytic Anemias

Pancytopenias (see below)

Pure red cell aplasia
- Destructive antibodies or lymphocytes → ineffective erythropoiesis
- Associated with thymoma and parvovirus infection
- Diagnostic studies: **lack of erythroid precursors on BM bx**, other lines normal
- Treatment: thymectomy if thymus enlarged; IVIg if parvovirus infection; immunosuppression if idiopathic; supportive care with PRBC transfusions

Sideroblastic anemias (see above)

Anemias of chronic disorders
- Anemia of chronic disease (see above)
- Renal failure: ↓ erythropoietin; usually normocytic; may see **burr cells**; treat with epo
- Liver disease: ? excess membrane cholesterol; often macrocytic; may see **target cells**; can also see hemolytic anemia associated with **spur cells**
- Endocrine deficiencies: hypometabolism and ↓ O_2 demand with thyroid, pituitary, adrenal, or parathyroid disease → ↓ erythropoietin; can be normocytic or macrocytic

Macrocytic Anemias

General
- Macrocytic anemias include megaloblastic and non-megaloblastic causes
- **Megaloblastic anemia**: **impaired DNA synthesis** → cytoplasm matures faster than nucleus → ineffective erythropoiesis and macrocytosis; due to **folate** or **B_{12} deficiency**

Diagnostic evaluation of megaloblastic anemia
- **Neutrophil hypersegmentation**, **macroovalocytes**, anisocytosis, poikilocytosis
- ↑ LDH and indirect bilirubin (due to ineffective erythropoiesis)
- ✓ **folate** and **vitamin B_{12}**

Folate deficiency
- Folate present in leafy green vegetables and fruit; total body stores sufficient for **2-3 mos**
- Etiologies: **malnutrition** (alcoholics, anorectics, elderly), ↓ absorption (sprue), impaired metabolism (methotrexate, pyrimethamine, trimethoprim), ↑ requirement (chronic hemolytic anemia, pregnancy, malignancy, dialysis)
- Diagnosis: ↓ folate (in addition to findings above)
- Treatment: folate 1-5 mg PO qd; *important to r/o B_{12} deficiency* (see below)

Vitamin B_{12} deficiency
- B_{12} present only in foods of animal origin; total body stores sufficient for **2-3 years**
- Binds to **intrinsic factor** (IF) secreted by gastric parietal cells; absorbed in terminal ileum
- Etiologies: malnutrition (alcoholics, vegetarians), **pernicious anemia** (autoimmune disease against gastric parietal cells, associated with polyglandular endocrine insufficiency and ↑ risk of gastric carcinoma), other causes of ↓ absorption (gastrectomy, sprue, Crohn's disease), ↑ competition (intestinal bacterial overgrowth, fish tapeworm)
- Special clinical manifestations: **neurologic** changes (**subacute combined degeneration**) affecting peripheral nerves, posterior and lateral columns of the spinal cord, and cortex → numbness, paresthesias, ↓ vibratory and positional sense, ataxia
- Diagnosis: ↓ B_{12}; Schilling test can distinguish between different causes of deficiency
- Treatment: 1 mg B_{12} IM qd × 7 d → q wk × 4-8 wks → q month for life
  neurologic abnormalities are reversible if treated within 6 mos
  folate can reverse *hematologic* abnormalities of B_{12} deficiency but not *neurologic* changes

Non-megaloblastic macrocytic anemias
- Liver disease (may see target and spur cells)
- Alcoholism (BM suppression & macrocytosis independent of folate/B_{12} defic. or liver dis.)
- Hypothyroidism
- Reticulocytosis
- Some patients with aplastic anemia, MDS, or sideroblastic anemia
- Drugs that impair DNA synthesis (e.g., zidovudine, 5-FU, hydroxyurea)

PANCYTOPENIA

Etiologies
- Hypocellular bone marrow: **aplastic anemia**, hypoplastic MDS
- Cellular bone marrow: **MDS**, aleukemic leukemia, PNH, severe megaloblastic anemia
- Marrow replacement (myelophthisis): **myelofibrosis**, metastatic solid tumors, granulomas
- Systemic diseases: hypersplenism, sepsis, alcohol

Clinical manifestations
- Anemia → fatigue
- Neutropenia → recurrent infections
- Thrombocytopenia → mucosal bleeding

Aplastic anemia (stem cell failure; *NEJM* 1997;336:1365)
- Epidemiology: 2-5 cases/10^6/yr; biphasic (major peak in adolescents, 2nd peak in elderly)
- Etiologies
  - **idiopathic** (1/2-2/3 of cases)
  - **radiation, chemotherapy, chemicals** (e.g., benzene)
  - idiosyncratic reaction to **medications** (e.g., chloramphenicol, NSAIDs, sulfa drugs)
  - **viruses** (HHV-6, HIV, EBV, parvovirus B19), **immune disorders** (SLE, GVHD, thymoma)
  - PNH (see below), Fanconi's anemia (congenital disorder characterized by pancytopenia, ↑ incidence of malignancy, and multiple congenital physical anomalies)
- Treatment and prognosis
  - **immunosuppression** (CsA, ATG): 70-80% respond, with 80-90% 5-yr survival in responders; 15-20% 10-yr incidence of clonal disorders (mostly MDS, AML, PNH)
  - **allogeneic HSCT**: for young Pts with matched donor; 80% long-term survival and significantly ↓ risk of malignant evolution with transplant in this group
  - G-CSF and epo in some refractory cases; supportive care (transfusions, antibiotics)

Myelodysplastic syndromes (MDS)
- Definition: acquired clonal stem cell disorder → ineffective hematopoiesis → **cytopenias, dysmorphic blood cells and precursors**, variable risk of **leukemic transformation**

Comparison of FAB and WHO Classification Systems for MDS		
FAB Classification	**Marrow**	**WHO Classification Modifications**
Refractory anemia (RA)	<5% blasts <15% RS	RA: isolated erythroid dysplasia Refractory cytopenia with multilineage dysplasia (RCMD): dysplasia in ≥2 lines
Refractory anemia with RS (RARS)	<5% blasts ≥15% RS	RARS: RA with ≥15% RS RCMD with RS: RCMD with ≥15% RS
Refractory anemia with excess of blasts (RAEB)	5-20% blasts	RAEB-1: 5-9% blasts in BM RAEB-2: 10-19% blasts in BM
RAEB in transformation (RAEB-T)	21-30% blasts	Reclassified: AML w/ multilineage dysplasia
Chronic myelomonocytic leukemia (CMML)	>1000/µl peripheral monocytes	MDS/MPD: new category for CMML, atypical CML, juvenile CML
RS = ringed sideroblasts; (*J Clin Oncol* 1999;17:3835)		5q- syndrome: isolated del(5q)

- Epidemiology: <100 cases/10^6/yr; median age ~ 65 years
- Mechanisms/etiologies: **idiopathic** or 2° to chemotherapy with **alkylating agents, topoisomerase inhibitors**; ↑ risk with radiation, benzene
- Clinical manifestations: **anemia** (85%), neutropenia (50%), thrombocytopenia (25%)
- Diagnosis: dysplasia (usually multilineage) in peripheral smear (ovalomacrocytes, **pseudo-Pelger-Huët anomaly**, Auer rods) and bone marrow (blasts ± RS)
- Treatment: intensity based on risk category (see below), age, and performance status (PS)
  - Any risk, poor PS → **supportive care** = transfusions, **hematopoietic growth factors**
  - Low/intermed. risk → biologic response modifier (e.g., thalidomide), low-intensity chemo
  - Intermediate/high risk → combination **chemotherapy** or **allogeneic HSCT** if age <60
  - Hypoplastic MDS → **immunosuppressive regimen** (CsA, ATG, prednisone)
- Prognosis: IPSS (see below) correlates with **survival** and **progression to AML**

International Prognostic Scoring System (IPSS)					
	Score				
	0	0.5	1.0	1.5	2.0
Blasts (%)	<5	5-10	–	11-20	21-30
Karyotype	Good	Int.	Poor	–	–
Cytopenias	0 or 1	2 or 3	–	–	–

Risk group	Total score	Median survival
Low	0	5.7 yrs
Int-1	0.5-1	3.5 yrs
Int-2	1.5-2.0	1.2 yrs
High	≥2.5	0.4 yrs

(*Blood* 1997;89:2079)

Paroxysmal nocturnal hemoglobinuria (PNH)

- Pathophysiology: *acquired* clonal stem cell disorder = inactivating somatic mutation of *PIG-A* gene → ↑ **RBC sensitivity to complement** → complement activation indirectly stimulates platelet aggregation and *hypercoagulability*
- Clinical manifestations: intravascular **hemolytic anemia, venous thrombosis** (intraabdominal, cerebral), **deficient hematopoiesis** (cytopenias); associated with aplastic anemia, MDS and evolution into AML
- Diagnosis: **flow cytometry** has largely replaced Ham's or sucrose hemolysis tests
- Treatment: supportive care; allogeneic HSCT for hypoplasia or severe thrombosis eculizumab (Ab that inactivates terminal complement) ↓ hemolysis (*NEJM* 2004;350:552)

Myelophthisic anemia (see "Agnogenic Myeloid Metaplasia with Myelofibrosis")

- Infiltration of bone marrow
- Etiologies: agnogenic myeloid metaplasia with myelofibrosis, tumors, granulomas

HEMOLYTIC ANEMIAS

Causes of Hemolytic Anemia by Mechanism			
Location	**Mechanism**	**Examples**	**Mode**
Intrinsic	Enzyme defects	G6PD deficiency	**Hereditary**
	Hemoglobinopathies	Sickle cell anemia	
	Membrane abnormalities	Hereditary spherocytosis	
		PNH	**Acquired**
Extrinsic	Immune-mediated	Autoimmune; drug-induced	
	Traumatic hemolysis	MAHA; prostheses	
	Infections	Malaria, babesiosis	
	Entrapment	Hypersplenism	

(*Lancet* 2000;355:1169 & 1260)

Diagnostic evaluation

- ↑ reticulocyte count (RI >2%), ↑ LDH, ↑ indirect bilirubin, ↓ haptoglobin
- Autoimmune hemolysis: Coombs' test = direct antiglobulin test (DAT) → ⊕ if agglutination occurs when antisera against immunoglobulins or C3 are applied to patient RBCs
- Intravascular: ↑↑ LDH, ↓↓ haptoglobin; hemoglobinemia, hemoglobinuria, hemosiderinuria
- Extravascular: splenomegaly
- Family h/o anemia, personal or family h/o cholelithiasis

Glucose-6-phosphate dehydrogenase (G6PD) deficiency (*NEJM* 1991;324:169)

- X-linked defect of metabolism causing ↑ susceptibility to oxidative damage
- Most common in males of African or Mediterranean descent
- Hemolysis precipitated by **drugs** (sulfa, antimalarials), **infection**, or **foods** (fava beans)
- Diagnosis: smear may show RBC **Heinz bodies** (oxidized Hb) that result in **bite cells** once removed by spleen; ↓ G6PD levels (*may be normal after acute hemolysis* as older RBCs have already lysed and young RBCs may still have near normal levels)

Sickle cell anemia (*NEJM* 1999;340:1021)

- Recessive β-globin mutation results in a structurally abnormal hemoglobin (HbS) ~8% of African-Americans are heterozygotes and ~1 in 400 are homozygotes for HbS
- Deoxygenated HbS sickles and polymerizes → ↓ RBC deformability → **hemolysis** and **microvascular occlusion**
- **Anemia**: chronic hemolysis ± acute aplastic (parvo. B19) or splenic sequestration crises
- **Vaso-occlusion and infarction**: painful crises, acute chest syndrome, CVA, splenic sequestration, hand-foot syndrome, renal papillary necrosis, aseptic necrosis, priapism
- **Infection**: splenic infarction → overwhelming infection by **encapsulated organisms**; infarcted bone → **osteomyelitis** (*Salmonella, Staph. aureus*)
- Diagnosis: sickle-shaped RBCs and Howell-Jolly bodies on smear; Hb electrophoresis

- Treatment: **hydroxyurea** causes ↑ HbF → ↓ painful crises, acute chest episodes (*NEJM* 1995;332:1317) and may ↓ mortality (*JAMA* 2003;289:1645); allogeneic HSCT may have a role in young patients with severe disease (*Blood* 2000;95:1918)
- Supportive care: folic acid qd; pneumococcal & *H. flu* vaccination; penicillin prophylaxis; crises treated with **hydration**, supplemental **oxygen**, and **analgesia**; simple or exchange transfusions in some cases

Hereditary spherocytosis (HS)
- Molecular defect in one of the cytoskeletal proteins of RBC membrane → membrane loss mutations in ankyrin, α- and β- spectrin, band 3, and pallidin have been identified
- Most common in Northern European populations
- Anemia, jaundice, splenomegaly, pigmented gallstones
- Diagnosis: spherocytes on smear, ⊕ osmotic fragility test
- Treatment: splenectomy

Paroxysmal nocturnal hemoglobinuria (PNH) (see above)

Autoimmune hemolytic anemia (AIHA)
- Acquired, antibody-mediated RBC destruction
- **Warm AIHA**: **IgG** Abs opsonize RBCs *at room temp* → removal by spleen
  Etiologies: idiopathic, lymphoproliferative disorders (CLL), autoimmune diseases (SLE), drugs (see below)
- **Cold AIHA**: **IgM** Ab bind to RBCs *at temp <37°C* → **complement fixation** → intravascular hemolysis and acrocyanosis upon exposure to cold
  Etiologies: idiopathic, lymphoproliferative disorders (monoclonal), ***Mycoplasma pneumoniae*** infection and infectious mononucleosis (polyclonal)
- Diagnosis: spherocytes on smear, ⊕ **Coombs'**; ✓ cold agglutinin titer
- Treatment: treat underlying disease; corticosteroids ± splenectomy for warm AIHA; cold avoidance for cold AIHA, with ? benefit from rituximab

Drug-induced hemolytic anemia
- Acquired, antibody-mediated, RBC destruction *precipitated by a medication*
  Hapten-induced: drug binds to RBC membrane protein and Ab binds to drug-protein complex; association can be stable (e.g., **penicillin**) or unstable (e.g., **quinidine**)
  Alteration of RBC membrane protein to make it antigenic (e.g., **methyldopa**)
- Diagnosis: ± Coombs'

Microangiopathic hemolytic anemia (MAHA)
- Intra-arteriolar fibrin which damages RBCs → acquired intravascular hemolysis
- Etiologies: **disseminated intravascular coagulation** (DIC), **hemolytic-uremic syndrome** (HUS), **thrombotic thrombocytopenic purpura** (TTP), malignancy, malignant hypertension, eclampsia, HELLP, some prosthetic cardiac valves, infected vascular prostheses
- Diagnosis: **schistocytes** ± thrombocytopenia ± abnormalities associated with specific disorders, i.e., DIC or HUS/TTP (see "Thrombocytopenia" and "Disorders of Coagulation")
- Treatment: treat underlying abnormality

Hypersplenism
- Splenomegaly → stasis and trapping in the spleen → macrophagic attack and remodeling of RBC surface → spherocytosis → hemolysis

Causes of Splenomegaly	
Etiology	**Comments**
Reticuloendothelial system hyperplasia	Hemolytic anemia, sickle cell disease, **thalassemia major**
Immune hyperplasia	Infection (HIV, EBV, CMV, TB, **malaria, kala-azar, *Mycobacterium avium* complex**), autoimmune disorders (SLE, RA with Felty's syndrome), sarcoidosis, serum sickness
Congestion	Cirrhosis, CHF, portal/splenic vein thrombosis, **schistosomiasis**
Infiltration (nonmalignant)	Lysosomal storage disorders (**Gaucher's,** Niemann-Pick), glycogen storage diseases, histiocytosis X, splenic cysts
Neoplasm	**MPD** (**CML, AMM/MF, PV,** ET), **leukemia/lymphoma (hairy cell leukemia, CLL)**, multiple myeloma, amyloid

(**boldface** = causes of massive splenomegaly)

• DISORDERS OF HEMOSTASIS •

Clinical Characteristics of Bleeding Disorders		
Feature	**Platelet/Vascular Defect**	**Coagulation Defect**
Site	Skin, mucous membranes	Deep in soft tissues (muscles, joints)
Lesions	Petechiae, ecchymoses	Hemarthroses, hematomas
Bleeding	After minor cuts: yes After surgery: immediate, mild	After minor cuts: unusual After surgery: delayed, severe

Ddx of purpura

- Definition: *non-blanching* purple/red lesions due to extravasation of RBCs into dermis
  key subdivision is *palpable* vs. *non-palpable*
- **Non-palpable** (macular; ≤3 mm in diameter = petechiae; >3 mm = ecchymoses)
  platelet disorder: thrombocytopenia, ↓ platelet function
  thromboemboli: DIC, TTP, cholesterol or fat emboli
  vascular fragility: amyloidosis, Ehlers-Danlos, scurvy
  trauma
- **Palpable** (papular)
  vasculitis: leukocytoclastic, HSP, PAN
  infectious emboli: meningococcemia, RMSF

Fig. 5-3. Approach to abnormal hemostasis

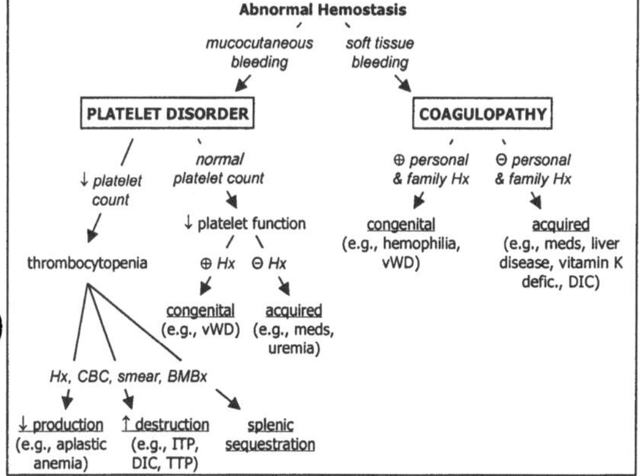

• PLATELET DISORDERS •

THROMBOCYTOPENIA

Definition
- Platelet count <150,000/µl

Thrombocytopenia and Risk of Bleeding	
Platelet count (cells/µl)	**Risk**
>100,000	No ↑ risk
50,000-100,000	Risk with major trauma; can proceed with general surgery
20,000-50,000	Risk with minor trauma or surgery
<20,000	Risk of *spontaneous* bleeding (less so with ITP)
<10,000	Risk of severe, life-threatening bleeding

Etiologies
- ↓ **production**
  hypocellular bone marrow: aplastic anemia (see "Aplastic anemia"), drugs (thiazides and alcohol can selectively suppress megakaryocytes)
  cellular bone marrow: MDS, leukemia, severe megaloblastic anemia
  marrow replacement: myelofibrosis, hematological and solid malignancies, granulomas
- ↑ **destruction**
  immune-mediated
  Primary (idiopathic): immune thrombocytopenic purpura (**ITP**, see below)
  Secondary: infections (HIV, herpes viruses, HCV), collagen vascular diseases (**SLE**), antiphospholipid syndrome, lymphoproliferative disorders (**CLL**, lymphoma), drugs (*many*, including **heparin**, quinidine, sulfa drugs), alloimmune (post-transfusion)
  non-immune-mediated: **MAHA** (DIC, HUS, TTP), vasculitis, preeclampsia and HELLP syndrome, cardiopulmonary bypass, IABP, cavernous hemangioma
- **Abnormal distribution or pooling**: splenic sequestration, dilutional, hypothermia

Diagnostic evaluation
- History and exam: especially medications, infections, underlying conditions, splenomegaly
- **CBC with differential**: isolated thrombocytopenia *vs.* multilineage involvement
- **Peripheral smear**
  ↑ destruction → look for large platelets, **schistocytes**
  ↓ production → rarely limited to platelets → look for **blasts**, hypersegmented PMNs, leukoerythroblastic Δs; rule out **pseudothrombocytopenia** due to platelet clumping

Fig. 5-4. Approach to thrombocytopenia

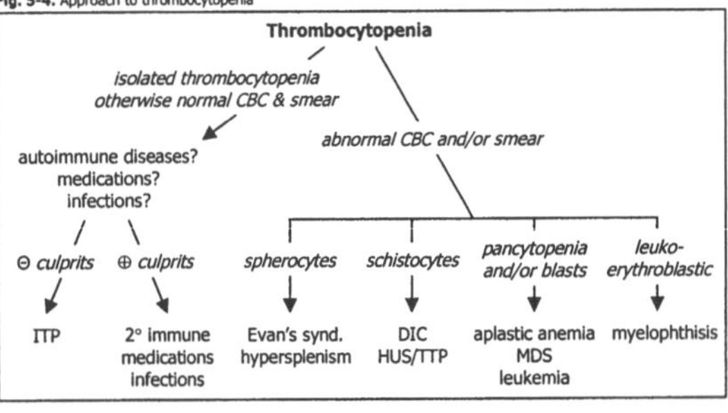

- Additional laboratory evaluations as indicated
  if anemia: ✓ reticulocyte count, LDH, haptoglobin, bilirubin to detect hemolysis
  if hemolytic anemia: ✓ PT, PTT, fibrinogen, D-dimer, Coombs', ANA
  BM bx for unexplained thrombocytopenia, especially if associated with **splenomegaly**

Immune thrombocytopenic purpura (ITP)

- Definition: ITP refers to *primary* immune platelet destruction; *a diagnosis of exclusion*
- Clinical manifestations: insidious onset of mucocutaneous bleeding; female:male = 3:1
- Diagnosis: *rule out other etiologies*
  CBC (usually isolated ↓ platelets; 10% have ITP + AIHA = Evan's syndrome) and peripheral smear (large platelets)
  BM bx: ↑ megakaryocytes; perform in adults >60 years to rule-out myelodysplasia
  consider ANA, viral serologies (e.g., HIV, EBV, hepatitis)
  antiplatelet antibody tests are not useful
- Treatment: treatment for active bleeding or consider if platelet count <20,000/µl (? higher threshold if coexisting bleeding risks)

Treatment of ITP in Adults		
Treatment	**Mechanism**	**Indication**
Prednisone 1-1.5 mg/kg/d PO, taper over wks	↓ Fc receptor on Mϕ ↓ anti-plt Ab production	1st-line Rx. Dexamethasone (40 mg PO x 4 d) may be an alternative (*NEJM* 2003;349:831).
Anti-Rh(D) Ig 75 µg/kg/d IV	Ab-coated RBCs overwhelm Mϕ Fc receptors	1st-line or for relapse; for Rh(D) ⊕ Pts only
Platelet transfusion	Minimal effect w/o IVIg or anti-Rh(D)	Bleeding
Methylprednisolone 1 g/d IV x 3 d	Same as prednisone	Bleeding
IVIg 1 g/kg/d IV x 2-3 d	Blocks Fc receptors on Mϕ ↓ anti-plt Ab production	Bleeding Platelets <5,000 despite steroids Relapse after steroids
Aminocaproic acid	Inhibits plasmin activation	Bleeding
Rituximab	Ab against B-cell CD20	Preliminary data encouraging
Splenectomy	↓ platelet clearance	Relapse after medical therapy
Danazol	↓ platelet clearance	Chronic refractory ITP
Vincristine	↓ platelet clearance	Chronic refractory ITP
Azathioprine **Cyclophosphamide**	Immunosuppressants ↓ anti-plt Ab production	Chronic refractory ITP
Autologous HSCT	Reconstitution after high dose immunosuppression	Chronic refractory ITP (investigational)

(*NEJM* 2002;346:995)

- Prognosis
  50-75% respond to steroids, but <20% have sustained remission after taper
  ~65% have long-term remission with splenectomy; response to IVIg predicts response to splenectomy (*NEJM* 1997;336:1494)

Heparin-induced thrombocytopenia (HIT)

Overview of Heparin-Induced Thrombocytopenia		
Feature	**Type I**	**Type II**
Mechanism	Direct effect of heparin	Immune (Ab)-mediated
Incidence	10-20%	1-3%
Onset	After 1 to 4 days of heparin therapy	After 5 to 10 days of heparin therapy Can occur earlier with h/o prior exposure within the last 120 days Can occur after heparin discontinuation
Platelet nadir	>100,000/µl	<50,000/µl, ↓ >50%
Clinical sequelae	None	Thrombotic events in ~20% Rare hemorrhagic complications
Management	Can continue with heparin and observe	**Discontinue heparin** Alternative anticoagulation

(*JACC* 1998;31:1449)

- Pathophysiology (type II): Ab binds heparin-PF4 → immune complex binds to platelets → **platelet activation**, further PF4 release → platelet aggregates removed from circulation → **thrombocytopenia**; procoagulants released by platelets and tissue factor released by endothelial cells damaged by HIT Abs → **prothrombotic state.**

- Diagnosis: need to meet clinical and pathologic criteria (*Annu Rev Med* 1999;50:129)
  Clinical: thrombocytopenia (plts <150,000 *or* ↓ 50% from baseline); or **venous** (DVT, PE) or **arterial** (limb ischemia, CVA, MI) thrombosis; or heparin-induced skin lesions
  Pathologic: ⊕ HIT Ab using a functional platelet aggregation assay (>90% specific) or ELISA using PF4-heparin as the substrate (~90% sensitive)
- Treatment of Type II (*Blood* 2003;101:31; *Archives* 2004;164:361)
  discontinue heparin *(including flushes, LMWH prophylaxis)*
  ⊕ thrombosis: alternative anticoagulation (lepirudin or argatroban), overlap w/ warfarin; treat for ≥3 mos
  ⊖ thrombosis: alternative anticoagulation until platelet count normal; no consensus on duration of subsequent anticoagulation

Hemolytic-uremic syndrome (HUS) & Thrombotic thrombocytopenic purpura (TTP)

- Definition: vascular occlusive disorders w/ systemic (TTP) or intrarenal (HUS) aggregation of plt → thrombocytopenia & mechanical injury to RBCs (MAHA) (*NEJM* 2002;347:589)
  HUS triad = thrombocytopenia + MAHA + renal failure
  TTP pentad = thrombocytopenia + MAHA ± Δ MS ± renal failure ± fever
- Pathophysiology: mechanism in most TTP cases is distinct from HUS (*NEJM* 1998;339:1578)
  TTP: ↓ ADAMTS13 protease activity → persistence of large multimers of vWF on endothelial surface → adhesion and aggregation of passing platelets → thrombosis
  HUS: Shiga toxin binds & activates renal endothelial cells & platelets → intrarenal thrombi
- Clinical manifestations and associations
  HUS: usually in children; prodrome of bloody diarrhea due to enterohemorrhagic *E. coli*
  TTP: usually in adults; **idiopathic, drugs** (CsA, gemcitabine, mitomycin C, ticlopidine/clopidogrel), HIV, pregnancy, HSCT, autoimmune disease, familial
- Diagnosis: unexplained thrombocytopenia + MAHA → *sufficient for dx*
  ⊕ **schistocytes**, ⊖ Coombs', normal PT/PTT & fibrinogen, ⊖ D-dimer
  ↑↑ LDH (tissue ischemia + hemolysis), ↑ indirect bili., ↓↓ haptoglobin, ↑ Cr (esp. in HUS)
  Skin biopsy: arterioles filled with platelet hyaline thrombi
  Ddx: DIC, vasculitis, malignant hypertension, preeclampsia/HELLP syndrome
- Treatment: **plasma exchange** in all adults with suspected TTP-HUS (*NEJM* 1991;325;393) ± glucocorticoids; *platelet transfusions are contraindicated* → ↑ microvascular thrombosis

Disseminated intravascular coagulation (DIC): see "Disorders of Coagulation"

Disorders of Platelet Function

Mechanisms and Etiologies of Platelet Function Abnormalities		
Function	**Inherited**	**Acquired**
Adhesion	Bernard-Soulier; vWD	Uremia; acquired vWD
Aggregation	Afibrinogenemia Glanzmann's thrombasthenia	Ticlopidine, clopidogrel, GP IIb/IIIa Dysproteinemias (myeloma)
Granule release	Chediak-Higashi syndrome Hermansky-Pudlak syndrome	Drugs (ASA, NSAIDs); liver disease; MPD; cardiopulmonary bypass

Tests of platelet function

- Bleeding time: global screen of platelet function; *not reliable and rarely used*
- Platelet aggregation tests: measure aggregation in response to agonists (e.g., ADP)

von Willebrand's disease (vWD)

- Most common inherited bleeding disorder.
- von Willebrand's factor (vWF) function = *platelet glue* + *plasma carrier of factor VIII*
- Classification of inherited vWD
  Type 1 (autosomal dominant; 70-80% of cases): partial quantitative deficiency in vWF
  Type 2 (autosomal dominant; 20-30% of cases): qualitative deficiency of vWF
  Type 3 (autosomal recessive; rare): near complete deficiency of vWF
- Acquired vWD: associated with many disorders (malignancy, autoimmune, hypothyroidism, drugs) and caused by different mechanisms (anti-vWF Abs, ↑ clearance, ↓ synthesis)
- Diagnosis: ↓ **vWF:Ag**, ↓ **vWF activity** (measured by ristocetin cofactor assay), ↓ **factor VIII**, ± ↑ PTT, ± ↓ platelets; confirm with **vWF multimer analysis**
- Treatment
  Desmopressin: ↑ release of vWF from endothelial cells; variable efficacy depending on disease type → need to ✓ response before use with subsequent bleeding or procedures
  vWF replacement: cryoprecipitate; factor VIII concentrates rich in vWF; recombinant vWF

• COAGULOPATHIES •

Screening Test Abnormalities in Inherited and Acquired Coagulopathies			
PT	PTT	Inherited	Acquired
↑	↔	Factor VII deficiency	Warfarin; vitamin K deficiency; liver disease; inhibitor of factor VII
↔	↑	Hemophilias vWD	Heparin; factor inhibitors; antiphospholipid Ab
↑	↑	Deficiency of prothrombin, fibrinogen, factors V or X; combined factor deficiencies	Heparin + warfarin; DIC; liver disease; inhibitor of prothrombin, fibrinogen, factors V or X

Further coagulation tests
- Mixing study: useful if ↑ PT or PTT; mix Pt's plasma 1:1 with normal plasma and retest
  PT/PTT normalizes → factor **deficiency**; PT/PTT remains elevated → factor **inhibitor**
- Coagulation factor levels: useful if mixing study suggests factor deficiency
  DIC → all factors consumed; ∴ ↓ factor V and VIII
  liver disease → ↓ all factors *except* VIII; ∴ ↓ factor V, normal factor VIII
  vitamin K deficiency → ↓ factors II, VII, IX, X (and protein C, S); ∴ normal V and VIII
- **DIC screen**: fibrinogen (consumed), fibrin degradation products (FDPs, ⊕ due to intense fibrinolysis), D-dimer (more specific FDP test that detects degradation of X-linked fibrin)

Hemophilias (*NEJM* 1994;330:38)
- Definition: X-linked **factor VIII** (hemophilia A) or **factor IX** (hemophilia B) **deficiency**
- Classification: mild (5-25% normal factor activity), moderate (1-5%), or severe (<1%)
- Diagnosis: ↑ PTT (normalizes with mixing study), normal PT and vWF, ↓ factor VIII or IX
- Treatment: purified or recombinant factor VIII or IX concentrate, desmopressin (for mild disease), ε-aminocaproic acid; recombinant factor VIIa for factor inhibitors (see below)

Coagulation factor inhibitors
- Etiologies: hemophilia (treated with factor replacement); postpartum, lymphoproliferative disorders and other malignancies, autoimmune diseases; most commonly anti-factor VIII
- Diagnosis: ↑ PTT (does *not* normalize with mixing study); Bethesda assay quantitates titer
- Treatment: high titer → **recombinant factor VIIa**, porcine factor concentrates, activated prothrombin complex; others → high purity human factor (massive doses to overcome inhibitor), plasmapheresis, immune tolerance induction

Disseminated intravascular coagulation (DIC)
- Etiologies: trauma, shock, infection, malignancy, obstetric complications
- Pathogenesis: *massive* activation of coagulation that overwhelms control mechanisms
  thrombosis in microvasculature → ischemia + microangiopathic hemolytic anemia
  acute consumption of coagulation factors and platelets → **bleeding**
  chronic DIC → able to replete factors and platelets → **thrombosis**
- Diagnosis: ↑ PT, ± ↑ PTT, **↓ fibrinogen**, **⊕ FDP/D-dimer**, ↓ platelets, ⊕ schistocytes, ↑ LDH, ↓ haptoglobin; *chronic* DIC: ⊕ FDP/D-dimer, variable platelets, other labs normal
- Treatment: treat underlying process; support with **FFP**, **cryoprecipitate** (maintain fibrinogen >100 mg/dl), and **platelets**; activated protein C in severe sepsis

Vitamin K deficiency
- Etiologies: malnutrition, ↓ absorption (**antibiotic**-suppression of vitamin K-producing intestinal flora or malabsorption), liver disease (↓ stores), **warfarin**
- Diagnosis: **↑ PT**, ± **↑ PTT**, ↓ factors II, VII, IX, X
- Treatment *(in addition to holding warfarin)*
  INR >5.0, but no bleeding: **vitamin K** 1-5 mg PO (superior to SC, Annals *2002*;137:251)
  Bleeding: **vitamin K** 10 mg IV **+ FFP** 2-4 units IV q 6-8 hrs

Heparin
- Diagnosis: ↑ **PTT**, ± ↑ PT
- Treatment: cessation of heparin → normalization within ~4-6 hours
  serious bleeding → **protamine sulfate** IV at 1 mg/100 U heparin (not to exceed 50 mg)
  (for infusions, dose protamine to reverse 2x the amount of heparin given per hour)
- LMWH reversal by protamine is **incomplete**; direct thrombin inhibitors have **no antidote**

Thrombolytics
- Diagnosis: ↓ **fibrinogen**, **⊕ FDP/D-dimer**, ± ↑ PTT
- Treatment for serious bleeding: **cryoprecipitate**, **FFP**, ± aminocaproic acid

• HYPERCOAGULABLE STATES •

Suspect in patients with venous or arterial thrombosis at young age or unusual locations, recurrent thromboses or pregnancy loss, ⊕ family history

Inherited Hypercoagulable States			
Risk factor	**Prevalence** (Caucasians)	**VTE risk**	**Comments**
Factor V Leiden	4%	7×	Activated protein C (APC) resist.
Prothrombin mutation	2%	2.8×	G20210A → ↑ prothrombin level
Hyperhomocysteinemia	5-10%	2.5×	Inherited or acquired
Protein C or S deficiency	0.3%	10×	Warfarin-induced skin necrosis risk
Antithrombin III deficiency	0.04%	25×	May be relatively heparin-resistant

	Vascular Beds Affected by Inherited and Acquired Hypercoagulable States	
	Venous	**Venous and arterial**
Inherited	Factor V Leiden Prothrombin mutation ↓ protein C, S, or AT III	? factor V Leiden + smoking Hyperhomocysteinemia (inherited or acquired) Dysfibrinogenemia
Acquired	Stasis: immobilization, surgery, CHF Malignancy Hormonal: OCPs, HRT, tamoxifen, pregnancy Nephrotic syndrome	Platelet defects: myeloproliferative disorders, HIT, PNH Hyperviscosity: polycythemia vera, Waldenström's macroglobulinemia, sickle cell, acute leukemia Vessel wall defects: vasculitis, trauma, foreign bodies Others: antiphospholipid syndrome, IBD

Diagnostic evaluation

- APC resistance screen; prothrombin PCR test; functional assays for protein C and S, AT III; homocysteine level; anticardiolipin and lupus anticoagulant antibody assays
- Proteins C and S, and AT III can be affected by acute thrombosis and anticoagulation; ∴ best assessed ≥2 weeks after completing anticoagulation course
- Age-appropriate malignancy screening (⊕ in 12% with "idiopathic" DVT; *Annals* 1996;125:785)

Treatment

- Thrombosis with inherited risk factor: see "Venous Thromboembolism"
- Asymptomatic patient with inherited risk factor: consider prophylactic anticoagulation when an acquired risk factor appears

Antiphospholipid syndrome (APS) (*NEJM* 2002;346:752)

- Definition: ≥1 clinical *and* ≥1 laboratory criteria
- Clinical: thrombosis (any) or complication of pregnancy (≥3 spontaneous abortions before 10 wks or ≥1 fetal loss after 10 wks or premature birth before 34 wks)
- Laboratory: ⊕ moderate-high titer anticardiolipin (ACL) or lupus anticoagulant (LA) antibodies on ≥2 occasions at least 6 wks apart
- Clinical manifestations: **DVT/PE/CVA**, **recurrent fetal loss**, **thrombocytopenia**, hemolytic anemia, livedo reticularis; "**catastrophic APS**" = widespread acute thrombotic microangiopathy with visceral damage → high mortality
- Etiologies: primary (idiopathic) or secondary due to **autoimmune syndromes** (e.g., SLE), **malignancy**, **infections**, drugs reactions
- Diagnosis: **antiphospholipid antibodies** are classified by method of detection
  ACL: Ab against cardiolipin, a mitochondrial phospholipid; IgG more specific than IgM
  LA: Ab that prolongs phospholipid-dependent coagulation reactions; ∴ ↑ **PTT** that does *not* correct with mixing study but does correct with excess phospholipids or platelets; standard PT is not affected because the reaction contains much more phospholipid
  false ⊕ VDRL: non-treponemal test for syphilis in which cardiolipin is part of Ag complex
- Treatment: lifelong warfarin after a thrombotic event; goal INR ≥3.0 (*NEJM* 1995;332:993) or 2.0-3.0 (*NEJM* 2003;349:1133); consider ASA prophylaxis for high-risk asx patient (e.g., SLE)

• DISORDERS OF LEUKOCYTES •

Neutrophilia (>7,500-10,000/μl)	
Etiology	**Comments**
Infection	Usually bacterial; ± toxic granulations, Döhle bodies
Inflammation	Burn, tissue necrosis, MI, PE, collagen vascular disease
Drugs and toxins	Corticosteroids, β-agonists, lithium, G-CSF; cigarette smoking
Stress	Release of endogenous glucocorticoids and catecholamines
Marrow stimulation	Hemolytic anemia, immune thrombocytopenia
Asplenia	Surgical, acquired (sickle cell), congenital (dextrocardia)
Neoplasm	Can be 1° (MPD) or paraneoplastic (e.g., carcinomas of lung, GI)
Leukemoid reaction	>50,000/μl + left shift, not due to leukemia; unlike CML, ↑ LAP

Lymphocytosis (>4000-5,000/μl)	
Etiology	**Comments**
Infection	Usually viral; "atypical lymphocytes" with mononucleosis syndromes Other: pertussis, toxoplasmosis
Hypersensitivity	Drug-induced, serum sickness
Stress	Cardiac emergencies, trauma, status epilepticus, post-splenectomy
Autoimmune	Rheumatoid arthritis (large granular lymphocytes), malignant thymoma
Neoplasm	Leukemia (ALL, CLL, others), lymphoma

Monocytosis (>500/μl)	
Etiology	**Comments**
Infection	Usually TB, SBE, *Listeria*, *Brucella*, rickettsiae, fungi, parasites
Inflammation	IBD, sarcoidosis, collagen vascular diseases
Neoplasm	Hodgkin's disease, leukemias, MPD, carcinomas

Eosinophilia (>500/μl)	
Etiology	**Comments**
Infection	Usually parasitic (helminths)
Allergic	Drugs; asthma, hay fever, eczema; ABPA
Collagen vascular disease	RA, Churg-Strauss syndrome, eosinophilic fasciitis, PAN
Endocrine	Adrenal insufficiency
Neoplasm	Hodgkin's disease, CML, mycosis fungoides, carcinomas
Atheroembolic disease	Cholesterol emboli syndrome
Hypereosinophilic syndrome	Multiorgan system involvement including heart and CNS

Basophilia (>150/μl)	
Etiology	**Comments**
Neoplasm	MPD, Hodgkin's disease
Alteration in BM or reticuloendothelial compartment	Hemolytic anemia, splenectomy
Inflammation or allergy	IBD, chronic airway inflammation

Lymphadenopathy	
Etiology	**Comments**
Viral	HIV, EBV, CMV, HSV, VZV, hepatitis, measles, rubella
Bacterial	Generalized (brucellosis, leptospirosis, TB, atypical mycobacteria, syphilis) Localized (streptococci, staphylococci, cat-scratch disease, tularemia)
Fungal and parasitic	Histoplasmosis, coccidioidomycosis, paracoccidioidomycosis Toxoplasmosis
Immunologic	Collagen vascular disease, drug hypersensitivity (phenytoin), serum sickness, histiocytosis X, Castleman's and Kawaski disease
Neoplasm	Lymphoma, leukemia, amyloidosis, metastatic carcinoma
Other	Sarcoidosis; lipid storage diseases
Factors that favor biopsy	Age (>40), size (>2 *vs.* <1 cm^2), location (supraclavicular is always abnormal), duration (>1 month). Consistency (hard *vs.* rubbery *vs.* soft) & tenderness are not reliable.

• TRANSFUSION THERAPY •

Blood Products	
Product	**Indications and comments**
Packed red blood cells (PRBCs)	Hb <7g/dl *or* higher threshold, (e.g., <10 g/dl) for active bleeding, coronary ischemia, cardiac/pulmonary comorbidities, advanced age (*NEJM* 1999;340:409 and 2001;345:1230). 1U PRBC → ↑ Hb by ~1g/dl
Platelets (plts)	Plts <10,000/µl *or* <20,000/µl with infection or ↑ bleeding risk *or* <50,000/µl with active bleeding or pre-procedure. *Contraindicated* in TTP/HUS, HELLP, HIT. Refractoriness caused by *alloimmunization* may require HLA-matched plts. 6U → ↑ plt count by ~30,000/µl
Fresh frozen plasma (FFP)	Contains all coagulation factors. For bleeding due to deficiency of multiple coagulation factors (e.g., DIC, TTP/HUS, liver disease, warfarin excess, dilution) *or* PT >17 sec pre-procedure.
Cryoprecipitate	Enriched for fibrinogen, vWF, VIII, and XIII. For bleeding in vWD, factor XIII deficiency or fibrinogen <100 mg/dl.
Irradiated	Prevents donor T-cell proliferation in recipient. For immunodeficient/immunosuppressed patients at risk for GVHD.
CMV-negative	CMV-seronegative pregnant women, transplant candidates/recipients, and SCID patients. All AIDS patients.
Leukoreduced	WBCs cause HLA alloimmunization and fever (cytokine release) and carry CMV. For chronically transfused patients, potential transplant recipients, h/o febrile nonhemolytic transfusion reaction, cases in which CMV-negative products are desired but unavailable.
Plasmapheresis and **cytapheresis**	Removes large molecular weight substances (e.g., cryoglobulinemia, Goodpasture's, Guillain-Barré, hyperviscosity syndrome, TTP) or cells (e.g., leukemia with hyperleukocytosis, symptomatic thrombocytosis, sickle cell syndromes), respectively, from plasma.
Intravenous immune globulin (IVIg)	Polyvalent IgG from >1,000 donors. For post-exposure prophylaxis (e.g., HAV), certain autoimmune disorders (e.g., ITP, Guillain-Barré), congenital or acquired hypogammaglobulinemia (e.g., CLL).

Transfusion Complications				
Noninfectious	**Risk (per unit)**		**Infectious**	**Risk (per unit)**
Febrile	1:100		CMV	common
Allergic	1:100		Hepatitis B	1:220,000
Delayed hemolytic	1:1000		Hepatitis C	1:1,600,000
Acute hemolytic	<1:250,000		HIV	1:1,800,000
Fatal hemolytic	<1:100,000		Bacteria (PRBCs)	1:500,000
TRALI	1:5000		Bacteria (platelets)	1:12,000

(*NEJM* 1999;340:438; *JAMA* 2003;289:959)

Transfusion reactions

- For all reactions (except minor allergic): **stop transfusion**; send remaining blood product and fresh blood sample to blood bank
- **Acute hemolytic**: fever, hypotension, flank pain, renal failure <24 hrs after transfusion
  Due to ABO incompatibility → preformed antibodies against donor RBCs
  Treatment: vigorous IVF, maintain UOP with diuretics, mannitol, or dopamine
- **Delayed hemolytic**: generally less severe than acute hemolytic; 5-7 d after transfusion
  Due to undetected alloantibodies against minor antigens → anamnestic response
  Treatment: usually no specific therapy required; dx is important for future transfusions
- **Febrile nonhemolytic**: fever and rigors 0-6 hrs after transfusion
  Due to antibodies against donor WBCs and cytokines released from cells in blood product
  Treatment: acetaminophen ± meperidine; rule out infection and hemolysis
- **Allergic**: urticaria; rarely, **anaphylaxis**: bronchospasm, laryngeal edema, hypotension
  Reaction to plasma proteins in the blood product; anaphylaxis is usually seen in IgA-deficient patients who have anti-IgA antibodies
  Treatment: urticaria → diphenhydramine; anaphylaxis → epinephrine ± glucocorticoids
- **Transfusion-related acute lung injury** (TRALI): noncardiogenic pulmonary edema
  Due to donor antibodies that bind recipient WBCs, which aggregate in the pulmonary vasculature and release mediators causing increased capillary permeability
  Treatment: see "ARDS"

• MYELOPROLIFERATIVE DISORDERS (MPD) •

Clonal expansion of multipotent hematopoietic stem cell → ↑ in ≥1 peripheral blood element

Polycythemia Vera (PV)

Definition
- ↑ in RBC mass ± ↑ granulocytes and platelets in the absence of physiologic stimulus

Etiologies of erythrocytosis
- *Relative* ↑ RBC (↓ plasma): dehydration; "stress" erythrocytosis (Geisböck's syndrome)
- *Absolute* ↑ RBC: 1° (PV, other MPD) or 2° due to **hypoxia**; **carboxyhemoglobinemia**; **inappropriate erythropoietin** (renal, hepatic, cerebellar tumors); Cushing's syndrome

Clinical manifestations
- Symptoms
  - **hyperviscosity** (erythrocytosis): headache, dizziness, tinnitus, blurred vision
  - **thrombosis** (hyperviscosity, thrombocytosis): TIA/CVA; Budd-Chiari; erythromelalgia = intense burning, pain and erythema of extremities due to microvascular thrombi
  - **bleeding** (abnormal platelet function): easy bruising, epistaxis, GI bleeding
  - ↑ histamine from basophils → **pruritus**, peptic ulcers; ↑ uric acid (cell turnover) → gout
- Signs: **plethora**, **splenomegaly**, hypertension, engorged retinal veins

Diagnostic evaluation
- ✓ Epo to rule out secondary causes of erythrocytosis; if epo ↓, PV likely
  if epo ↑, then ✓ S_aO_2 or P_aO_2, carboxyhemoglobin
- ± ↑ WBC, platelets, basophils; ↑ uric acid, leukocyte alkaline phosphatase, vitamin B_{12}
- Peripheral smear → no morphologic abnormalities; BM bx → hypercellular BM, usually with megakaryocytic hyperplasia; ↓ iron stores; absence of Philadelphia chromosome

Treatment
- **Phlebotomy** to moderate degree of Fe deficiency → Hct <45% (men) or <42% (women)
- **Low-dose ASA** in all patients (*NEJM* 2004;350:114)
- Add **hydroxyurea** if high risk of thrombosis (i.e., age ≥60, prior thrombosis)
- Anagrelide if symptomatic thrombocytosis (plt $>1.5 \times 10^6$/µl)
- Supportive: allopurinol (gout), H_2-blockers/antihistamines (pruritus)

Prognosis
- Median survival 9-12 yrs with transformation into acute leukemia in 2% of cases
- Post-PV myeloid metaplasia (spent phase) occurs in 15% of cases, usually after 10 yrs

Essential Thrombocytosis (ET)

Definition
- ↑ in platelets (>600,000/µl), ± ↑ RBC and granulocytes

Etiologies of thrombocytosis
- 1° = ET or other MPD; myelodysplastic syndromes (5q- syndrome)
- 2° = **reactive thrombocytosis**: inflammation (RA, IBD, vasculitis), infection, acute bleeding, iron deficiency, post-splenectomy, neoplasms (particularly Hodgkin's disease)
- Of patients w/ plt $>10^6$/µl, <1 in 6 will have ET

Clinical manifestations (see "Polycythemia Vera")
- Thrombosis with erythromelalgia, bleeding, pruritus; mild splenomegaly

Diagnostic evaluation
- Peripheral smear → large hypogranular platelets
- BM bx → megakaryocytic hyperplasia; absence of Philadelphia chromosome and lack of collagen fibrosis; normal iron stores

Treatment of ET			
Risk	**Features**	**Low-dose ASA**	**Cytoreduction**
Low	Age <60 *and* no h/o thrombosis *and* plt <1.5 x 10^6/µl *and* no CV risk factors	Consider for vasomotor symptoms	No
Int.	Neither low nor high risk	±	Consider if plt >1.5 x 10^6/µl
High	Age ≥60 *or* h/o thrombosis	⊕	**Anagrelide** or **hydroxyurea** (*NEJM* 1995;332:1132) Goal plt <400,000/µl

Prognosis
- Overall survival similar to control population with low rate of transformation into PV, AMM/MF or acute leukemia; ∴ low risk patients (see below) do not need treatment

Agnogenic Myeloid Metaplasia with Myelofibrosis (AMM/MF)

Definition
- Clonal myeloproliferation with reactive marrow fibrosis and extramedullary hematopoiesis

Etiologies of myelophthisis (marrow replacement)
- 1° = agnogenic myeloid metaplasia with myelofibrosis; post-PV/ET myeloid metaplasia
- 2° = hematologic (e.g., leukemia, MDS) or metastatic malignancies (e.g., breast, prostate)
  collagen vascular disorders (e.g., SLE)
  toxins (e.g., benzene, radiation)
  granulomas from infection (e.g., TB, fungal) or sarcoid
  deposition diseases (e.g., Gaucher's disease)

Clinical manifestations (*NEJM* 2000;342:1255)
- Ineffective erythropoiesis → anemia; extramedullary hematopoiesis → **massive splenomegaly** (abdominal pain, early satiety) ± hepatomegaly
- Tumor bulk and ↑ cell turnover → fatigue, weight loss, fever, sweats

Diagnostic evaluation
- Anemia with variable WBC and platelet counts
- Peripheral smear → **"leukoerythroblastic"** (**teardrop cells**, nucleated RBCs, immature WBCs); large abnormal platelets
- BM aspirate → **"dry" tap**; BM bx → **severe fibrosis**, replacement by reticulin & collagen

Treatment
- Allogeneic HSCT only potential cure → consider in young Pts with poor prognosis
- Supportive care: **transfusions**; inconsistent benefit from androgens or epo; splenectomy for blood counts refractory to transfusion or painful splenomegaly
- Hydroxyurea for significant leukocytosis or thrombocytosis

Complications and prognosis
- Median survival ~5 yrs; transformation into AML occurs at a rate of ~ 8%/yr
- Worse prognosis with Hb <10 g/dL or with either WBC >30,000/µL or WBC <4,000/µL

Chronic Myelogenous Leukemia

see "Leukemia"

• LEUKEMIA •

Acute Leukemia

Definition

- Clonal proliferation of hematopoietic precursor with ↓ ability to differentiate into mature elements → ↑ blasts in bone marrow and periphery → ↓ RBCs, platelets, and neutrophils
- Termed acute myelogenous (AML) or acute lymphocytic (ALL) leukemia based on whether malignant clone is of **myeloid** or **lymphoid** lineage, respectively

Epidemiology and risk factors

- AML: ~10,500 cases/yr; median age 65 yrs; >80% of adult acute leukemia cases
- ALL: ~3,600 cases/yr; median age 10 yrs; bimodal with 2nd peak in elderly
- Environmental: **radiation, chemotherapy** (alkylating agents and topoisomerase inhibitors), benzene, smoking
- Acquired hematopoietic diseases: MPD (especially CML), MDS, aplastic anemia, PNH
- Inherited: Down's & Klinefelter's, Fanconi's anemia, Bloom syndrome, ataxia telangiectasia

Clinical manifestations

- Cytopenias → **fatigue** (anemia), **infection** (neutropenia), **bleeding** (thrombocytopenia)
- More common in **AML:**
  - **leukostasis** (seen when WBC >100,000/μl): occluded microcirculation → local hypoxemia and hemorrhage → headache, blurred vision, TIA/CVA, dyspnea, hypoxia; look for *hyperviscosity retinopathy* (vascular engorgement, exudates, hemorrhage)
  - DIC (especially with M3 subtype)
  - leukemic infiltration of skin, gingiva (especially with monocytic subtypes M4 and M5)
  - chloroma: extramedullary tumor of leukemic cells, virtually any location
- More common in **ALL:**
  - bone pain, lymphadenopathy, hepatosplenomegaly (also seen in monocytic AML)
  - CNS involvement (~15%): cranial neuropathies, nausea and vomiting, headache
  - anterior mediastinal mass (especially in T-cell ALL)
  - tumor lysis syndrome (see "Oncologic Emergencies")

Diagnostic evaluation

- **Peripheral smear**: anemia, thrombocytopenia, variable WBC (50% present with ↑ WBC, 50% present with normal or ↓ WBC) + circulating **blasts** (seen in >95%)
- **Bone marrow**: hypercellular with ≥30% (FAB criteria) or ≥20% (WHO criteria) blasts morphology, cytochemistry, cytogenetics, flow cytometry, and molecular studies
- Electrolyte disarray: ↑ UA, ↑ LDH, ↑ K, ↑ PO_4, ↓ Ca from rapid cell turnover, tumor lysis
- Coagulation studies to r/o DIC: PT, PTT, fibrinogen, D-dimer
- Lumbar puncture for *all* ALL Pts (CNS is sanctuary site) and for AML Pts w/ CNS symptoms
- CXR; TTE if prior cardiac history or prior use of anthracyclines
- **HLA typing** of patient, siblings, and parents for potential allogeneic HSCT candidates

Acute Myelogenous Leukemia (AML)

Classification (*NEJM* 1999;341:1051)

- Features used to confirm myeloid lineage and subclassify AML to guide treatment:
  - morphology: ⊕ **granules**, ± **Auer rods** (eosinophilic needle-like inclusions)
  - cytochemistry: ⊕ **myeloperoxidase** (MPO) (or Sudan black) and/or **non-specific esterase** (NSE); FAB classification utilizes cytochemistry and morphology (see below)
  - immunophenotype: CD13 and CD33 are myeloid antigens; ⊕ CD41 associated with M7
  - cytogenetics: important for prognosis, e.g., t(15;17) associated with M3 subtype

FAB Classification of AML

Subtype	Freq.	Common name	MPO	NSE
M0	<5%	Minimally differentiated	–	–
M1	20%	Myeloblastic without maturation	±	–
M2	25%	Myeloblastic with maturation	⊕	–
M3	10%	Promyelocytic (APML)	⊕⊕	–
M4	20%	Myelomonocytic; M4Eo = eosinophilic variant	±	⊕
M5	20%	Monocytic	–	⊕
M6	5%	Erythroleukemia	±	–
M7	<5%	Megakaryoblastic	–	–

WHO Classification of AML	
Subtype	**Examples**
With recurrent genetic abnormalities	t(8;21); inv(16); t(15;17); 11q23 anomalies
With multilineage dysplasia	With or without antecedent MDS or MPD
Therapy-related	Alkylating agents or topoisomerase inhibitors
Not otherwise categorized	Other entities as defined in FAB system

Treatment

- **Induction chemotherapy**: "3+7" = idarubicin/daunorubicin × 3 d and cytarabine × 7 d
- ✓ for complete remission (CR) = normal peripheral counts & BM cellularity, <5% BM blasts
  CR ≠ cure; ∴ always f/u induction with **consolidation Rx**
- ⊕ CR → consolidation therapy based on risk stratification: chemotherapy *or* allogeneic *or* autologous HSCT (*NEJM* 1995;332:217, *Lancet* 1998;351:700, *NEJM* 1998;339:1649)
  allo HSCT indicated for younger patients with high-risk cytogenetics and matched donor
- ⊖ CR or relapse after CR → allogeneic or autologous HSCT or salvage chemotherapy
- M3 subtype = APML: biologically distinct; responds to **all-*trans*-retinoic acid (ATRA)**, which induces differentiation; daily PO ATRA added to induction chemotherapy improves outcome; both untreated and refractory M3 AML also respond to arsenic
- Supportive care: hydration + allopurinol for tumor lysis prophylaxis; electrolyte correction; transfusions ± erythropoietin and G-CSF; antibiotics for fever and neutropenia; hydroxyurea ± leukopheresis for leukostasis

Prognosis

- 60-80% achieve CR; up to 40-60% *cure* rates with chemo or HSCT (but <15% if age >60)
- Poor prognostic factors: **age >60**, unfavorable cytogenetics (e.g., monosomy or deletion of chromosome 5 or 7, complex karyotype), poor performance score, 2° to MDS/MPD
- APML is the most favorable subtype because of response to ATRA

ACUTE LYMPHOCYTIC LEUKEMIA (ALL)

Classification (*NEJM* 1998;339:605)

- Features used to exclude myeloid lineage and subclassify ALL to guide treatment:
  morphology: *no granules*
  cytochemistry: ⊕ terminal deoxynucleotidyl transferase (TdT) in 95% of ALL
  immunophenotype: based on markers of B and T cell maturation (see below)
  cytogenetics: t(9;22) = Philadelphia chromosome (Ph) in ~25% of adults w/ ALL
- FAB subtypes based on morphology (L1 = small, L2 = large, and L3 = undifferentiated cells) generally do not correlate with clinico-pathologic entities; ∴ not clinically useful
- Immunohistochemistry can distinguish 3 major entities, as recognized by the WHO/REAL classification of lymphoid malignancies (see "NHL")

Immunophenotype Classification of ALL				
Type	**Freq.** (adults)	**FAB subtype**	**WHO/REAL designations**	**Immunohistochemistry**
Pre-B cell	75%	L1, L2	Precursor B-cell ALL/lymphoma	⊕ TdT, ⊕ CD19; variable CD10, CD20
T-cell	20%	L1, L2	Precursor T-cell ALL/lymphoma	⊕ TdT, ⊕ acid phosphatase, ⊖ CD10, ⊕ T-cell Ag (e.g., CD7)
B-cell	5%	L3	Burkitt's lymphoma	⊖ TdT, ⊕ surface Ig

Treatment

- **Induction chemotherapy**: e.g., cyclophosphamide, daunorubicin, vincristine, prednisone (≈ CHOP), ± asparaginase
- **CNS prophylaxis**: intrathecal MTX ± either cranial irradiation *or* systemic MTX
- **Postremission therapy** options:
  consolidation/intensification chemotherapy followed by maintenance chemotherapy
  high-dose chemo w/ allo or auto HSCT; survival benefit in high-risk Pts w/ allo HSCT
- If relapse → chemotherapy *vs.* allogeneic or autologous HSCT
- Emerging therapies: imatinib for Ph ⊕ ALL; monoclonal Abs against lymphoid antigens

Prognosis

- CR achieved in >90% of children, 60-80% of adults
- Predictors of good outcome: younger age, WBC <30,000/µl, T-cell immunophenotype, absence of Ph chromosome or t(4;11), early attainment of CR
- Good prognostic factors → cure rate 50-70%; poor prognostic factors → cure rate 10-30%

Chronic Myelogenous Leukemia (CML)

Definition (*NEJM* 1999;340:1330)
- **Myeloproliferative disorder** with overproduction of myeloid cells that can differentiate
- **Philadelphia chromosome** (Ph) = t(9;22) → **Bcr-Abl** fusion → ↑ Abl kinase activity

Epidemiology and risk factors
- ~4,300 new cases/yr in U.S.; median age ~50 at presentation; 15% of adult leukemias
- ↑ risk with irradiation; no clear relation to cytotoxic drugs

Clinical manifestations
- Triphasic clinical course; 85% present in the chronic phase
- **Chronic phase** (~3-4 yrs): often asx but common features are fatigue, malaise, weight loss, night sweats, abdominal fullness (**splenomegaly**, 50%)
- **Accelerated phase**: refractory leukocytosis and worsening symptoms → fever, weight loss, progressive splenomegaly, bone pain, bleeding, infections, pruritus (basophilia)
- **Blastic phase** ≈ acute leukemia → severe constitutional symptoms, infection, bleeding, and **leukostasis** (see "Acute Leukemia")

Diagnostic evaluation
- **Peripheral smear**: **leukocytosis** (often >100,000/μl), left-shifted with *all stages of maturation* seen; anemia, thrombocytosis, basophilia; <5% blasts (chronic phase)
- **Bone marrow**: hypercellular, ↑ myeloid to erythroid ratio, <5% blasts (chronic phase)
- Accelerated phase: leukocytosis refractory to therapy; progressive BM myelofibrosis
- Blast phase: acute leukemia with ≥20-30% blasts in peripheral blood or BM and extramedullary leukemic infiltrates; 25% lymphoid, 75% myeloid or undifferentiated
- ↓ **leukocyte alkaline phosphatase (LAP)**
- Detection of the **Philadelphia chromosome** or the Bcr-Abl product is required for dx
  atypical CML (Ph-negative): ~5% with clinical features of CML lack Bcr-Abl and show poor response to therapy with ↓ survival; likely a distinct entity related to MDS

Treatment (*NEJM* 2003;349:1451)
- **Allogeneic HSCT** is the only known curative therapy and should be offered up front to good candidates with available donor who present in chronic phase.
- **Imatinib**, a selective inhibitor of the Bcr-Abl tyrosine kinase, is 1st-line medical therapy
  significantly higher response rates (68% complete cytogenetic response, and in those, 57% w/ 3 log ↓ Bcr-Abl transcripts) than prior standard of IFN + ara-C, but durability of response unknown (*NEJM* 2003;348:994 & 1423)
  active in chronic, accelerated and blastic phases
  imatinib resistance is associated with Bcr-Abl mutation or amplification
- Hydroxyurea ± leukopheresis for rapid ↓ of WBC count and palliation of symptoms
- Failure to respond to imatinib → allo HSCT if candidate *vs.* hydroxyurea *vs.* experimental
- Accelerated or blast phase → allo HSCT if chronic phase achieved with medical therapy

Prognosis
- Available statistics reflect management in the pre-imatinib era
- Median survival 4-6 yrs overall; <1 yr for accelerated phase; months for blastic phase
- 5-yr survival = 60-80% with allo HSCT in chronic phase
- Poor prognostic factors = ↑ age, ↑ platelet count, ↑ spleen size, and ↑ percentage of blasts

CHRONIC LYMPHOCYTIC LEUKEMIA (CLL)

Definition (*NEJM* 1995;333:1052)
- Malignant monoclonal accumulation of immunologically incompetent mature B-lymphocytes
- CLL and small lymphocytic lymphoma (SLL) are the same disease at different stages

Epidemiology and risk factors
- ~7,300 new cases/yr; median age at dx is 65 yrs; most common adult leukemia
- ↑ incidence in 1st-degree relatives; no known association with radiation, chemicals, or drugs

Clinical manifestations
- Symptoms: **often asymptomatic** and identified when CBC reveals lymphocytosis; 10-20% present with fatigue, malaise, night sweats, weight loss (i.e., lymphoma "B" symptoms)
- Signs: **lymphadenopathy** (80%) and **hepatosplenomegaly** (50%)
- **Autoimmune hemolytic anemia** (AIHA) or **thrombocytopenia** (ITP)
- Hypogammaglobulinemia ± neutropenia → ↑ susceptibility to **infections**
- Bone marrow failure
- Monoclonal gammopathy in ~5%
- Aggressive transformation: ~5% develop **Richter's syndrome** = transformation into high-grade lymphoma (usually DLBCL) and sudden clinical deterioration

Diagnostic evaluation (see "Lymphoma" for general approach)
- **Peripheral smear: lymphocytosis** (>5000/µl, mature-appearing small cells) **"smudge"** cells from damage by shear stress of making blood smear
- **Bone marrow**: normo- or hypercellular; infiltrated with small B-cell lymphocytes (≥30%)
- **Lymph nodes**: infiltrated with small lymphocytic or diffuse small cleaved cells = SLL
- **Flow cytometry**: extremely low levels of surface Ig (sIg); ⊕ ≥1 B-cell antigen; ⊕ CD5

Staging of CLL

Rai System		Median survival	Binet System	
Stage	**Description**		**Description**	**Stage**
0	Lymphocytosis *only*	>10 yrs	<3 node areas	A
I	⊕ lymphadenopathy	7 yrs	>3 node areas	B
II	⊕ hepatosplenomegaly			
III	⊕ anemia (not AIHA)	1-2 yrs	Anemia or thrombocytopenia	C
IV	⊕ thrombocytopenia (not ITP)			

Treatment (*NEJM* 2000;343:1799)
- Treatment is *palliative* → early stage disease can be followed without specific therapy
- Indications for anti-leukemia treatment: Rai stages III/IV, Binet stage C, disease-related symptoms, progressive disease, AIHA or ITP refractory to steroids, recurrent infections
- Initial treatment: equivalent overall survival with available single agents fludarabine (higher response rate) or chlorambucil (better tolerated) (*NEJM* 2000;343:1750) ± monoclonal Ab against CD20 (rituximab) or CD52 (alemtuzumab)
- Radiation for compression symptoms due to bulky lymphoid masses
- Splenectomy for marked splenomegaly and refractory cytopenias
- Role of autologous and allogeneic HSCT being studied
- Supportive care
  corticosteroids for AIHA or ITP
  IVIg for recurrent major infections

• LYMPHOMA •

Definition
- Malignant disorder of lymphoid cells that reside predominantly in lymphoid tissues
- **Hodgkin's disease** (HD) is distinguished from **non-Hodgkin's lymphoma** (NHL) by the presence of **Reed-Sternberg** (RS) **cells**

Clinical manifestations
- **Lymphadenopathy**
  HD: nontender superficial (usually **cervical/supraclavicular**) ± mediastinal lymphadenopathy; **nodal** disease with **orderly, anatomic spread** to adjacent nodes
  NHL: nontender diffuse lymphadenopathy; **nodal and extranodal** disease with **non-contiguous spread**; symptoms reflect involved sites (abdominal fullness, bone pain)
- Constitutional ("B") symptoms: **fever** (>38°), **sweats**, **weight loss** (>10% over 6 mos)
  HD: periodic, recurrent fever is called "Pel-Ebstein;" 10-15% have pruritus
  NHL: "B" symptoms less common than in HD

Diagnostic and staging evaluation
- History: document "B" symptoms
- Physical exam: lymph nodes, liver/spleen size, Waldeyer's ring; testes (1% of NHL), skin
- Pathology: **excisional lymph node bx** (need surrounding architecture, ∴ FNA *seldom* sufficient) with immunophenotyping and cytogenetics; **BM bx** (except in HD clinical stage IA/IIA with favorable features); LP if CNS involvement is clinically suspected
- Laboratory tests: CBC, BUN/Cr, LFTs, ESR, LDH, uric acid, Ca, albumin; for NHL add β2-microglobulin and SPEP; consider HIV, HBV, HCV, HTLV, EBV, connective tissue diseases
- Imaging: **chest/abdomen/pelvic CT** (but don't reliably detect spleen/liver involvement)
  ∴ need 2nd modality: **gallium** or PET scans
  head CT and bone scan based on clinical suspicion
  staging laparatomy no longer used
- Ann Arbor staging system was developed for HD and can be applied to NHL. However, grade is more important for NHL because ~90% present at an advanced stage.

Ann Arbor Staging System	
Stage	**Features**
I	Single lymph node (LN) region
II	≥2 LN regions on the same side of the diaphragm
III	LN regions on both sides of the diaphragm
IV	Disseminated involvement of one or more extralymphatic organs
Modifiers: A=no symptoms; B=fever, night sweats or weight loss; X=bulky disease; E=involvement of single contiguous extranodal site	

HODGKIN'S DISEASE (HD)

Epidemiology and risk factors
- ~7,500 cases/yr; bimodal distribution (15-35 & >50 yrs); male predom.; ? role for EBV

Pathology
- Affected nodes show small minority (<1%) of RS cells in background of nonneoplastic cells
- Classic RS cells have a bilobed nucleus and prominent nucleoli with surrounding clear space ("owl's eyes"). RS cells are now known to be **clonal B-cells**.

Rye Histologic Classification of Classical HD		
Type	**Freq.**	**Histologic and clinical features**
Lymphocyte predominance	5%	Abundant normal-appearing lymphocytes; mediastinal LAN uncommon; male predominance; good prognosis
Nodular sclerosis	60-80%	Collagen bands; frequent mediastinal LAN; young adults; female predominance; usually stage I/II at dx
Mixed cellularity	15-30%	Pleomorphic; older age; male predominance; ≥50% stage III/VI at presentation; intermediate prognosis
Lymphocyte depletion	<1%	Diffuse fibrosis and large numbers of RS cells; older, male patients; disseminated at dx; seen in HIV; worst prognosis

Treatment (*Lancet* 2003;361:943)

- Stage I and II: 4-6 cycles of ABVD (doxorubicin= Adriamycin, bleomycin, vinblastine, dacarbazine) followed by involved field radiation; however, added radiation ↑ risk of late 2nd malignancy with unclear benefit (*NEJM* 2003;348:2396)
- Stage III and IV: ABVD for 2 cycles beyond best response (min. 6 cycles) with radiation for bulky disease and/or incomplete regression. Regimen involving ↑ dose BEACOPP (bleomycin, etoposide, doxorubicin, cyclophosphamide, vincristine, procarbazine, and prednisone) achieved >90% 5-yr survival in Pts w/ adv. disease (*NEJM* 2003;348:2386).
- Relapsed disease: chemotherapy or high-dose chemotherapy plus autologous HSCT

Prognosis

- Long-term survival: limited disease → ~80%; advanced disease → 50-70% (with "B" symptoms) or >75% (w/o "B" symptoms)
- **Second malignancies**: **acute leukemia**, NHL, lung cancer (related to both radiation and chemotherapy), breast cancer (mantle radiation)

NON-HODGKIN'S LYMPHOMA (NHL)

Epidemiology and risk factors

- ~53,000 new cases/yr; median age at diagnosis ~ 65 yrs; male predominance
- ↑ incidence since 1950s, partially attributed to HIV epidemic
- Associated conditions: immunodeficiency (e.g., HIV, post-transplant); autoimmune disorders (e.g., Sjögren's, RA, SLE); infection (e.g., EBV, HTLV-I, *H. pylori*)
- Burkitt's: (1) endemic or African (jaw mass, 80-90% EBV-related); (2) sporadic or American (20% EBV-related); (3) HIV-related

WHO/REAL Classification System	
Aggressiveness	**Lymphomas** (90% B cell, 10% T cell or NK cell)
Indolent (35-40% of NHL)	**follicular lymphoma** **small lymphocytic lymphoma (SLL) / B-cell CLL** plasma cell myeloma, marginal zone lymphoma (includes MALT), mantle cell lymphoma, lymphoplasmacytic lymphoma (= Waldenström's), hairy cell leukemia, T-cell/NK cell tumors (mycosis fungoides, T-cell large granular lymphocyte leukemia, T-cell prolymphocytic leukemia, NK cell large granular lymphocyte leukemia)
Aggressive (~50% of NHL)	**diffuse large B-cell lymphoma** (DLBCL) follicular lymphoma (grade III) peripheral T-cell lymphoma, anaplastic large cell lymphoma
Highly aggressive (~5% of NHL)	**Burkitt's lymphoma** precursor B lymphoblastic leukemia (= pre B-ALL) / lymphoma precursor T lymphoblastic leukemia (= T-ALL) / lymphoma adult T-cell lymphoma/leukemia

Treatment

- Treatment and prognosis determined by histopathologic classification rather than stage
- Indolent: goal of treatment is symptom management (bulky disease, cytopenias, "B" sx)
  Options include radiation for localized disease, single agent chemotherapy (chlorambucil, cyclophosphamide, fludarabine), combination chemotherapy, and rituximab.
- Aggressive: goal of treatment is cure
  Combination chemotherapy, with radiation added for localized or bulky disease
  CHOP (cyclophosphamide, doxorubicin=hydroxydaunorubicin, vincristine=Oncovorin, prednisone) is mainstay; addition of **rituximab** beneficial in DLBCL (*NEJM* 2002;346:235)
  CNS prophylaxis with intrathecal methotrexate if large cells found in bone marrow
  Relapse → high-dose chemotherapy + autologous HSCT

Prognosis

- Indolent: ↓ response to chemotherapy, but long median survival
- Aggressive: ↑ chance of cure, but overall worse prognosis

International Prognostic Index		
Factors: age >60, stage III/IV, ≥2 extranodal sites, performance status ≥2, LDH >250		
# factors	**Complete remission**	**Disease-free survival at 5 yrs**
0-1	87%	70%
2	67%	50%
3	55%	43%
4-5	44%	26%

(*NEJM* 1993;329:987)

• PLASMA CELL DYSCRASIAS •

MULTIPLE MYELOMA (MM)

Definition

- Malignant proliferation of **plasma cells** producing a monoclonal Ig = "**M component**"

Epidemiology

- ~14,600 new cases and ~10,900 deaths/yr in U.S.; median age at diagnosis is 66 yrs
- African-American:Caucasian ratio ≈ 2:1

Clinical manifestations

- **Anemia** (normocytic) due to myelophthisis, ↓ bone marrow production, autoimmune Ab
- **Bone pain** and **hypercalcemia** due to ↑ osteoclast activity → lytic lesions, pathologic fx
- **Recurrent infections** due to hypogammaglobulinemia (excluding M component)
  pneumonia and pyelonephritis are the most common infections
- **Renal disease**: multiple mechanisms
  toxic effect of filtered light chains → **renal failure** (cast nephropathy) or **type II RTA**
  amyloidosis or light chain deposition disease → **nephrotic syndrome**
  hypercalcemia, urate nephropathy, pyelonephritis, type I cryoglobulinemia
- Neurologic: cord compression; POEMS (polyneuropathy, organomegaly, endocrinopathy, M protein, skin changes) syndrome
- Amyloidosis (see "Amyloidosis")
- Hyperviscosity: usually when IgM >4 g/dl, IgG3 >5 g/dl, or IgA >7 g/dl
- Coagulopathy: inhibition of or Ab against clotting factor; Ab-coated platelets

Diagnostic and staging evaluation

- **Criteria** = marrow plasmacytosis >10% (or presence of a plasmacytoma) *and one of following:* lytic bone lesions *or* M component in either serum (usually >3 g/dL) or urine
- **Variants:**
  smoldering MM (asx w/ M >3 g/dL and/or plasmacytosis >10%)
  solitary bone plasmacytoma (single lytic lesion w/o marrow plasmacytosis)
  extramedullary plasmacytoma (usually upper respiratory tract)
  plasma cell leukemia (plasma cell count >2,000/µl)
  nonsecretory MM (marrow plasmacytosis & lytic lesions, but no M component)
- Ddx of M component: MM, MGUS (see below), CLL, lymphoma, cirrhosis, sarcoidosis, RA
- CBC, peripheral smear (rouleaux); calcium, albumin, Cr; ↓ anion gap, ↑ globulin,↑ ESR
- **Protein electrophoresis and immunofixation**
  serum protein electrophoresis (SPEP): quantitates M component; ⊕ in ~80% of patients
  urine protein electrophoresis (UPEP): detects the ~20% of Pts who secrete only light chains (= Bence Jones proteins), which are filtered rapidly from the blood
  immunofixation: shows component is monoclonal and identifies Ig type → IgG (50%), IgA (20%), IgD (2%), IgM (0.5%), light chain only (20%), nonsecretors (<5%)
- **Bone marrow biopsy**
- **Skeletal survey** (plain radiographs) to identify lytic bone lesions and areas at risk for pathologic fracture; *bone scan is not useful for detecting lytic lesions*
- **Staging**: Durie-Salmon system is based on an assessment of total-body tumor burden
- ↑ β_2**-microglobulin** (>4 µg/ml) is the most powerful independent poor prognostic factor

Durie-Salmon Staging System		
Stage	**Criteria**	**Median survival**
I	*all of the following:* Hb >10 g/dl Ca ≤12 mg/dl 0-1 lytic bone lesions IgG <5 g/dl or IgA <3 g/dl or urine light chain <4 g/24 hr	61 mos
II	fulfilling criteria for neither I nor III	55 mos
III	*any of the following:* Hb <8.5 g/dl Ca >12 mg/dl >5 lytic bone lesions IgG >7 g/dl or IgA >5 g/dl or urine light chain >12 g/24 h	30 mos for IIIA 15 mos for IIIB
Subclassification by serum Cr: A <2.0 mg/dl; B ≥2.0 mg/dl		

(*Cancer* 1975;36:842)

Treatment (*NEJM* 1997;336:1657)

- Treatment not indicated for smoldering MM or asymptomatic stage I disease
- **Systemic chemotherapy**: ↑ median survival, but not curative
  - initial regimen = alkylating agent (e.g., **melphalan**) + **prednisone**
    - avoid alkylating agents if auto HSCT considered → Rx w/ vincristine, adriamycin, dex
  - **thalidomide** (*NEJM* 1999;341:1565) and **bortezomib,** a proteasome inhibitor (*NEJM* 2003;348:2609), have shown benefit for relapsed disease in phase II trials
- High-dose chemotherapy + **autologous HSCT**: not curative, but ↑ survival compared to conventional chemo (*NEJM* 1996;335:91 & 2003;348:1875); ∴ offer to good candidates <70 yrs
  - *double* auto HSCT offers ↑ survival, espec. if poor response to 1st auto (*NEJM* 2003;349:2495)
- Local radiation for solitary or extramedullary plasmacytoma
- Adjunctive treatment
  - bone: **bisphosphonates** ↓ skeletal complic. (*NEJM* 1996;334:488); XRT for sx bony lesions
  - renal: *avoid NSAIDs and IV contrast*; consider plasmapheresis for acute renal failure
  - hyperviscosity syndrome: plasmapheresis
  - infections: consider IVIg for recurrent infections

Monoclonal Gammopathy of Uncertain Significance (MGUS)

Definition

- M component <3 g/dl, no urinary Bence Jones proteins, marrow plasmacytosis <10%, and no lytic bone lesions, anemia, hypercalcemia, or renal insufficiency

Epidemiology

- Prevalence ~1% in population >50 yrs of age, ~10% in population >75 yrs of age

Management

- CBC, calcium, Cr, SPEP and UPEP with immunofixation to exclude multiple myeloma
- Close observation (i.e., repeat SPEP in 6 months and then yearly thereafter if stable)

Prognosis

- ~25% progress to MM, WM, amyloidosis or a malignant lymphoproliferative disease over 20 yrs (*NEJM* 2002:346:564)
- No reliable predictors of which patients will progress

Waldenström's Macroglobulinemia (WM)

Definition (*Lancet Oncology* 2003;4:679)

- Low grade malignant proliferation of lymphoplasmacytoid cells that secrete IgM
- *No evidence of bone lesions* (IgM M component + lytic bone lesions = "IgM myeloma")

Clinical manifestations

- **Tumor infiltration**: BM (cytopenias), hepatomegaly, splenomegaly, lymphadenopathy
- **Circulating IgM**
  - **hyperviscosity syndrome** (~15%)
    - neurologic: blurred vision ("sausage" retinal veins on funduscopy), HA, dizziness, Δ MS
    - cardiac: congestive heart failure
    - pulmonary: pulmonary infiltrates
  - type I **cryoglobulinemia** → **Raynaud's phenomenon**
  - anemia (prominent **rouleaux**; 10% Coombs' ⊕ = AIHA)
  - mucosal bleeding due to abnormalities in platelet fxn
- **IgM deposition**
  - **peripheral neuropathy**: may be due to IgM against myelin-associated glycoprotein
  - amyloidosis
  - glomerulopathy

Diagnostic evaluation

- SPEP + immunofixation with IgM >3 g/dl; only 20% have ⊕ UPEP
- Bone marrow biopsy: ↑ plasmacytoid lymphocytes
- **Relative serum viscosity**: defined as ratio of viscosity of serum to H_2O (normal ratio 1.8)
  - hyperviscosity syndrome when relative serum viscosity >5-6

Treatment

- **Plasmapheresis** for hyperviscosity
- **Systemic chemotherapy**: chlorambucil, fludarabine or cladribine
- Rituximab, thalidomide, and HSCT are investigational modalities

• HEMATOPOIETIC STEM CELL TRANSPLANTATION (HSCT) •

Definitions

- Transplantation of donor pluripotent cells that can reconstitute all recipient blood lineages

Categories of Stem Cell Transplantation		
Feature	**Allogeneic (Allo)**	**Autologous (Auto)**
Donor-recipient relationship	Immunologically distinct	Donor is also recipient
Graft-versus-host disease (and ∴ need for posttransplant immunosuppression)	Yes	No
Graft-versus-tumor effect	Yes	No
Risk of graft contam. w/ tumor	No	Yes
Relapse risk (leukemia)	Lower	Higher
Transplant-related mortality	Higher	Lower

- **Graft-versus-host disease (GVHD)**: *undesirable* side effect of allo HSCT; allogeneic T cells view host cells as foreign; ↑ incid. w/ mismatch or unrelated donors
- **Graft-versus-leukemia (GVL) effect**: *desirable* consequence of allo HSCT; allogeneic T cells attack host tumor cells

Indications

- **Nonmalignant disease**: allo HSCT to replace an abnormal lymphohematopoietic system with one from normal donor (e.g., immunodeficiencies, aplastic anemia, hemoglobinopathies, ? autoimmune disorders)
- **Malignant disease**:
  - **Auto HSCT** to allow **higher doses of chemo** by rescuing hematopoietic system (e.g., lymphoma, multiple myeloma, testicular cancer)
  - **Allo HSCT** to produce **graft-versus-leukemia** (GVL) effect, in addition to above mech. (e.g., AML, ALL, CML; ? CLL, ? MDS)

Transplantation procedure

- **Preparative regimen**: *eradication of disease* for which transplant is being performed and *immunosuppression* to prevent rejection of transplanted graft (allo only)
  - myeloablative (traditional): chemotherapy and/or total body irradiation
  - nonmyeloablative: low-intensity conditioning regimens → ↓ toxicity yet induce sufficient host immunosuppression to allow donor engraftment and thus a GVT effect
- **Sources of stem cells**: bone marrow (BM) vs. peripheral blood stem cells (PBSC)
  - faster engraftment and immunologic recovery with PBSC than BM
- **Peripheral blood counts** reach nadir several days to a week posttransplant due to preparative regimen; cells produced by the transplanted stem cells then begin to appear
- **Absolute neutrophil count (ANC)** recovers to 500/μl w/in ~3 wks w/ BM and ~2 wks w/ PBSC. G-CSF accelerates recovery by 3-5 d in both scenarios.

Complications

- Either **direct chemoradiotoxicites** associated with preparative regimen or consequences of **interaction between donor and recipient immune systems**

Timing and Mechanism of Non-infectious Complications of HSCT			
Timing	**<30 days**	**30-90 days**	**>90 days**
Regimen-related	Pancytopenia		Growth failure
	Mucositis, rash, alopecia		Hypogonadism/infertility
	Nausea, vomiting, diarrhea		Hypothyroidism
	Peripheral neuropathies		Cataracts
	Hemorrhagic cystitis		Avascular necrosis of bone
	Veno-occlusive disease		Second malignancy
	Interstitial pneumonitis		
Immune-mediated	Acute GVHD		Chronic GVHD
	Primary graft failure	Secondary graft failure	

- **Veno-occlusive disease** of the liver (**VOD**; incidence ~10%, mortality ~30%)
  Mech: direct cytotoxic injury to hepatic venules → *in situ* thrombosis
  Symptoms: tender hepatomegaly, ascites, jaundice, fluid retention
  with severe disease → progressive liver failure, encephalopathy, hepatorenal syndrome
  Diagnosis: ↑ ALT/AST, ↑ bilirubin; ↑ PT with severe disease;
  Doppler U/S w/ reversal of portal vein flow, ↑ hepatic wedge pressure, abnl liver bx
  Treatment: supportive; prophylaxis with **ursodiol** or low-dose heparin; defibrotide
- **Idiopathic interstitial pneumonitis** (**IIP**, up to 70% mortality)
  Mech: alveolar injury due to direct toxicity → fever, hypoxia, diffuse pulmonary infiltrates
  Diffuse alveolar hemorrhage (DAH): subset of IIP; more common with auto than allo
  Diagnosis: bronchoscopy to exclude infection; ↑ bloody lavage fluid seen with DAH
  Treatment: high-dose corticosteroids (limited data)
- **Acute GVHD** (w/in 3 mos of transplant)
  Clinical grade I-IV based on scores for **skin** (severity of maculopapular rash), **liver** (bilirubin level), and **GI** (volume of diarrhea) disease; bx supports dx
  Prevention: **immunosuppression** (MTX + CsA or tacrolimus) ± T-cell depletion of graft
  Treatment: grade I not clinically significant; grade II-IV associated with ↓ survival and ∴ treated with immunosuppressants (corticosteroids, CsA, tacrolimus, rapamycin, etc.)
- **Chronic GVHD** (developing or persisting beyond 3 mos post-transplant)
  Clinical features: malar rash, sicca syndrome, arthritis, obliterative bronchiolitis, bile duct degeneration and cholestasis
  Treatment: immunosuppressants as above, with prophylactic TMP-SMX; photopheresis
- **Graft failure**
  Primary = persistent neutropenia without evidence of engraftment
  Secondary= delayed pancytopenia after initial engraftment; either immune-mediated due to attack by immunocompetent host cells in the allogeneic setting (termed **graft rejection**) or non-immune mediated (e.g., CMV infection)
- **Infectious complications**
  due to regimen-induced pancytopenia and immunosuppression
  auto HSCT recipients do not require immunosuppression and ∴ remain at ↑ risk only during the preengraftment and immediate postengraftment phases
  both primary infections and reactivation events occur (e.g., CMV, HSV, VZV)

Infectious Complications Following Allogeneic HSCT

Class of pathogen and associated prophylaxis	Time after transplant and associated risk factors: Days 0 to 30 (Mucositis, Organ dysfunction, Neutropenia)	Days 30-90 (Acute GVHD, ↓ cellular immunity)	>90 days (Chronic GVHD, ↓ cellular & humoral immunity)
Viral acyclovir to d 30 (for HSV) or d 365 (VZV); ganciclovir to d 100 (CMV)	Respiratory and enteral viruses		
	HSV*	CMV*, HHV 6 & 7	
		EBV-related lymphoma	
			VZV*, BK/JC
Bacterial antibiotics (e.g., fluoroquinolone) while neutropenic	Gram ⊕ cocci (coagulase-negative staph., *S. aureus*, *S. viridans*) GNRs (*Enterobacteriaceae*, *Pseudomonas*, *Legionella*, *S. maltophilia*)		Encapsulated bacteria
Fungal fluconazole to d 75 for *Candida*	*Candida* spp.		
	Aspergillus spp.		
Parasitic TMP-SMX to d 180 (or off immunosuppression) for PCP		*T. gondii* *P. carinii* *S. stercoralis*	*T. gondii* *P. carinii*

*Primarily among persons who are seropositive before transplant

• LUNG CANCER •

Epidemiology and risk factors

- Most common cause of cancer-related death for both men and women in U.S.
- ~172,000 new cases and ~157,000 deaths/yr
- **Cigarette smoking**: 85% of all lung cancers occur in smokers
  risk proportional to total pack-years; ↓ risk after quitting, but not to baseline
  squamous & small cell almost exclusively in smokers
  adenocarcinoma most common type in non-smokers
- Asbestos: when combined with smoking, synergistic ↑ in risk of lung cancer
- Radon: risk to general population unclear

Pathology

- **Non-small cell lung cancer (NSCLC)**
  Adenocarcinoma: ~35% of lung cancers; ↑ incidence worldwide; typically peripheral
  Squamous cell carcinoma: ~30% of lung cancers; typically central
  Large cell carcinoma: ~10% of lung cancers; typically peripheral
- **Small cell lung cancer (SCLC)**: ~25% of lung cancers; typically central

Clinical manifestations

- ~10% are asymptomatic at presentation and detected incidentally by imaging.
- **Endobronchial growth** of 1° tumor: **cough**, **hemoptysis**, **dyspnea**, wheezing, post-obstructive pneumonia; more common with squamous or small cell (central location)
- **Regional spread**
  pleural effusion, pericardial effusion, hoarseness (recurrent laryngeal nerve palsy), dysphagia (esophageal compression), stridor (tracheal obstruction)
  Pancoast's syndrome: apical tumor → brachial plexus involvement (C8, T1, T2) → Horner's syndrome, shoulder pain, rib destruction, atrophy of hand muscles
  superior vena cava syndrome: central tumor → SVC compression → dyspnea, headache, facial swelling, venous distention of neck and chest wall
- **Extrathoracic metastases**: brain, bone, liver, adrenal, skin
- **Paraneoplastic syndromes**
  Endocrine
  ACTH (small cell) → **Cushing's syndrome**
  PTH-rP (squamous cell) → **hypercalcemia**
  ADH (small cell) → **SIADH**
  Skeletal: digital clubbing (non-small cell), **hypertrophic pulmonary osteoarthropathy** (adenocarcinoma) = symmetric polyarthritis and proliferative periostitis of long bones
  Neurologic (usually small cell): **Eaton-Lambert**, periph. neuropathy, cerebellar degen.
  Cutaneous: acanthosis nigricans, dermatomyositis
  Hematologic: hypercoagulable state (adenocarcinoma), DIC, marantic endocarditis

Screening

- No proven benefit to screening CXR or sputum cytology, even in high-risk subgroups
- In *observational* studies, **spiral CT** is more sensitive than CXR and most of the detected cancers are early stage; RCTs to assess mortality benefit are underway (*Chest* 2003;123:72S)

Diagnostic and staging evaluation

- **Imaging** in all patients: **CXR**, **chest CT** (must include liver and adrenal glands)
- **Tissue**
  bronchoscopy (for central lesions) or **CT-guided needle biopsy** (for peripheral lesions or accessible sites of suspected metastasis)
  mediastinoscopy (for lymph node bx), VATS (for evaluation of pleura and peripheral lesions), thoracentesis (cell block for cytology), or sputum cytology (for central lesions)
- **Staging**
  NSCLC: TNM staging system (see below)
  SCLC: limited (disease is confined to ipsilateral hemithorax) *vs.* extensive
- Intrathoracic staging: mediastinoscopy or VATS; thoracentesis if pleural effusion
- Extrathoracic staging
  PET scan or integrated PET-CT more sens. than CT alone for detecting mediastinal and distant metastases (*NEJM* 2000;343:254 & 2003;348:2500)
  brain MRI, bone scan: for all SCLC patients and for NSCLC patients with localizing sx or lab abnormalities; consider for asx stage III NSCLC if potentially resectable
- CBC and chemistries (including Cr, calcium, Aϕ, LDH, LFTs)
- PFTs with quantitative V/Q if planned treatment includes surgical resection

NSCLC treatment

- **Stages I and II**: **surgical resection**; ? benefit from chemotherapy (*NEJM* 2004;350:351)
- **Stage III**: optimal **combo/sequence of chemo, radiation, & surgery** unknown
  IIIA has been viewed as potentially resectable and IIIB as unresectable
  neoadjuvant chemoradiation may convert unresectable → resectable
- **Stage IV**: **chemotherapy** prolongs survival compared to best supportive care
  standard is a platinum-based doublet (e.g., carboplatin + paclitaxel)
  no single regimen is superior (*NEJM* 2002;346:92)
  palliative radiation used to control local symptoms caused by tumor or metastasis
  solitary brain metastasis: surgical resection + whole brain irradiation may ↑ survival

<table>
<tr><th colspan="6">TNM Staging System for NSCLC</th></tr>
<tr><td rowspan="2">T stage</td><td>N stage</td><td>N0</td><td>N1</td><td>N2</td><td>N3</td></tr>
<tr><td>Definition</td><td>no ⊕ nodes</td><td>ipsilateral hilar</td><td>ipsilateral mediastinal</td><td>contralateral or supraclavicular</td></tr>
<tr><td>T1</td><td>Tumor ≤3 cm</td><td>IA</td><td>IIA</td><td rowspan="2"></td><td rowspan="3"></td></tr>
<tr><td>T2</td><td>Tumor >3 cm</td><td>IB</td><td>IIB</td></tr>
<tr><td>T3</td><td>Direct invasion of chest wall, diaphragm, mediastinal pleura, pericardium</td><td>IIB</td><td colspan="2">IIIA</td></tr>
<tr><td>T4</td><td>Malignant pleural effusion; invasion of mediastinum, heart, great vessels, trachea, esophagus, vertebral body, carina</td><td colspan="4">IIIB</td></tr>
</table>

NSCLC Simplified Staging Schema and Treatment				
Stage	**% at dx**	**Definition**	**Treatment**	**5-yr survival**
I	10%	Isolated lesion	Surgery ± chemo	>60%
II	20%	Hilar node spread	Surgery ± radiation ± chemo	40-50%
IIIA	15%	Mediastinal spread, but resectable	Neoadjuvant chemotherapy ± radiation → surgical resection	25-30%
IIIB	15%	Unresectable	Chemotherapy ± radiation ± surgery (selected cases)	10-20%
IV	40%	Metastatic	Chemotherapy and/or supportive care Palliative radiation	1%

(*NEJM* 2004;350:379)

SCLC Treatment

- SCLC usually *disseminated at presentation*, but *responsive to chemoradiation*
- **Chemotherapy** (platinum + etoposide) is primary treatment modality
- **Thoracic radiation** added to chemotherapy improves survival in limited stage disease
- **Prophylactic cranial irradiation** (PCI) improves survival for limited stage disease in complete remission (*NEJM* 1999;341:476)

SCLC Staging Schema and Treatment				
Stage	**% at dx**	**Definition**	**Treatment**	**Median survival**
Limited	30-40%	Confined to ipsilateral hemithorax within one radiation port	Radiation + chemotherapy ± PCI	1-2 yrs
Extensive	60-70%	Beyond one radiation port	Chemotherapy	~1 yr

• BREAST CANCER •

Epidemiology and risk factors

- Most common cancer in U.S. women; 2nd most common cause of cancer death in women
- ~213,000 new cases and ~40,000 deaths/yr in the U.S.; lifetime risk = 1 in 8
- Age: incidence rates ↑ with age, with decrease in slope at age of menopause
- **Genetics** (*NEJM* 2003;348:2339): 15-20% have ⊕ FHx
  Risk depends on # of affected 1st-degree relatives and their age at dx
  ~45% of cases of familial cases are associated with known germline mutations
  BRCA1/2: 50-85% lifetime risk of breast cancer & ↑ risk of **ovarian cancer**; ? ↑ colon & prostate cancer; BRCA2: ↑ risk of *male* breast cancer and ? ↑ pancreatic cancer
- Endogenous or exogenous **estrogen**: ↑ risk with early menarche, late menopause, late parity or nulliparity; ↑ risk with prolonged HRT (RR=1.24 after 5.6 yrs, *JAMA* 2003;289:3243); *no* ↑ risk shown with OCP use (*NEJM* 2002;346:2025)
- Benign breast conditions: ↑ risk with proliferative lesions (hyperplasia, sclerosing adenosis, complex fibroadenoma, intraductal papillomas); *no* ↑ risk with fibrocystic changes
- Radiation

Clinical manifestations

- Breast mass: hard, irregular, fixed, nontender
- Nipple discharge: higher risk if unilateral, limited to one duct, bloody, associated with mass
- Special types: **Paget's** disease → unilateral nipple eczema + nipple discharge;
  Inflammatory breast cancer → skin erythema and edema *(peau d'orange)*
- Metastases: lymph nodes, bone, liver, lung, brain

Screening

- **Self breast exam** (SBE): *no* proven mortality benefit (*JNCI* 2002;94:1445)
- **Clinical breast exam** (CBE): benefit independent of mammography not established
- **Mammography**: ~20-30% ↓ **in breast cancer mortality** (with smaller absolute benefit in women under 50) (*Lancet* 2001;358:1340 & 2002;359:909; *Annals* 2002;137:347)
  suspicious lesions: clustered **microcalcifications, spiculated** or **enlarging** masses
- Most U.S. groups recommend annual mammography + CBE beginning at age 40
  For women at ↑ risk, begin screening earlier: at age 25 in BRCA1/2 carrier (also consider screening **MRI**), 5-10 yrs before earliest index case in woman with ⊕ FHx, 8-10 yrs after thoracic irradiation, and upon dx of LCIS or atypical hyperplasia
- Women with strong family histories should be evaluated for possible genetic testing

Diagnostic evaluation

- **Palpable breast mass:**
  Age <30 yrs → can observe for resolution over 1-2 menstrual cycles
  Age <30 yrs, unchanging mass → **U/S** → aspiration if mass not simple cyst
  Age >30 yrs *or* solid mass on U/S *or* bloody aspirate *or* recurrence after aspiration → **mammography** (detect other lesions) *and* **fine-needle aspir.** or **core-needle bx**
  Clearly cancerous on exam or indeterminate read/atypia on needle bx → **excisional bx**
- **Suspicious mammogram** with normal exam: stereotactically-guided bx

Staging

- **Anatomic**: tumor size, chest wall invasion, axillary LN mets (*strongest prognostic factor*)
- **Histopathologic**: type (little prognostic relevance) and grade; lymphatic/vascular invasion
  In situ carcinoma: no invasion of surrounding stroma
    Ductal (DCIS): ↑ risk of invasive cancer in *ipsilateral* breast (~30%/10 yrs)
    Lobular (LCIS): marker of ↑ risk of invasive cancer in *either* breast (~1%/yr)
  Invasive carcinoma: infiltrating ductal (70-80%); invasive lobular (5-10%); tubular, medullary and mucinous (10%, better prognosis); papillary (1-2%); other (1-2%)
  Inflammatory breast cancer (see above): not a histologic type but a clinical reflection of tumor invasion of dermal lymphatics; very poor prognosis
  Paget's disease: ductal cancer invading nipple epidermis ± associated mass
- **Biologic**: estrogen and progesterone receptor (ER/PR) status; HER2/*neu* over-expression
- Metastatic workup: CBC, LFTs, bilateral mammography, CXR; include bone scan and abdomen/pelvis CT for stage III or symptoms or ↑ Aϕ
- Gene expression profiling outperforms standard prognostic criteria (*NEJM* 2002;347:1999)

Simplified Staging System for Breast Cancer			
Stage	**Characteristics**	**Description**	**5-yr surv**
I	Tumor ≤2 cm	Operable locoregional	90%
IIA	Tumor >2 cm or *mobile* axillary nodes		80%
IIB	Tumor >5 cm		65%
IIIA	Internal mammary or *fixed* axillary nodes	Locally advanced	50%
IIIB	Direct extension to chest wall or skin	Inoperable locoregional	45%
IIIC	Infraclavicular or supraclavicular nodes		40%
IV	Distant metastases	Metastatic	15%

Treatment modalities

- **Local control: surgery and radiation therapy (RT)**
  - *Breast-conserving therapy* [**lumpectomy + breast RT** + axillary lymph node dissection (ALND)] equivalent to *mastectomy* + ALND (*NEJM* 2002;347:1227 & 1233)
    - contraindications to breast-conservation: multicentric disease, diffuse malignant-appearing microcalcifications on mammo, prior RT, pregnancy, ? tumor >5 cm
  - *Radiation therapy* (RT) after mastectomy for ≥4 ⊕ LN, tumor >5 cm or ⊕ surgical margins → ↓ locoregional recurrence and ↑ survival
- **Systemic therapy: chemotherapy and hormonal therapy**
  - *Chemotherapy:* typically **anthracycline**-based (e.g., CAF (cyclophosphamide, adriamycin, fluorouracil) or AC) + **taxanes** (e.g., paclitaxel) for advanced disease, HER-2/neu ⊕, or node ⊕ tumors
  - High-dose chemotherapy + HSCT: *no survival benefit* in high-risk stage II/III (≥4 ⊕ lymph nodes) (*NEJM* 2003;349:7 & 17) or stage IV disease (*NEJM* 2000;342:1069)
  - *Hormonal therapy*
    - 1st-line = **selective estrogen receptor modulators** (e.g., tamoxifen; *NEJM* 2003;348:618); **aromatase inhibitors** (e.g., anastrozole, letrozole, exemestane) for *postmenopausal* women (*NEJM* 2003;348:2431); ? letrozole after adjuvant tamoxifen × 5 yrs (*NEJM* 2003;349:19); ? exemestane after tamoxifen × 2-3 yrs (*NEJM* 2004;350:1081)
    - 2nd-line = LHRH agonists (e.g., goserelin) if *premenopausal*; oopherectomy if *premenopausal*; pure antiestrogens (e.g., fulvestrant) if *postmenopausal*
  - *Monoclonal antibodies:* trastuzumab is directed against the HER2/*neu* protein

Treatment of Carcinoma *in situ* and Invasive Carcinoma of the Breast	
Stage	**Treatment**
LCIS	Close surveillance ± chemoprevention preferred Consider prophylactic bilateral mastectomy
DCIS	Mastectomy or lumpectomy + breast RT ALND *not* indicated unless invasive cancer found Offer chemoprevention
I or II	Surgery + RT Adjuvant chemotherapy for higher-risk disease = tumor >1 cm *or* ⊕ LN *or* ER/PR ⊖ (*Lancet* 1998;352:930) Tamoxifen x 5 yrs added for ER/PR ⊕ tumors (*Lancet* 1998; 351:1451); if postmenopausal may benefit from further Rx w/ letrozole (*NEJM* 2003;349:19)
III	Neoadjuvant chemotherapy → surgery + RT ± adjuvant chemotherapy Tamoxifen x 5 yrs for ER/PR ⊕ tumors ± letrozole in postmenopausal women
IV	ER/PR ⊕: hormonal therapy (see above) ER/PR ⊖, HER2/*neu* over-expressed: trastuzumab ± chemotherapy ER/PR ⊖, HER2/*neu* not over-expressed: chemotherapy Bony metastases: bisphosphonates ↓ skeletal complic. (*NEJM* 1998;339:357)

Prevention

- **Selective estrogen receptor modulators (SERMs):**
  - Tamoxifen: ↓ risk of contralateral breast cancer in adjuvant setting;
    - risk-benefit unclear when given as 1° prevention in women at ↑ risk: ↓ invasive breast cancer, but possible ↑ in all-cause mortality (*JNCI* 1998;90:1371; *Lancet* 2002;360:817)
  - Raloxifene: ↓ breast cancer in retrospective analysis in women treated for osteoporosis; prospective comparison with tamoxifen as 1° prevention is underway
- BRCA1/2 carriers: several options, including intensified surveillance as described above
  - Prophylactic surgery: bilateral mastectomy (*NEJM* 2001;345:159) and bilateral salpingo-oopherectomy (↓ risk of ovarian *and* breast cancer; *NEJM* 2002;346:1609) are effective
  - Chemoprevention: limited data supports use of tamoxifen for risk reduction

• PROSTATE CANCER •

Epidemiology and risk factors (*NEJM* 2003;349:366)

- Most common cancer in U.S. men; 2nd most common cause of cancer death in men
- Lifetime risk of prostate cancer dx ~16%; lifetime risk of dying of prostate cancer ~3%
- ~220,000 new cases and ~29,000 deaths/yr in U.S.
- Age: rare before age 45, with rapid increase in incidence thereafter
- Ethnicity: ~2-3x ↑ risk in African Americans; lowest risk in Asians
- Genetics: ~2x ↑ risk with one and ~5x ↑ risk with two affected 1st-degree relatives

Clinical manifestations

- Usually asymptomatic at presentation
- **Obstructive sx** (more common with BPH): hesitancy, ↓ stream, retention, nocturia
- **Irritative sx** (also seen with prostatitis): frequency, dysuria, urgency
- Periprostatic spread: hematuria, hematospermia, new onset erectile dysfunction
- Metastatic disease: bone pain, spinal cord compression, cytopenias

Screening (*NEJM* 2001;344:1373)

- Mortality benefit from screening has not been established (*Annals* 2002;137:915 & 917)
- **Digital rectal exam** (DRE): size, consistency, lesions
- **PSA**: neither sensitive nor specific; can ↑ with BPH, prostatitis, acute retention, after bx or TURP, and ejaculation (*no significant ↑ after DRE, cystoscopy*); ↓ free PSA %, ↑ PSA velocity, ↑ PSA density and age-adjusted PSA reference ranges may ↑ utility of test
- PSA = 4 ng/ml used as upper limit of normal (? verification bias, *NEJM* 2003;349:335)
- Offer DRE + PSA screening to men age ≥50 (≥45 if high risk) with life expectancy ≥10 yrs

Diagnostic and staging evaluation

- **Transrectal ultrasound** (TRUS) **guided biopsy**, with six to twelve core specimens
- **Histology**: **Gleason grade** (2-10; low grade ≤6) = sum of the differentiation score (1 = best, 5 = worst) of the two most prevalent patterns in the bx; correlates with prognosis
- **Imaging**: to evaluate extraprostatic spread
  bone scan: for PSA >10 ng/ml, high Gleason grade, or clinically advanced tumor
  abdomen-pelvis CT: inaccurate for detecting extracapsular spread and lymph node mets
  endorectal coil MRI: improves assessment of extracapsular spread

Jewett-Whitmore Staging System and Treatment of Prostate Cancer		
Stage	**Definition**	**Treatment**
A	Incidental, non-palpable tumor	**Radical prostatectomy** (± radiation and/or hormonal therapy if high risk features found at surgery) *or* **Radiation** (external beam or brachytherapy) *or* **Watchful waiting** (consider for those with limited life expectancy and low Gleason score)
B	Tumor confined within the prostate	
C	Tumor extends beyond prostate capsule	**Radiation** + neoadjuvant hormonal Rx (*NEJM* 1997;337:295)
D	Lymph node or distant metastases	**Hormonal therapy** orchiectomy **LHRH analogues** (leuprolide, goserelin) antiandrogens (flutamide, megestrol acetate) 2nd-line: androgen synthesis inhibitors (ketoconazole, aminoglutethimide) and estrogens ± chemotherapy for hormone-refractory disease **Bisphosphonates**, palliative radiation for bone mets

Prognosis

- PSA level, Gleason grade, and age are predictors of metastatic disease
- In surgically treated patients, 5-yr relapse-free survival >90% with disease confined to organ, ~75% with extension through capsule, and ~40% with seminal vesicle invasion
- Compared to watchful waiting, surgery ↓ prostate cancer mortality but not overall mortality (*NEJM* 2002;347:781); comparisons of surgery and radiation are underway
- Metastatic disease: median survival ~24-30 mos; all progress to androgen independence

Prevention

- Finasteride ↓ total prostate cancers detected by bx, but is associated with ↑ number of high Gleason grade tumors (*NEJM* 2003;349:215)

• COLORECTAL CANCER (CRC) •

Epidemiology and risk factors

- 3rd most common cancer in U.S men and women; 2nd leading cause of cancer death overall
- ~148,000 new cases (of which 42,000 = rectal) and ~57,000 deaths/yr; lifetime risk ~5%
- Age: rare before 40, with 90% of cases occurring after age 50
- **Genetics:** up to 25% of patients have ⊕ FHx → risk depends on number of 1st-degree relatives (with CRC *or* polyp) and age at dx; ~5% have an identifiable germline mutation
  Familial adenomatous polyposis (FAP): mutation of APC tumor suppressor → 100s to 1000s of polyps at young age → ~100% lifetime risk; ↑ risk of thyroid, stomach, and small intestine cancers; variants = attenuated FAP (<100 polyps), Gardner's (⊕ bone & soft tissue tumors, e.g., desmoid tumors) and Turcot's (⊕ brain tumors) syndromes
  Hereditary non-polyposis colorectal cancer (HNPCC): mutations in DNA mismatch repair genes → ↑ tumor progression → ~80% lifetime risk; predom. **right-sided** tumors; ↑ risk of **endometrial**, ovarian, stomach, small bowel cancers
- **Inflammatory bowel disease**: ↑ risk with ↑ extent and duration of disease
- Drugs: ↓ risk w/ NSAIDs & HRT; ASA ↓ risk of recurrent adenomas (*NEJM* 2003;348:883 & 891)

Pathology

- **Adenoma → carcinoma sequence** reflects accumulation of multiple genetic mutations ↑ risk of malignancy with large (>2.5 cm), villous, sessile adenomatous polyps
- Lymphovascular invasion and poorly differentiated histology are poor prognostic features
- ~50% of colon tumors are proximal to splenic flexure

Clinical manifestations

- Distal colon: Δ **bowel habits**, **obstruction**, colicky abdominal pain, **hematochezia**
- Proximal colon: **iron deficiency anemia**, dull vague abdominal pain; obstruction atypical due to larger lumen, liquid stool, and polypoid tumors (*vs.* annular distal tumors)
- Metastases: nodes, **liver**, lung, peritoneum → RUQ tenderness, ascites, supraclavicular LN
- Associated with *Streptococcus bovis* bacteremia and *Clostridium septicum* sepsis

Screening (*NEJM* 2002;346:40)

- **Fecal occult blood test** (FOBT): ↓ mortality in RCTs (e.g., *NEJM* 1993;328:1365)
- **Endoscopy**
  flexible sigmoidoscopy shown to ↓ distal CRC mortality (*NEJM* 1992;326:653)
  colonoscopy examines entire colon; ~½ of Pts w/ advanced proximal neoplasms have no distal polyps (*NEJM* 2000;343:162 & 169)
- Imaging: double-contrast barium enema (DCBE) less sensitive than colonoscopy; virtual colonoscopy is being studied (*NEJM* 2003;349:2191)
- **Average risk**, age >50: q5 yr flex sig + q1 yr FOBT *or* q10 yr colonoscopy *or* q5 yr DCBE
- ↑ **risk**: earlier (at age 40 if ⊕ FHx) and/or more frequent screening based on risk factor

Diagnostic and staging evaluation

- **Colonoscopy** + biopsy/polypectomy: best test for dx & examining entire colon for staging
- LFTs, CXR
- Abdomen/pelvis CT: inaccurate for assessing depth of invasion and malignant lymph nodes
- **Intraoperative staging** is essential for evaluating extracolonic spread
- Tumor markers: baseline **CEA** in a *patient with known CRC* has prognostic significance and is useful to follow response to therapy and detect recurrence; *not* a screening tool

Treatment based on TNM and Modified Dukes Staging of Colorectal Cancer

Stage		Criteria	5-year survival	Treatment
TNM	Dukes			
I	A	Into submucosa	95%	Surgery alone
I	B1	Into muscularis	90%	
IIA	B2	Into serosa	80%	Surgery; no established role for adjuvant chemotherapy*
IIB	B2	Direct invasion	70%	
IIIA/B	C	≤4 ⊕ lymph nodes	65%	Surgery + chemotherapy* (**5-FU + leucovorin**)
IIIC	C	≥4 ⊕ lymph nodes	35%	
IV	D	Distant metastases	5%	Chemotherapy (5-FU + leucovorin ± irinotecan; *NEJM* 2000;343:905) ± palliative surgery†

*For stage II or III **rectal cancer**, adjuvant treatment = **combined chemoradiation**
† Surgical resection of **isolated liver or lung metastases** may prolong survival

• PANCREATIC CANCER •

Epidemiology and risk factors
- 4th leading cause of cancer death in U.S. men and women
- ~30,700 new cases and ~30,000 deaths/yr
- Acquired risk factors: **smoking**, obesity, chronic pancreatitis, ? diabetes mellitus
- Hereditary risk factors: genetic susceptibility may play a role in 5-10% of cases
  Hereditary chronic pancreatitis: mutation in cationic trypsinogen gene
  Familial cancer syndromes and gene mutations with ↑ risk: Peutz-Jeghers (LKB1), familial atypical multiple mole melanoma syndrome (p16), and ataxia-telangiectasia (ATM); hereditary colorectal cancer and BRCA2 mutations may also ↑ risk

Clinical manifestations
- **Pain** (radiating to back), **weight loss**, *painless* **jaundice** (w/ head of pancreas mass)
- New-onset atypical diabetes mellitus; unexplained pancreatitis
- Migratory thrombophlebitis (Trousseau's sign)
- Physical exam: abdominal mass; nontender, palpable gallbladder (Courvoisier's sign); hepatomegaly; ascites; left supraclavicular (Virchow's) node; palpable rectal shelf
- Laboratory tests may show ↑ bilirubin, ↑ Aϕ, anemia

Diagnostic and staging evaluation
- **CT scan** is test of choice in patient with suspected pancreatic mass
  if no lesion seen→ EUS, ERCP or MRCP may reveal mass or malignant ductal strictures
- Determine **resectability** (see below) → initial staging study is **helical CT with contrast**
  candidates for resection can be further evaluated with MRI, EUS or laparascopy
- Poor surgical candidates or metastatic disease → must establish tissue dx by bx
- Tumor markers: ↑ CA 19-9; may be useful to follow disease postoperatively

Clinical (Radiologic) Staging of Pancreatic Cancer

Stage	Criteria	% at dx
I = Resectable	No extrapancreatic disease Patent SMV-portal vein confluence No involvement of the celiac axis or SMA	15-20%
II = Locally advanced	No distant metastases Venous occlusion or involvement of celiac axis/SMA	40%
III = Metastatic	Typically to liver and peritoneum, occasionally lung	40%

Pathology
- ≥95% of malignant pancreatic neoplasms arise from **exocrine** (ductal or acinar) cells
- ~60% arise in head, 15% in body, 5% in tail; in 20% tumor diffusely involves whole gland

Treatment
- Resectable: surgery ± adjuvant (neoadjuvant or postoperative) therapy
  pancreaticoduodenectomy: **Whipple procedure** = resection of pancreatic head, duodenum, 1st 15 cm of jejunum, CBD and gallbladder + partial gastrectomy
  adjuvant therapy: ? ↑ survival w/ **postoperative 5-FU chemoradiation**
- Locally advanced: **5-FU chemorad** ↑ survival over chemo or XRT alone; ? gemcitabine
- Metastatic: **gemcitabine** improves survival over 5-FU (*J Clin Onc* 1997;15:2403)
- Palliative and supportive care:
  obstructive jaundice or gastric outlet obstruction: endoscopic stenting or surgical bypass
  pain: opiates, celiac plexus neurolysis, radiation therapy
  weight loss: pancreatic enzyme replacement for suspected fat malabsorption

Prognosis
- Resectable: 10-20 month median survival
  Nodal status most important factor: 5-yr survival ~10% if ⊕ *vs.* 25-30% if ⊖
  Other favorable factors: tumor <3 cm, ⊖ margins, well-differentiated tumors
- Locally advanced: 8-12 month median survival
- Metastatic: 3-6 month median survival

• ONCOLOGIC EMERGENCIES •

FEVER AND NEUTROPENIA (FN)

Definitions
- **Fever**: single oral temperature ≥38.3°C (101°F) or ≥38.0°C (100.4°F) for ≥1 hour
- **Neutropenia**: ANC <500 cells/µl or <1000 cells/µl with predicted nadir <500 cells/µl
- Absolute neutrophil count (ANC) = WBC x (% neutrophils + % bands)

Pathophysiology and microbiology
- Predisposing factors: catheters, skin breakdown, mucositis throughout GI tract, obstruction (lymphatics, biliary tract, GI, urinary tract), immune defect associated with malignancy
- Majority of episodes thought to result from seeding of bloodstream by flora in GI tract
- GNRs (especially *P. aeruginosa*) historically most common
- Gram ⊕ infections have recently become more common (60-70% of identified organisms)
- Fungal superinfection common with prolonged neutropenia and antibiotic use

Diagnostic evaluation
- Exam: skin, oropharynx, lung, perirectal area, surgical & catheter sites; avoid DRE
- Labs: CBC with differential, electrolytes, BUN/Cr, LFTs, u/a
- Micro: blood (peripheral & through each indwelling catheter port), urine, & sputum cx; for localizing signs or symptoms → stool, peritoneal, CSF or skin biopsy cultures
- Imaging: CXR; for localizing signs or sx → CNS, sinus, chest, or abdomen/pelvis imaging
- Caveats: neutropenia → impaired inflammatory response → *exam and radiographic findings may be subtle*; absence of neutrophils by Gram stain does not rule out infection

Risk stratification
- Factors that predict lower risk
  - History: age <60, no symptoms, no major comorbidities, cancer in remission, solid tumor, no h/o fungal infection or recent antifungal therapy
  - Exam: temp <39°, no tachypnea, no hypotension, no Δ MS, no dehydration
  - Studies: ANC >100 cells/µl, anticipated duration of neutropenia <10 d, normal CXR

Initial antibiotic therapy
- Any empiric regimen should include a drug with **anti-pseudomonal activity**
- PO abx can be used in low-risk Pts: cipro + amoxicillin-clavulanate (*NEJM* 1999;341:305 & 312)
- IV antibiotics: no clearly superior regimen; monotherapy or 2-drug regimens can be used
  - Monotherapy: ceftazidime, cefepime, imipenem-cilastatin or meropenem
  - 2-drug therapy: aminoglycoside + anti-pseudomonal β-lactam
- **Vancomycin** added in selected cases (e.g., hypotension, suspected catheter-related infection, severe mucositis, colonization with MRSA, h/o quinolone prophylaxis) discontinue when cultures ⊖ x 48 hr

Modifications to initial antibiotic regimen
- Low-risk patients who become afebrile within 3-5 d can be switched to PO antibiotics
- Abx are optimized for ⊕ cultures; however, *broad spectrum coverage must be maintained*
- Empiric antibiotics are changed for fever >3-5 d with progressive disease
- Antifungal therapy is added for fever >5-7 d without expected imminent ↑ ANC amphotericin B or voriconazole (*NEJM* 2002;346:225)

Duration of therapy
- Known source: complete at least standard course (i.e., 14 d for *S. aureus* bacteremia)
- No known source: ideally continue antibiotics until afebrile *and* ANC >500 cells/µl
  - Afebrile and ANC >500 for 48 h: stop antibiotics; some recommend minimum 7 d course
  - Afebrile but ANC <500: stop antibiotics after afebrile for 14 d and reassess
  - Febrile but ANC >500: stop antibiotics 4-5 d after ANC reaches >500 and reassess
  - Febrile and ANC <500: reassess after 14 d abx; stop if stable with no identifiable disease

Role of hematopoietic growth factors (*J Clin Onc* 2000;18:3558)
- Granulocyte (G-CSF) and granulocyte-macrophage (GM-CSF) colony-stimulating factors can be used as 1° prophylaxis when expected FN incidence >40% or as 2° prophylaxis after FN has occurred in a previous cycle (to maintain dose-intensity for curable tumors)
- Colony-stimulating factors can be considered as adjuvant therapy in high-risk FN patients

Spinal Cord Compression

Pathophysiology
- Metastases located in vertebral body extend and cause epidural spinal cord compression

Clinical manifestations
- **Prostate**, **breast**, and **lung** cancer are the most common causes, followed by renal cell carcinoma, NHL and myeloma
- Site of involvement: **thoracic** (70%), lumbar (20%), cervical (10%)
- Signs and symptoms: **pain** (96%), **weakness**, **autonomic dysfunction** (urinary retention, ↓ anal sphincter tone), **sensory loss**

Diagnostic evaluation
- Always take back pain in patients with solid tumors very seriously
- Do *not* wait for neurologic signs to develop before initiating evaluation b/c duration & severity of neurologic dysfunction before Rx are best predictors of neurologic outcome
- **Urgent MRI is the study of choice**

Treatment
- **Dexamethasone** (10 mg IV followed by 4 mg IV or PO q6 hrs)
  initiate immediately while awaiting imaging if patient has back pain + neurologic deficits
- Emergent radiation or surgical decompression if spinal cord compression is confirmed

Tumor Lysis Syndrome

Definition
- Large tumor burden or a rapidly proliferating tumor → spontaneous or chemotherapy-induced release of intracellular electrolytes and nucleic acids

Clinical manifestations
- Most common with treatment of high-grade lymphomas (**Burkitt's**) and leukemias (**ALL**); rare with solid tumors; rarely due to spontaneous necrosis
- Electrolyte abnormalities: ↑ K, ↑ uric acid, ↑ PO_4 → ↓ Ca
- **Renal failure** (urate nephropathy)

Treatment
- If anticipated → prophylaxis with allopurinol and hydration for ≥2 days prior to treatment
- Allopurinol + aggressive IV hydration ± diuretics to ↑ UOP
- ± Alkalinization of urine w/ $NaHCO_3$ (e.g., 3 amps $NaHCO_3$ in 1 L of D_5W) to ↑ solubility of uric acid and ↓ risk of urate nephropathy
- Treat hyperkalemia, hyperphosphatemia, and hypocalcemia as indicated
- Hemodialysis may be necessary

• PEFORMANCE STATUS •

ECOG Performance Status	
Score	**Definition**
0	Fully active, able to carry on all predisease performance without restriction
1	Slightly impaired but able to carry out light or sedentary work
2	Up and about >50% of waking hours; capable of all self-care
3	Confined to bed or chair >50% of waking hours; only limited self-care
4	Totally confined to bed or chair; cannot carry on any self-care

• PNEUMONIA •

Microbiology of Pneumonia	
Clinical Setting	**Etiologies**
Community-acquired (*NEJM* 2002;347:2039)	***S. pneumoniae*** *Mycoplasma, Chlamydia,* viral (espec. in young & healthy) *H. influenzae, M. catarrhalis* (espec. in COPD'ers) *Legionella* (espec. in elderly, smokers, ↓ immunity) *Klebsiella* & other GNR (especially in alcoholics & aspirators) *S. aureus* (espec. post-viral infection) (no organism identified in 40-60% cases)
Hospital-acquired	GNR including *Pseudomonas, Klebsiella, Enterobacter, Serratia, Acinetobacter,* and *S. aureus*
Immunocompromised	*All of the above* + PCP, fungi, *Nocardia,* atypical mycobacteria, CMV, HSV
Aspiration (*NEJM* 2001;334:665)	*Pneumonitis* due to aspiration of sterile gastric contents *Pneumonia* due to inhalation of oropharyngeal microbes outpatients = typical oral flora (*Strep, Staph,* anaerobes) inpatients or chronically ill = GNR and *S. aureus*

Clinical manifestations

- "Typical": acute onset of fever, cough productive of purulent sputum, consolidation on CXR
- "Atypical": insidious onset of dry cough, extrapulmonary symptoms (nausea, vomiting, diarrhea, headache, myalgias, sore throat), patchy interstitial pattern on CXR
- Although distinction used clinically, differences do *not* reliably implicate "typical" (*S. pneumoniae, H. influenzae*) vs. "atypical" (*Mycoplasma, Chlamydia*) pathogens

Diagnostic studies

- **Sputum gram stain**: utility debated, but sens. up to 85% if well-performed
  Is it a good sample (i.e., sputum or spit)? → should be <10 squamous epithelial cells/lpf
  Is it a purulent sample? → should be >25 PMNs/lpf
- **Sputum culture**: (sample should be transported to laboratory w/in 1-2 hrs of collection)
- Blood cultures (*before antibiotics!*): ⊕ in ~10% of hospitalized patients
- **CXR** (PA and lateral); effusions should be tapped
- $\mathbf{S_aO_2}$ or P_aO_2
- Other laboratory evaluation: CBC with differential, electrolytes, BUN/Cr, glucose, LFTs
- Special microbiologic studies:
  previous tests for *Mycoplasma* (cold agglutinins, sens. 30-60%), *Chlamydia* (acute and convalescent titers), and *Legionella* (urine Ag, sens. <70%) now being replaced by *PCR*
  MTb: sputum for acid-fast stain and mycobacterial cx *and patient in respiratory isolation*
  HIV ⊕ or known immunosuppression: induced sputum for PCP
  viruses: nasal washings or swabs for EIA or DFA
  HIV test if Pt 15-54 yrs and hospital has >1 new HIV dx per 1000 discharges
- Bronchoscopy: consider if Pt immunosuppressed, critically ill, or failing to respond, or if suspect MTb or PCP and need adequate samples, or if Pt has had a chronic pneumonia

P.O.R.T. Score, Prognosis, and Recommended Triage			
Class	**Score**	**Mortality**	**Suggested Triage**
I	age <50, no comorbidities	<1.0%	Outpatient
II	≤70	<1.0%	Outpatient
III	71-90	2.8%	? Brief inpatient
IV	91-130	8.2%	Inpatient
V	>130	29.2%	ICU
Variables	**Points**		
Demograph.	Men (age in yrs), women (age - 10), nursing home resident (+10)		
Coexist. probs	Neoplasm (+30), liver disease (+20), CHF (+10), CVA (+10), renal disease (+10)		
Exam	Δ MS (+20), RR >30 (+20), SBP <90 (+20), Temp <35° or >40° (+15), HR >125 (+10)		
Laboratory	pH <7.35 (+30), BUN >30 (+20), Na <130 (+20), glc >250 (+10), Hct <30 (+10), P_aO_2 <60 or S_aO_2 <90 (+10), pleural effusion (+10)		

(*NEJM* 1997;336:243)

Treatment	
Clinical scenario	**Empiric treatment guidelines**
Outpatient	Macrolide *or* anti-pneumococcal FQ *or* doxycycline
Community-acquired, hospitalized	[3rd gen. ceph. ± macrolide] *or* broad-spectrum FQ
Community-acquired, hospitalized, ICU	[3rd gen. ceph. *or* broad-spectrum FQ] + macrolide
Hospital-acquired	[Anti-pseudomonal penicillin *or* 3rd gen. ceph.] and [anti-pseudomonal aminoglycoside (AG) *or* FQ] + macrolide *if* suspect *Legionella* + vancomycin *if* suspect MRSA
Immunocompromised	As above + TMP-SMX ± steroids to cover PCP
Aspiration, outpatient	FQ
Aspiration, inpatient	FQ or 3rd gen. Ceph.
Route of therapy	Inpatients should initially be treated with IV antibiotics Δ to PO when clinically responding and able to take PO's

(When possible, organism-directed therapy, guided by *in vitro* susceptibilities or local patterns of drug resistance should be utilized. *CID* 2000:31:347. For ventilator-associated pneumonia, 8 ≈ 15 d of Rx, except for *Pseudomonas* and other non-fermenting GNR; *JAMA* 2003;290:2588)

Prognosis (also see PORT score above)
- Patients usually stabilize in 2-3 d (*JAMA* 1998;279:1452)
- For low-risk Pts, can discharge immediately after switching to PO abx (*Chest* 1998;113:142)
- CXR resolves in 50% by 2 wks, in 75% by 6 wks; important to document complete resolution to r/o underlying malignancy

FUNGAL INFECTIONS

Histoplasmosis
- Epidemiology: central & SE U.S. (especially in areas w/ bird & bat droppings)
- Clinical manifestations
  acute pulmonary: often subclinical; granulomas, calcification & scarring
  chronic pulmonary: ↑ productive cough, wt loss, night sweats, infiltrates, cavitation
  acute disseminated (immunocompromised): fever, HSM w/ hepatitis, LAN, oral ulcers
- Treatment: itraconazole; amphotericin if severe or disseminated

Coccidioidomycosis
- Epidemiology: SW U.S. (San Joaquin or Valley fever)
- Clinical manifestations
  acute pulmonary: often subclinical; pleural effusion; granulomas, calcification & scarring
  chronic pulmonary: cough, hemoptysis, fever, night sweats, wt loss
  chronic disseminated (in immunocompromised, pregnant, & diabetics): fever, malaise, hilar adenopathy, bone, skin, & meningeal involvement
- Treatment of disseminated or high-risk 1° pulmonary: itraconazole; amphotericin if severe

Blastomycosis
- Epidemiology: south central U.S.
- Clinical manifestations
  acute pulmonary: often subclinical
  chronic disseminated: fever, wt loss, verrucous, ulcerated skin lesions, bone involvement
- Treatment: itraconazole; amphotericin if severe

Aspergillus (*Chest* 2002;121:1988)
- **Saprophytic**: colonize diseased bronchial tree
- **ABPA**: see "Interstitial Lung Disease"
- **Hypersensitivity pneumonitis**: see "Interstitial Lung Disease"
- **Aspergilloma**: usually in Pts w/ pre-existing cavity (from TB, etc.); most asx, but can lead to hemoptysis; sputum cx ⊕ in <50%; CT → mobile intracavitary mass with air crescent
  Rx: anti-fungals w/o benefit; embolization or surgery for persistent hemoptysis
- **Necrotizing tracheitis**: white necrotic pseudomembranes in Pts w/ AIDS
- **Chronic necrotizing (semi-invasive)**: seen in Pts w/ COPD or mild immunosuppression present w/ sputum, fever, wt loss over months; CT shows infiltrate ± fungus ball ± pleural thickening; lung bx → invasion; Rx = amphotericin or voriconazole
- **Invasive**: seen if immunocompromised (neutropenia, s/p transplant, glucocorticoid Rx, AIDS); clinical: s/s pneumonia including *chest pain* and *hemoptysis*; CT shows nodules, halo sign, air crescent sign; BAL spec. but not sens.; lung bx if prior testing inconclusive
  Rx: amphotericin or voriconazole

• URINARY TRACT INFECTIONS (UTI) •

Definitions

- Anatomic
  - **lower**: urethritis, cystitis (superficial infection of bladder), prostatitis
  - **upper**: pyelonephritis (inflammatory process of the renal parenchyma), renal abscess
- Clinical
  - **uncomplicated**: cystitis in nonpregnant women w/o underlying structural or neurological disease
  - **complicated**: upper tract infection in women *or* any UTI in men or pregnant women *or* UTI with underlying structural or neurological disease

Microbiology

- Uncomplicated UTI: ***E. coli*** (80%), *Proteus, Klebsiella, S. saprophyticus*
- Complicated UTI: *E. coli* (30%), enterococci (20%), *Pseudomonas* (20%), *S. epidermidis* (15%), other GNR
- Catheter-associated UTI: **yeast** (30%), *E. coli* (25%), other GNR, enterococci, *S. epi*
- Urethritis: *Chlamydia trachomatis, Neisseria gonorrhoeae*

Clinical manifestations

- **Cystitis**: **dysuria, urgency, ↑ frequency**, Δ in urine color/odor, suprapubic pain; fever generally *absent*
- **Urethritis**: may be identical to cystitis except for *urethral discharge*
- **Prostatitis**: similar to cystitis except *symptoms of obstruction* (hesitancy, weak stream)
- **Pyelonephritis**: fever, shaking chills, flank or back pain, nausea, vomiting, diarrhea
- **Renal abscess** (intrarenal or perinephric): identical to pyelonephritis except *persistent fever despite appropriate antibiotics*

Diagnostic studies

- **Urinalysis: pyuria + bacteriuria** ± hematuria
  - significant bacterial counts: $\geq 10^5$ CFU/ml in asymptomatic women, $\geq 10^3$ CFU/ml in men, $\geq 10^2$ CFU/ml in symptomatic or catheterized patients
  - sterile pyuria → urethritis, renal tuberculosis, foreign body
- **Urine gram stain and cx** (from clean-catch midstream or straight-cath specimen)
- Pregnant women & those undergoing urologic surgery *screen for asymptomatic bacteriuria*
- Blood cultures: consider in complicated UTIs
- DNA detection/cx for *C. trachomatis/N. gonorrhoeae* in sexually active Pts or sterile pyuria
- First-void and midstream urine specimens, prostatic expressate, and post-prostatic massage urine specimens in cases of suspected prostatitis
- Abdominal CT to rule-out abscess in patients with pyelo who fail to defervesce after 72 hrs
- Urologic workup (renal U/S, abdominal CT, voiding cystography) if recurrent UTIs in men

Treatment of UTIs

Clinical scenario	Empiric treatment guidelines
Cystitis	TMP-SMX *or* FQ PO × 3 d (uncomplic.) or × 10-14 d (complicated) Asymptomatic bacteriuria in pregnant women or prior to urologic surgery → antibiotics × 3 d
Urethritis	Treat for both *Neisseria* and *Chlamydia* *Neisseria:* ceftriaxone 125 mg IM × 1 *or* levofloxacin 500 mg PO × 1 *Chlamydia:* doxy 100 mg PO × 7 d *or* azithromycin 1 g PO × 1
Prostatitis	TMP-SMX *or* FQ PO × 14-28 d (acute) or 6-12 wks (chronic)
Pyelonephritis	Outpatient: FQ *or* amoxicillin/clav *or* 1st gen. ceph. PO × 14 d Inpatient: [amp IV + gent] *or* ampicillin/sulbactam *or* FQ × 14 d (Δ IV → PO when Pt improved clinically and afebrile × 24-48 hrs and then complete 14 d course)
Renal abscess	Drainage + antibiotics as for pyelonephritis

(When possible, organism-directed therapy, guided by *in vitro* susceptibilities or local patterns of drug resistance should be utilized.)

• SOFT TISSUE AND BONE INFECTIONS •

CELLULITIS

Definition
- Infection of superficial and deep dermis and subcutaneous fat

Microbiology (*NEJM* 2004;350:904)
- *Streptococcus* and *Staphylococcus* (less commonly a cause)
- Dog bite: *P. multocida, C. canimorsus, Fusobacterium, Bacteroides*
- Penetrating injury: *Pseudomonas*
- Fish spine: *E. rhusiopathiae, V. vulnificus*

Clinical manifestations
- Erythema, edema, warmth, pain (rubor, tumor, calor, dolor)
- ± Lymphadenitis (proximal red streaking) and regional lymphadenopathy

Diagnosis
- Largely clinical diagnosis; needle aspiration and blood cultures have yield <5%

Treatment
- **Antibiotics** (1st gen. ceph. or penicillinase-resistant penicillin; erythromycin if allergic) + **limb elevation** (erythema may get *worse* after initiation of abx b/c bacterial killing → release of inflammatory enzymes)

"DIABETIC FOOT"

Definition
- Infected neuropathic foot ulcer
  mild = superficial, no bone or joint involvement
  limb or life-threatening = deep, bone/joint involvement, systemic tox., limb ischemia

Microbiology
- Mild: usually *S. aureus* or aerobic streptococci
- Limb or life-threatening: *polymicrobial* with aerobes + anaerobes
  aerobes = staphylococci, streptococci, enterococci, and GNR (including *Pseudomonas*)
  anaerobes = anaerobic streptococci, *Bacteroides, Clostridium* (rare)

Clinical manifestations
- Ulcer with surrounding erythema and warmth ± purulent drainage
- Tenderness may be absent due to neuropathy
- ± Crepitus (indicating gas and ∴ mixed infection w/ GNR & anaerobes or *Clostridium*)
- ± Underlying osteomyelitis
- ± Systemic toxicity (fever, chills, leukocytosis, hyperglycemia)

Diagnostic studies
- Superficial swabs from ulcers *not* helpful (only yield superficial colonizing organisms)
- Wound cx (e.g., curettage at base of ulcer after débridement) has ↑ sens. for pathogens
- Blood cultures (should be obtained in all patients, ⊕ in 10-15%)
- **Osteomyelitis should always be ruled out** (see below for specific imaging tests)
  probing to bone (ability to reach bone via ulcer/tract) has high spec. but low sens.
  bone biopsy specimens are most reliable

Treatment (*NEJM* 1994;331:854)
- Bedrest, elevation, non-weight-bearing status
- Antibiotics

Severity of infection	Empiric antibiotics
Mild	1st gen. ceph. *or* penicillinase-resistant penicillin
Limb-threatening	[FQ + clindamycin] *or* ampicillin-sulbactam *or* ticarcillin-clavulanate *or* cefoxitin *or* cefotetan
Life-threatening	Imipenem *or* [vancomycin + aztreonam + metronidazole] *or* [ampicillin-sulbactam + AG]

- **Surgery**: early, aggressive, and repeated surgical débridement; revascularization or amputation may be necessary

Necrotizing Fasciitis

Definition

- Infection and necrosis of superficial fascia, subcutaneous fat, and deep fascia (necrosis of arteries and nerves in subcutaneous fat → gangrene)
- Fournier's gangrene: necrotizing fasciitis of the male genitalia (used by some to describe involvement of male or female perineum)

Epidemiology

- ↑ risk in patients with diabetes, PVD, alcohol abuse, IVDA, immunosuppression, cirrhosis
- Can also affect healthy individuals

Microbiology

- Group I (abd wall/perineum): polymicrobial (anaerobe + facultative anaerobe + GNR)
- Group II (extremities): *Streptococcus pyogenes* ± staphylococci
- Group III: marine *Vibrio* infection

Clinical manifestations

- Most common sites: extremities, abdominal wall, and perineum, but can occur anywhere
- **Cellulitic skin Δs** with poorly defined margins + **rapid spread** + **systemic toxicity**
- **Pain out of proportion** to degree of apparent cellulitis; skin hyperesthetic or anesthetic
- **Bullae formation** (serous → hemorrhagic); darkening of skin to bluish-gray → **cutaneous gangrene** ± **crepitus** or radiographically-visible gas

Diagnostic signs

- Need *high degree of clinical suspicion* because of nonspecific physical exam
- Aspiration of necrotic center; blood cultures; gram stain; ✓ CK for tissue necrosis
- Imaging studies: plain radiographs → soft tissue gas; CT → extent of infection, soft tissue gas; MRI → best tissue contrast
- Clinical diagnosis enough to initiate **urgent surgical exploration**

Treatment

- Definitive treatment is **surgical débridement** of necrotic tissue and fasciotomy
- **Broad antibiotics** to cover skin flora, enterococci, enteric gram negatives, and anaerobes (e.g., clindamycin + penicillin + AG)
- **Hyperbaric oxygen**: useful adjunct, but should not delay definitive surgical treatment

Prognosis

- Generally fatal if untreated; reported mortality 20-50%

Clostridial Myonecrosis (Gas Gangrene)

Definition

- Life-threatening, fulminant clostridial infection of skeletal muscle
- Usually **muscle trauma** + **wound contamination** with clostridial spores
- Occasionally *C. perfringens*, *septicum*, or *histolyticum* + malignancy (heme or GI)

Clinical manifestations

- Incubation period 6 hrs to 2-3 d
- Acute onset with sense of heaviness or pain that rapidly ↑'s with marked systemic toxicity
- Bronze discoloration of skin, tense bullae, serosanguinous or dark fluid and necrotic areas
- **Crepitus** present but not prominent (gas is in muscle) may be obscured by edema

Diagnostic studies

- Gram stain of discharge: **large, gram positive bacilli with blunt ends,** very few polys
- Clostridial bacteremia in ~15%
- Plain radiographs: gas dissecting into muscle

Treatment

- **Surgical exploration with débridement** of involved muscles, fasciotomies, and amputation if necessary
- **Antibiotics**: high-dose **penicillin G** 24 MU IV divided q 2-3 hrs + **clinda** 900 mg IV q 8 h
- ? Hyperbaric oxygen

OSTEOMYELITIS

Definition

- Infection of bone due to hematogenous seeding or direct spread from contiguous focus

Microbiology (*NEJM* 1997;336:999)

- Hematogenous: ***S. aureus;*** mycobacterial infection of vertebral body = Pott's disease
- Contiguous focus due to an open fracture, orthopedic surgery, etc.: ***S. aureus*** and ***S. epi***
- Contiguous focus + vascular insufficiency (e.g., diabetic foot): **polymicrobial** (aerobic+ anaerobic GPC and GNR)

Clinical manifestations

- Surrounding soft-tissue compromise ± fistula to superficial skin
- Vertebral osteomyelitis (common manifestation in adults over 50 yrs): back pain + fever
- ± Fever, malaise, and night sweats (more common in hematogenous than contiguous)

Diagnostic studies

- Identification of the causative organism is key
- **Culture data from tissue** (surgical sampling/needle biopsy) *not* swabs of ulcers/fistulae
- **Blood cultures** (more often ⊕ with acute hematogenous osteomyelitis)
- Imaging
  plain radiographs: normal early in disease; lytic lesions seen after 2-6 wks
  CT: can demonstrate periosteal reaction and cortical and medullary destruction
  MRI: can detect very early changes
  radionuclide imaging: very sens. but not spec. (false ⊕ if soft-tissue inflammation)

Treatment

- **Antibiotics** (based on cx data) × 4-6 wks
- **Surgery** should be considered for any of the following: acute osteo that fails to respond to medical therapy; chronic osteo; complications of pyogenic vertebral osteo (e.g., cord compression, spinal instability, epidural abscess); or infected prosthesis

EPIDURAL ABSCESS

Etiology

- Hematogenous spread (2/3): skin infection, soft tissue (dental abscess), or endocarditis
- Direct extension (1/3): vertebral osteomyelitis, sacral decubitus ulcer, spinal anesthesia or surgery, lumbar puncture
- Risk factors: diabetes, renal failure, alcoholism, IVDA, immunosuppression
- ***S. aureus*** most common pathogen

Clinical manifestations

- **Back pain** (midline or radicular) + **fever** + **progressive weakness**

Diagnostic studies

- **MRI**
- Blood cultures ⊕ in <25%

Treatment

- **Antibiotics + surgery** (decompressive laminectomy and débridement)

• MENINGITIS •

Acute Bacterial Meningitis

Definition
- Bacterial infection of the subarachnoid space

Microbiology in Adult Meningitis	
Etiology	**Comments**
S. pneumoniae (30-50%)	Most common cause in adults. Look for distant infection (e.g., Osler's triad = meningitis, pneumonia, endocarditis). Drug-resistant *S. pneumoniae* (DRSP): ~40% PCN-resistant (15% intermed.; 15-20% high) ~10% 3rd gen. ceph.-resistant (5% intermed.; <5% high) *even intermed. resistance problematic for Rx of meningitis*
N. meningitidis (10-35%)	Primarily in children and young adults; may be associated with petechiae or purpura. Deficiencies in terminal complement predispose to recurrent meningococcemia &, rarely, meningitis.
H. influenzae (<5%)	↓ incidence in children because of *H. influenzae* type b vaccine. Look for predisposing factors in adults (e.g., CSF leak, recent neurosurgical procedure, trauma, mastoiditis).
L. monocytogenes (5-10%)	Seen in elderly, alcoholics, or patients with malignancy, immunosuppression, or iron overload. Outbreaks associated with contaminated milk, cheese, coleslaw, raw vegetables. Despite name, often associated with *poly-predominant* pleocytosis.
GNRs (1-10%)	Usually nosocomial or post-procedure or in elderly or immunosuppressed.
Staphylococci (5%)	Seen with indwelling CSF shunt (*S. epidermidis*) or following neurosurgery or head trauma (*S. aureus*).
Mixed infection	Suspect parameningeal focus.

Clinical manifestations (*NEJM* 1993;328:21)
- **Fever** (95%)
- **Headache, stiff neck** (88%), and **photosensitivity**
- **Δ MS** (78%) including delirium, ↓ consciousness, confusion, lethargy; **seizures** (23%)
- Presentation may be *atypical* in elderly, with primarily lethargy and confusion, and no fever

Physical exam
- **Nuchal rigidity** (sens. 30%), **Kernig's sign** (Pt supine, hip flexed at 90°, knee flexed at 90°; ⊕ if passive extension of knee results in resistance), **Brudzinski's sign** (Pt supine and limbs supine; ⊕ if passive neck flexion → involuntary hip and/or knee flexion); note, Kernig's and Brudzinski's signs ⊕ in only ~5% of Pts (*CID* 2002;35:46)
- ± Focal neuro findings (28%; hemiparesis, aphasia, visual field cuts, cranial nerve palsies)
- ± Fundoscopic findings: papilledema, absent venous pulsations
- ± Rash: macular-papular, petechial, or purpuric

Diagnostic studies
- **Blood cultures**
- *Consider* **head CT** to r/o mass effect before LP *if* presence of high-risk feature (age >60 yrs, immunocompromised, h/o CNS disease, recent seizure, Δ MS, focal neuro findings); absence of all these has NPV 97%; however, should be noted that in Pts w/ mass effect herniation may occur even w/o LP and may not occur even w/ LP (*NEJM* 2001;345:1727)
- **Lumbar puncture**: CSF gram stain has 60-90% sens. and culture has 70-85% sens.
  opening pressure >25 cm carries risk of herniation, ∴ remove only CSF in manometer,
    infuse IV mannitol 20% solution (0.25-0.5 g/kg) over 20-30 min, consult neurosurgery

CSF Findings in Meningitis					
Condition	**Appearance**	**Pressure (cm)**	**WBC/mm^3** ***predom type***	**Glc (mg/dl)**	**TP (mg/dl)**
Normal	clear	9-18	0-5 *lymphs*	50-75	15-40
Bacterial	cloudy	18-30	100-10,000 *polys*	<45	100-1000
TB	cloudy	18-30	<500 *lymphs*	<45	100-200
Fungal	cloudy	18-30	<300 *lymphs*	<45	40-300
Aseptic	clear	9-18	<300 *polys* $\rightarrow$ *lymphs*	50-100	50-100

- Additional CSF studies depending on clinical suspicion: acid-fast smear and culture, India ink preparation, cryptococcal antigen (CRAg), fungal culture, PCR (e.g., of HSV), cytology

Fig. 1-1. Nomogram for estimating probability of acute bacterial (ABM) *vs.* acute viral (AVM) meningitis

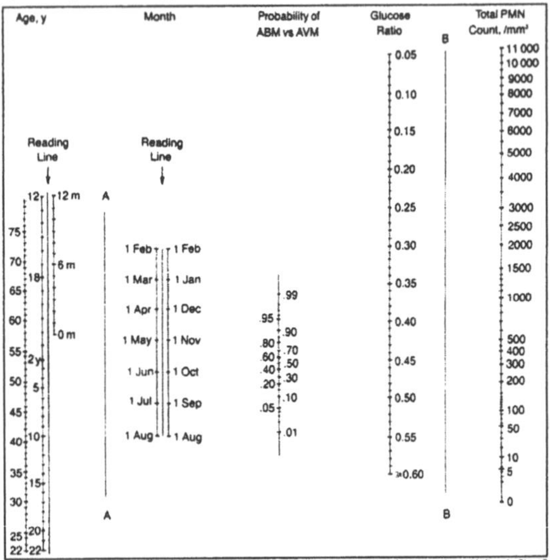

(Step 1, place ruler on reading lines for Pts age and month of presentation and mark intersection with line A. Step 2, place ruler on values for glc and total PMN count in CSF and mark intersection with line B. Step 3, use ruler to join marks on lines A and B, then read probability of ABM vs. AVM. Used with permission from Spanos, A., Harrell, F.E. Jr., Durack, D.T. Differential diagnosis of acute meningitis. *JAMA* 262:2700, 1989. © 1989, AMA.)

Treatment of Meningitis	
Clinical scenario	**Empiric treatment guidelines**
Normal adult	**Ceftriaxone 2 g IV q 12 hrs + Vancomycin 1 g IV q 12 hrs** (n.b., Cftx in case PCN-resistant *S. pneumo*; Vanco, which has poorer CSF penetration, in case Cftx-resistant *S. Pneumo*) + Ampicillin 2 g IV q 4 hrs if suspect *Listeria* Chloramphenicol + TMP/SMX + vancomycin if β-lactam allergic
Immuno-compromised	Ampicillin + ceftazidime ± vancomycin +acyclovir
CSF shunts, recent neurosurgery, or head trauma	Vancomycin + ceftazidime
Empiric antibiotics should be started as soon as possible. If concerned about ↑ ICP, obtain BCx → start empiric abx → obtain head CT → LP (if not contraindicated); yield of CSF fluid unlikely to be changed if obtained w/in ~4 hrs of initiation of abx.	
Corticosteroids: Dexamethasone 10 mg IV q 6 hrs x 4 d → ↓ neurologic disability & mortality by ~50% particularly w/ *S. pneumo.* (*NEJM* 2002;347:1549)	
Prophylaxis: rifampin (600 mg PO bid × 2 d) or ciprofloxacin (750 mg PO × 1) for close contacts of patient with meningococcal meningitis.	

(When possible, organism-directed Rx, guided by suscept. or local patterns of drug resistance should be used.)

Prognosis
- In-hospital mortality 25% for community-acquired; 35% for nosocomial meningitis

Aseptic Meningitis

Definition
- **Negative bacterial microbiologic data**, CSF pleocytosis *without* poly predominance
- Misnomer as "aseptic" only in sense that less likely to be acute bacterial meningitis, but can be due to both infectious and noninfectious etiologies

Etiologies
- **Viral**: enteroviruses (75%), HIV, HSV (type 2 more common than 1), mumps, lymphocytic choriomeningitis virus, encephalitis viruses, adenovirus, CMV, EBV
- **Parameningeal focus of infection** (e.g., brain abscess, epidural abscess, septic thrombophlebitis of dural venous sinuses, or subdural empyema)
- **Tuberculosis, fungal, spirochetal** (Lyme disease, syphilis, leptospirosis), **rickettsial**, *Coxiella*, *Ehrlichia*
- Partially treated bacterial meningitis
- **Medications**: TMP/SMX, NSAIDs, penicillin, isoniazid
- **Systemic illness**: SLE, sarcoidosis, Behçet's, Sjögren's syndrome, rheumatoid arthritis
- **Neoplasms**: intracranial tumors (or cysts), lymphomatous or carcinomatous meningitis

Empiric treatment
- No abx if suspect viral (cell count <500 w/ >50% lymphs, TP <80-100 mg/dl, normal glc, ⊖ gram stain, not elderly/immunocompromised); o/w start empiric abx, wait for cx data

Viral Encephalitis

Definition
- Viral infection of the brain parenchyma

Etiologies (*Lancet* 2002;359:507)
- **HSV-1**
- **Arboviruses**: Eastern equine, Western equine, West Nile, St. Louis
- **Enteroviruses**: Coxsackie, echo
- Others: CMV, EBV, VZV, HIV, rabies, adenoviruses
- Non-viral etiologies that mimic: abscess, toxo, TB, toxins, vasculitis, subdural hematoma

Clinical manifestations
- **Fever, H/A, Δ MS**, ± seizures and focal neuro findings (latter atypical for viral *meningitis*)

Diagnostic studies
- **Lumbar puncture**: lymphocytic pleocytosis; PCR; ELISA for viral Ags; serologies
- **MRI**

Treatment
- HSV: acyclovir 10 mg/kg IV q 8 hrs (recovery related to promptness of Rx)

• BACTERIAL ENDOCARDITIS •

Definition

- Infection of endothelium of heart (including but not limited to the valves)
- Acute (ABE): infection of normal valves with a virulent organism (e.g., *S. aureus*)
- Subacute (SBE): indolent infection of abnormal valves with a less virulent organism (e.g., *S. viridans*)

Predisposing conditions

- **Abnormal valve**
  high-risk: prior endocarditis, rheumatic valvular disease, aortic valve disease, complex cyanotic lesions, prosthesis (1.5-3% at 12 mos, 3-6% at 5 yrs)
  medium-risk: mitral valve disease (including MVP w/ MR or leaflet thickening), HCMP
- **Abnormal risk of bacteremia**: IVDA, indwelling venous catheters (20% of bacteremias shown to have endocarditis), poor dentition, hemodialysis, diabetes mellitus

Modified Duke Criteria	
Major	**Minor**
• **Sustained bacteremia** by an organism known to cause endocarditis • **Endocardial involvement** document by *either* ⊕ **echocardiogram** (vegetation, abscess, prosthetic dehiscence) *or* **new valvular regurgitation**	• Predisposing condition (see above) • Fever • **Vascular phenomena**: septic arterial or pulmonary emboli, mycotic aneurysms, ICH, Janeway lesions • **Immune phenomena**: ⊕ RF, GN, Osler's nodes, Roth spots • ⊕ **blood cx** not meeting major criteria
Definitive (i.e., highly probable) diagnosis if 2 major, or 1 major + 3 minor, or 5 minor criteria	

(*CID* 2000;30:633)

Microbiology of Endocarditis				
	Native valve endocarditis (NVE)		**Prosthetic valve endocarditis (PVE)**	
Etiology	**non-IVDA**	**IVDA**	**early** (<6 mos post)	**late** (>6 mos post)
S. viridans et al.	**40%**	**10%**	<10%	**35%**
Enterococcus	**10%**	10%	<5%	10%
S. aureus	**30%**	**60%**	**25%**	**20%**
S. epidermidis	5%	<5%	**40%**	**20%**
GNR	5%	**10%**	**10%**	<5%
Other	<5%	<5%	10%	10%
Culture ⊖	5%	<5%	<5%	5%
Culture ⊖ = nutritionally-deficient streptococci, HACEK (*Haemophilus parainfluenzae* & *aphrophilus, Actinobacillus, Cardiobacterium, Eikenella,* and *Kingella*), *Bartonella, Coxiella, Chlamydia, Legionella, Brucella*				

(Adapted from Braunwald, E, ed., *Heart Disease*, 5th ed., 1997.)

Clinical manifestations (*NEJM* 2001;345:1318)

- **Persistent bacteremia**: **fever** (80-90%), anorexia, weight loss, night sweats, fatigue
- **Valvular or perivalvular infection**: new murmur, CHF, conduction abnormalities
- **Septic emboli**: systemic emboli (e.g., to periphery, CNS, kidneys, spleen, or joints), pulmonary emboli (if right-sided), mycotic aneurysm, MI (coronary artery embolism)
- **Immune complex phenomena**: arthritis, glomerulonephritis, ⊕ RF, ↑ ESR

Physical exam

- HEENT: **Roth spots** (retinal hemorrhage + pale center), **petechiae** (conjunctivae, palate)
- Cardiac: **valvular regurgitation** ± thrill (fenestrated valve or ruptured chordae), muffled prosthetic valve sounds, pericardial rub. *Frequent examinations* for changing murmurs.
- Abdomen: tender splenomegaly

- Extremities *(seen in SBE not ABE)*
  Janeway lesions (septic emboli → nontender, hemorrhagic macules on palms or soles)
  Osler's nodes (immune complexes → tender nodules on pads of digits)
  proximal nail bed splinter hemorrhages
  clubbing

Diagnostic studies

- **Blood cultures** (*before initiation of antibiotics*): at least 3 sets (aerobic & anaerobic bottles) from different sites, ideally spaced at least one hour apart. ✓ surveillance blood cultures (at least 2 sets) after appropriate antibiotics have been initiated to document clearance; repeat every 24-48 hrs until ⊖. Recheck at completion of Rx.
- CBC with differential, ESR, rheumatoid factor, BUN, Cr, U/A & UCx
- **ECG** (on admission and at regular intervals): to assess for new conduction abnormalities
- **Echocardiogram**: obtain TTE; TEE if (1) intermediate pretest probability (4-60%), (2) prosthetic valve, (3) TTE non-diagnostic, (4) TTE ⊖ but endocarditis strongly suspected, or (5) suspect progressive or invasive infection (e.g., persistent bacteremia or fever, new conduction abnormality, intracardiac shunt, etc.) (*NEJM* 2001;345:1318)

Method	Sensitivity		
	NVE	PVE	Abscess
Transthoracic (TTE)	~65%	~25%	28%
Transesophageal (TEE)	>90%	~90%	87%

(*Chest* 1991;100:351; *NEJM* 1991;324:795; *JACC* 1991;18:391; *AJC* 1993;71:201)

Treatment

- Obtain culture data first
  ABE → antibiotics should be started promptly after culture data obtained
  SBE → if patient hemodynamically stable, antibiotics may be delayed in order to properly obtain adequate blood culture data, especially in the case of prior antibiotic treatment
- **Suggested empiric therapy**
  native valve ABE: [naf + gent] ***or*** **[vanco + naf + gent] if high prev. of MRSA**
  native valve SBE: penicillin/ampicillin + gentamicin
  prosthetic valve: vancomycin + gentamicin + rifampin
- Adjust antibiotic regimen based on organism and sensitivities
- Repeat blood cultures qd until patient defervesces; usually 2-3 days
- Fever may persist up to one week after appropriate antibiotic therapy instituted
- Systemic anticoagulation relatively *contraindicated* given risk of hemorrhagic transformation of cerebral embolic strokes (however, in absence of cerebral emboli, can continue anticoagulation for pre-existing indication)
- Duration of therapy is usually **4-6 wks** (with the AG used only for the first 2 wks), except in cases of uncomplicated right-sided endocarditis, in which 2 wks of therapy may have comparable outcomes

Indications for surgery

- In general, try to deliver as many days of antibiotics as possible, in hopes of ↓ incidence of recurrent infection in the prosthesis, as well as to improve the structural integrity of the tissue that will receive the prosthesis.
- Cerebral septic embolism often considered *contraindication* to immediate surgery as risk of hemorrhagic conversion during cardiopulmonary bypass high during the first 10-14 days
- Indications for surgery
  refractory CHF (i.e., despite maximal, ICU-level medical therapy)
  persistent or refractory infection (e.g., ⊕ BCx after 1 wk of appropriate IV abx)
  invasive infection (ring abscess, worsening conduction; seen in 15% native, 60% prosthetic)
  prosthetic valve, especially with valve malfunction *or* dehiscence *or S. aureus* infection
  hard to eradicate infections (e.g., *Pseudomonas*, fungi)
  ? recurrent systemic emboli or large (>10 mm) or growing vegetations

Prognosis

- Non-IVDA ABE w/ *S. aureus* → 55-70% survival
- IVDA ABE w/ *S. aureus* → 85-90% survival
- SBE → 85-90% survival

Endocarditis Prophylaxis	
Cardiac conditions	**High risk**: prosthetic valve, previous endocarditis, complex cyanotic CHD, surgically constructed systemic pulmonic shunts or conduits **Moderate risk**: most other CHD, acquired valvular heart disease, bicuspid Ao valve, MVP with leaflet thickening or regurgitation, HCMP
Procedures	**Dental**: extractions, periodontal procedures, implants, root canal, cleanings **Respiratory**: surgery on respiratory mucosa, rigid bronchoscopy **GI**: sclerotherapy, esophageal dilatation, ERCP with biliary obstruction, biliary tract or intestinal surgery **GU**: prostate surgery, cystoscopy, urethral dilatation
Regimens	**Dental, respiratory, or esophageal procedures** amoxicillin 2 g 1 hr before (clindamycin 600 mg if penicillin-allergic) **GI/GU + moderate-risk condition** amoxicillin 2 g 1 hr before or ampicillin 2 g IM/IV within 30 min of procedure (vancomycin 1 g IV if penicillin-allergic) **GI/GU + high-risk condition** ampicillin 2 g IM/IV + gentamicin 1.5 mg/kg within 30 min of procedure followed by ampicillin 1 g IM/IV or amoxicillin 1 g PO 6 hrs later (vancomycin 1 g IV + gentamicin as above if penicillin-allergic)

(*JAMA* 1997;277:1794)

• TUBERCULOSIS •

Epidemiology

- U.S. prevalence 10-15 million people; worldwide prevalence ~1.7 billion people
- ↑ incidence in U.S. from 1984-1992 due to HIV, poverty, homelessness, immigration
- **High-risk populations**
  ↑ risk of exposure: contact with Pt w/ active TB, health care worker at facility w/ TB Pts
  ↑ risk of TB infection: immigrants from high-prevalence areas, homeless or medically underserved, resident or worker in long-term care facility or jail
  ↑ risk of active TB once infected: HIV ⊕ or other immunodeficiencies, chronic renal failure, diabetes mellitus, IVDA, alcoholics, malnourished, malignancy, s/p gastrectomy

Microbiology and natural history

- Transmission of *Mycobacterium tuberculosis* via small-particle aerosols (i.e., droplet nuclei)
- 90% of infected normal hosts will never develop clinically evident TB, 10% will
- Localized disease: healing & calcification *or* progressive 1° TB
- Hematogenous spread: latent infection ± reactivation TB *or* progressive disseminated TB
- Two-thirds of TB is due to reactivation; risk is ~2%/yr for first 2-3 yrs after infection

Screening for prior infection

- **Whom to screen**: high risk populations (HIV ⊕ Pts should have PPD testing as part of initial baseline laboratory evaluation and annually thereafter)
- **How to screen**: Mantoux tuberculin test (i.e., purified protein derivative or PPD) inject 5-TU (0.1 ml) intermediate strength PPD intradermally → wheal; examine 48-72 h
- **How to interpret**: determine maximum diameter of induration by palpation

Size of reaction	Persons considered to have ⊕ test
>5 mm	HIV ⊕ or immunosuppressed (e.g., prednisone 15 mg/d × >1 mo) Close contacts with Pt w/ active TB CXR c/w prior TB
>10 mm	All other high-risk populations Recent conversion (↑ in induration by >10 mm in past 2 yrs)
>15 mm	Everyone else
False ⊖	Faulty application, anergy, acute TB (2-10 wks to convert), acute non-TB infections, malignancy
False ⊕	Improper reading, cross-reaction with atypicals, w/in 2 yrs of BCG vaccination (although usually <10 mm)
Booster effect	↑ induration b/c immunologic boost provided by prior skin test in previously sensitized (i.e., infected) individual. Test goes from ⊖ → ⊕, but does *not* represent true conversion due to *recent* infection. 2nd test is Pt's true baseline. Can be seen 1 yr after initial skin test.

(*NEJM* 2002;347:1860)

- IFN-γ assays may be comparable or even superior (*Lancet* 2001;357:2017 & *JAMA* 2001;286:1740)

Clinical manifestations

- **Primary tuberculous pneumonia**: middle or lower lobe **consolidation**, ± effusion, ± cavitation
- **Tuberculous pleurisy**: can occur with primary or reactivation disease. Due to breakdown of granuloma with spilling of contents into the pleural cavity and local inflammation. **Pulmonary effusion** ± pericardial and peritoneal effusions (tuberculous polyserositis).
- **Reactivation tuberculous pulmonary disease**: apical scarring + cavitation
- **Miliary tuberculosis**: acute or insidious; wide dissemination due to hematogenous spread, usually in immunocompromised, diabetic, alcoholic, or malnourished patients. **Constitutional symptoms** (fever, night sweats, weight loss) are prominent. Pulmonary disease with small millet seed-like lesions (2-4 mm) on CXR.
- **Extrapulmonary tuberculosis**: lymphadenitis, pericarditis, peritonitis, meningitis, nephritis, osteomyelitis (vertebral = Pott's disease), hepatitis, cutaneous.
- **Tuberculosis and HIV infection**: HIV-infected and other immunosuppressed patients are at increased risk for reactivation and progressive uncontrolled primary infection.

Diagnostic studies of active TB *(high index of suspicion is key!)*

- **Acid-fast smear** (rapid diagnosis) and **culture** (more sensitive and allows susceptibility testing) of sputum, bronchoscopic alveolar lavage, pleura, or other clinical specimens.
- PCR: 94-97% sens. when compared to smear; 40-77% sens. when compared to culture
- CXR: fibrocavitary apical disease in reactivation; middle & lower lobe consolidation in 1° TB

Preventive therapy

- **Rule out active disease** in any Pt w/ suggestive signs or symptoms, before starting INH
- Appropriate prophylaxis reduces incidence of subsequent disease by 65-75%
- Treat Pts who are ⊕ based on screening guidelines listed above

Scenario	Regimen
Likely INH-sensitive	INH 300 mg PO qd + pyridoxine 25 mg po qd × 9 mos
Abnormal CXR or HIV ⊕	INH 300 mg PO qd + pyridoxine 50 mg po qd × 12 mos
Contact case INH-resistant	RIF + PZA × 4 mos
Contact case known or suspected to have multi-drug resistant TB	No proven regimen: ? PZA + ETB, ? PZA + FQ

(INH = isoniazid, RIF = rifampin, PZA = pyrazinamide, ETB = ethambutol, FQ = fluoroquinolone)

- **Monitor for hepatitis**: if aminotransferases 5× normal *or* symptomatic → d/c current anti-TB medications and re-evaluate

Treatment of active tuberculosis (*Lancet* 2003;362:887)

- Isolate patient
- Use regimens containing multiple drugs to which the organism is susceptible
- Promote adherence to therapy; directly-observed therapy (DOT) cost-effective for Pts at high risk for non-adherence

Anti-Tuberculous Medications		
Drug	**Dose**	**Adverse effects**
Isoniazid (INH)	300 mg po qd	Hepatitis, peripheral neuropathy (prevented by concomitant pyridoxine), lupus-like syndrome
Rifampin (RIF)	600 mg po qd	Orange discoloration or urine/tears, hepatitis, GI upset, hypersensitivity, fever
Pyrazinamide (PZA)	25 mg/kg po qd	Hepatitis, hyperuricemia, arthritis
Ethambutol (EMB)	15-25 mg/kg po qd	Optic neuritis
Streptomycin (SM)	15 mg/kg IM qd	Ototoxicity, nephrotoxicity
Amikacin (AMK)	15 mg/kg IM qd	Ototoxicity, nephrotoxicity
Ciprofloxacin (CIP)	750 mg po bid	GI upset

Anti-Tuberculous Regimens	
Scenario	**Regimen**
Pulmonary TB ≥4% INH-resist. in community (includes most of U.S.)	INH + RIF + PZA + (EM or ETB) until suscept. known If *sensitive* to INH & RIF → INH + RIF + PZA × 2 mos, *then* → INH + RIF × 4 mos If *resistant*, see next row
Drug-resistant TB (INH-, RIF-, or multidrug resistant)	*Consult ID specialist*
Extrapulmonary TB	*Consult ID specialist*
TB in HIV ⊕ patient	*Consult ID specialist*

• HIV/AIDS •

Definitions

- AIDS: HIV + CD4 count <200/mm³ or opportunistic infection (OI) or malignancy

Epidemiology

- ~1 million Americans infected with HIV; leading cause of death in 25-44 year old age group
- ~34 million individuals infected worldwide
- Routes: sexual (0.3% for male-to-male, 0.2% for male-to-female, and 0.1% for female-to-male transmission), IVDA, transfusions, needle sticks (0.3%), vertical (15-35%)

Acute retroviral syndrome (ARS)

- Occurs in ~40% of HIV ⊕ patients ~4 wks after infection; ⊖ ELISA, ⊕ viral load
- Manifestations: mononucleosis-like syndrome ± salmon-colored maculo-papular rash

Diagnostic studies

- **ELISA** for HIV-1 Ab: ⊕ 1-12 wks after acute infection; 99% sens. & spec.; 1° screen test
- **Western blot**: ⊕ if ≥2 bands from diff regions of HIV genome; confirmatory after ⊕ ELISA
- **PCR (viral load)**: detects HIV-1 RNA in plasma; 3-4 fold (0.5-0.75 log) Δ considered signif
- **CD4 count**: not a dx test *per se*, as may be HIV ⊕ and have a normal CD4 count or may have a low CD4 count and *not* be HIV ⊕; acute illness may ↑ or ↓ CD4 count

Initial approach to HIV ⊕ patient

- **Document HIV infection** (if adequate documentation is not available, repeat dx studies
- **H & P** (evidence of OIs, malignancies, STDs); **review all meds**
- **Laboratory evaluation**: CD4 count, viral load (use same assay each time), CBC with diff., Cr, LFTs, TB skin test, syphilis, toxoplasmosis, CMV, and hepatitis serologies, baseline CXR, Pap smear in women

Antiretrovirals			
Drug	**Type**	**Dose**	**Adverse Effects**
Zidovudine (AZT) *Retrovir*	NRTI (Group A)	200 mg tid 300 mg bid	**bone marrow suppression** GI intol, HA, insomnia, hepatitis
Stavudine (d4T) *Zerit*	NRTI (Group A)	40 mg bid	**peripheral neuropathy** pancreatitis, hepatitis (rare)
Didanosine (ddI) *Videx*	NRTI (Group B)	200 mg bid	**pancreatitis, peripheral neuro** GI intolerance, hepatitis (rare)
Zalcitabine (ddC) *Hivid*	NRTI (Group B)	0.75 mg tid	**peripheral neuropathy** stomatitis, hepatitis (rare)
Abacavir Ziagen	NRTI (Group B)	300 mg bid	Fatal hypersensitivity 3% lactic acidosis; hepatitis
Lamivudine (3TC) *Epivir*	NRTI (Group B)	150 mg bid	*minimal toxicity* hepatitis (rare)
Nevirapine *Viramune*	NNRTI	200 mg bid	rash, hepatitis *induces* CYP_{450}
Delavirdine *Rescriptor*	NNRTI	400 mg tid	rash, headache *inhibits* CYP_{450}
Efavirenz *Sustiva*	NNRTI	600 mg qhs	CNS effects, rash, hepatitis *mixed inducer/inhibit* of CYP_{450}
Indinavir *Crixivan*	PI	800 mg tid (fasting)	**nephrolithiasis**, GI intol., ↑ LFTs fat redistrib., *inhibits* CYP_{450}
Ritonavir *Norvir*	PI	600 mg bid (with meals)	**GI intol., paresthesias,** ↑ LFTs, DM, fat redistrib., *inhibits* CYP_{450}
Saquinavir *Fortovase*	PI	1200 mg tid (w/ meals)	GI intol., headache, ↑ LFTs, fat redistrib. DM, *inhibits* CYP_{450}
Nelfinavir *Viracept*	PI	1250 mg bid (w/ meals)	diarrhea, DM, fat redistrib. *inhibits* CYP_{450}
Amprenavir *Agenerase*	PI	1200 mg bid	rash, GI intol., fat redistrib. *inhibits* CYP_{450}
Lopinavir/Ritonavir *Kaletra*	PI	3 cap. bid (w/ meals)	GI intol., HA, fat redistrib., pancreatitis, *inhibits* CYP_{450}

(NRTI = nucleoside reverse transcriptase inhibitor; NNRTI = non-nucleoside RTI; PI = protease inhibitor)

- ***Use of antiretrovirals should be done in consultation with an HIV specialist*** as recommendations continue to be in flux and many of these drugs are potent inhibitors or inducers of CYP_{450}, necessitating the discontinuation or redosing of other drugs. Below are merely some guidelines. (*JAMA* 2002;288:222)
- Indications for initiation of therapy (HAART)
  AIDS or **symptomatic HIV** (e.g., thrush, unexplained fevers)
  asymptomatic + high viral load (>10-20,000 copies/ml) *or* **low CD4** (<350/mm^3)
- Regimens: **[PI (± low-dose ritonavir) + 2 NRTI]** *or* [NNRTI + 2 NRTI] *or* 3 NRTI
  monotherapy and dual therapy *not* recommended
  ? addition of *fusion inhibitor* (e.g., enfurvitide) to optimal regimens in Pts w/ drug-resistant HIV (TORO 1 & TORO 2, *NEJM* 2003;348:2175 & 2186)
- Viral load should ↓ 3-4 fold (0.5-0.75 log) w/in 2-8 wks and continue to ↓ thereafter
  goal is undetectable viral load at 6 mos
  6-month CD4 count and viral load predict outcome (*Lancet* 2003;362:679)
- Initiation of antiretrovirals may *transiently worsen* existing OIs for several wks b/c ↑ immune response
- If Rx needs to be interrupted, *stop all antiretrovirals* to minimize development of resistance
- Failing regimen = unable to achieve undetectable viral load, ↑ viral load, ↓ CD4 count, or clinical deterioration (consider resistance testing)

OI Prophylaxis		
OI	**Indication**	**1° Prophylaxis**
Tuberculosis	⊕ PPD (≥5 mm) *or* high-risk exposure (✓ PPD annually)	INH + vitamin B_6 × 9 mos *or* RIF + PZA × 2 mos
PCP	CD4 count <200/mm^3 *or* thrush	TMP-SMX DS or SS qd or DS tiw *or* dapsone 100 mg qd *or* atovaquone 1500 mg qd *or* pentamidine 300 mg q 4 wks
Toxoplasmosis	CD4 count <100/mm^3 *and* ⊕ *Toxoplasma* serology	TMP-SMX DS qd *or* dapsone 200 mg qd + pyrimethamine 75 mg qd + leucovorin 25
MAC	CD4 count <50/mm^3	azithro 1200 mg q wk *or* clarithro 500 mg bid
If OI has occurred, usually require lifelong 2° prophylaxis PCP: same as 1° prophylaxis Toxoplasmosis: sulfadiazine 500-1000 mg qid + pyrimethamine 25-50 mg qd + leucovorin 10-25 mg qd MAC: clarithro 500 mg bid + ethambutol 15 mg/kg qd ± rifabutin 300 mg qd		
1° or 2° prophylaxis for PCP, toxoplasmosis, and MAC may be interrupted if CD4 count above initiation threshold × ≥3 mos while Pt is on HAART.		

(*MMWR* June 14, 2002)

Complications of HIV/AIDS

CD4 count	Complications
<500	Constitutional symptoms Seborrheic dermatitis, oral hairy leukoplakia, Kaposi's sarcoma Oral, esophageal, and recurrent vaginal candidiasis Recurrent bacterial infections Pulmonary and extrapulmonary tuberculosis HSV, VZV
<200	*Pneumocystis carinii* pneumonia (PCP), *Toxoplasma* *Cryptococcus, Histoplasma, Coccidioides* *Bartonella*
<50-100	CMV, MAC Invasive aspergillosis, bacillary angiomatosis (disseminated *Bartonella*) CNS lymphoma, PML

Fever

- Etiologies (*CID* 1999;28:341)
  infections (88%): MAC, CMV, early PCP, TB, histoplasmosis, sinusitis, endocarditis
  lymphoma
  drug reaction
- Workup: CBC, extended chemistries, LFTs, BCx, CXR, UA, review medications, ? ✓ abd CT
  CD4 <200 → serum cryptococcal Ag, LP, urinary *Histo* Ag, mycobacterial isolators, CMV
  pulmonary s/s → CXR; ABG; sputum for bacterial culture, PCP, AFB; bronchoscopy
  diarrhea → stool for fecal leukocytes, culture, O&P, AFB; endoscopy
  abnormal LFTs → abdominal CT, liver biopsy
  cytopenias → bone marrow biopsy

Cutaneous

- Seborrheic dermatitis; eosinophilic folliculitis; HSV and VZV infections
- **Molluscum contagiosum**: 2-5 mm pearly papules with central umbilication
- **Kaposi's sarcoma:** red-purple non-blanching nodular lesions
- **Bacillary angiomatosis** (disseminated *Bartonella*): friable vascular papules

Ophthalmologic

- **CMV retinitis** (CD4 count <50): Rx = ganciclovir, foscarnet, or cidofovir
- *Pneumocystis, Toxoplasma, Histoplasma*

Oral

- Aphthous ulcers
- **Thrush** (oral candidiasis): curdlike patches that reveal raw surface when scraped off
- **Oral hairy leukoplakia**: caused by EBV; *adherent* white coating on *lateral* tongue
- Kaposi's sarcoma

Cardiac

- Dilated cardiomyopathy, pulmonary hypertension

Pulmonary

Radiographic pattern	Common causes
Normal	PCP
Diffuse interstitial infiltrates	PCP, TB, viral and disseminated fungal pneumonias Kaposi's sarcoma
Focal consolidation or masses	Bacterial or fungal pneumonias, TB, Kaposi's sarcoma
Cavitary lesions	TB, aspergillosis and other fungal pneumonias Bacterial pneumonias (including *Nocardia* and *Rhodococcus*)
Pleural effusion	TB, bacterial or fungal pneumonias Kaposi's sarcoma, lymphoma

- ***Pneumocystis carinii* pneumonia (CD4 <200)**
  constitutional symptoms, fever, night sweats, dyspnea on exertion, nonproductive cough
  CXR w/ interstitial pattern, ↓ P_aO_2, ↑ A-a ∇, ↑ LDH, ⊕ PCP sputum stain
  Rx if P_aO_2 >70: **[TMP 5 mg/kg PO tid + dapsone 100 mg PO qd]** *or* TMP-SMX DS 2 tabs PO 8 hrs *or* [clindamycin + primaquine] *or* atovaquone
  Rx if P_aO_2 <70: **prednisone** (40 mg PO bid then ↓ after 5 d; start *before* TMP/SMX; *NEJM* 1990;323:1444 & 1451); **TMP-SMX 15 mg of TMP/kg IV divided q 6-8 hrs** *or* [clindamycin + primaquine] *or* pentamidine *or* trimetrexate

Gastrointestinal

- **Esophagitis**: *Candida*, CMV, HSV, HIV, pill-induced
  upper endoscopy if no thrush or unresponsive to empiric antifungal therapy
- Enterocolitis
  bacterial (usually acute): *Salmonella, Shigella, Campylobacter, Yersinia, C. difficile*
  protozoal (usually chronic): *Giardia, Entamoeba, Cryptosporidium, Isospora, Microsporidium, Cyclospora*
  viral (CMV, adenovirus), MAC, AIDS enteropathy
- **GI bleeding**: CMV, Kaposi's sarcoma, lymphoma
- **Proctitis**: HSV, CMV, *Chlamydia*, gonococcal

Hepatobiliary

- **Hepatitis**: HBV, HCV, CMV, MAC, drug-induced
- **AIDS cholangiopathy**: often in association with CMV or *Cryptosporidium*

Renal

- AIDS nephropathy, heavy proteinuria, echogenic kidneys

Hematologic

- **Anemia**: anemia of chronic disease, bone marrow involvement, drug toxicity, hemolysis
- Leukopenia
- **Thrombocytopenia**: bone marrow involvement, ITP
- ↑ globulin

Oncologic

- **Non-Hodgkin's lymphoma**: ↑ frequency regardless of CD4 count
- **CNS lymphoma**: CD4 count <50
- **Kaposi's sarcoma**: can occur at any CD4 count; caused by HHV-8
  usually occurs in *homosexual men*
  mucocutaneous: red-purple nodular lesions
  pulmonary: bilateral lower lobe infiltrates + effusion
  GI: GI bleeding, obstruction, obstructive jaundice
  Rx: limited disease → XRT, cryo, or intralesional vinblastine; systemic → chemotherapy
- Cervical cancer

Endocrine

- Hypogonadism
- Abnormal thyroid function
- Adrenal insufficiency
- Wasting syndrome
- Lipodystrophy: central obesity, wasting of the extremities, dyslipidemia, hyperglycemia
- Lactic acidosis: nausea, vomiting, abdominal pain; ? mitochondrial toxicity of AZT/NRTI

Neurologic

- **Meningitis**: ***Cryptococcus***, bacterial (incl. *Listeria*), viral (HSV, CMV, HIV), tuberculosis, lymphomatous
- Neurosyphilis: meningitis, cranial nerve palsies, dementia
- **Space-occupying lesions**: may present as headache, focal deficits, or Δ MS
  workup: MRI, stereotactic brain biopsy if suspect non-*Toxoplasma* etiology or if Pt fails to respond to a 2-week trial of empiric toxoplasmosis therapy (of those who ultimately respond, 50% do so by day 3, 86% by day 7, 91% by day 14, *NEJM* 1993;329:995)

Etiology	Appearance	Diagnostic studies
Toxoplasmosis	enhancing lesions (can be multiple)	⊕ *Toxoplasma* serology
CNS lymphoma	enhancing lesion (usually single)	⊕ CSF PCR for EBV ⊕ SPECT or PET scan
Progressive multifocal leukencephalopathy (PML)	multiple non-enhancing lesions	⊕ CSF PCR for JC virus
Other: bacterial abscess, nocardiosis, cryptococcoma, or tuberculoma	variable	biopsy

- **AIDS dementia complex**: memory loss, gait disorder, spasticity
- **Myelopathy**: **infection** (CMV, HSV), **cord compression** (epidural abscess, lymphoma), **vacuolar** (HIV)
- Peripheral neuropathy: HIV, CMV, demyelinating, medication-induced

***Mycobacterium avium* complex (MAC)**

- Clinical manifestations: fever, night sweats, weight loss, lymphadenopathy, abdominal pain, hepatosplenomegaly, diarrhea, pancytopenia
- Treatment: clarithromycin + ethambutol ± rifabutin

Cytomegalovirus (CMV)

- Clinical manifestations: retinitis, esophagitis, colitis, hepatitis, neuropathies
- Treatment: ganciclovir, foscarnet, or cidofovir

• LYME DISEASE •

Microbiology
- Infection with **spirochete** *Borrelia burgdorferi* (5% coinfection w/ *Ehrlichia, Babesia*)
- Transmitted by **ticks** (*Ixodes*); animal hosts include deer and mice
- Infection usually requires **tick attachment >36-48 hrs**

Epidemiology
- Lyme disease most common vector-borne illness, incidence only ~4 per 100,000 pop
- Peak incidence is in the summer months (May-Aug)
- Majority of cases in NY, NJ, CT, RI, CT, MN, WI, PA, VA, OR, CA
- Humans contact ticks usually in fields with low brush near wooded areas

Clinical Manifestations	
Stage	**Manifestations**
Stage 1 = early localized wks after infection	Due to local effects of spirochete *General:* **flu-like illness** *Dermatologic* (~80%): **erythema chronicum migrans** (ECM) = macular, erythematous lesion with central clearing, usually found on thigh, groin or axilla, ranging in size from 6-38 cm; lymphocytomas; regional lymphadenopathy
Stage 2 = early dissem. wks to mos after infection	Due to spirochetemia and immune response *General:* fatigue, malaise, LAN, HA; fever uncommon *Derm:* **multiple (1-100) annular lesions ≈ ECM** *Rheumatologic* (~10%): **migratory arthralgias** (knee & hip) **& myalgias**, oligoarthritis *Neurologic* (~15%): **Bell's palsy** (or other cranial neuropathies), aseptic meningitis, mononeuritis multiplex (may be painful), transverse myelitis *Cardiac* (~8%): **heart block**, myocarditis
Stage 3 = late persistent mos to yrs after infection	Due to chronic infection *or* autoimmune response *Derm:* **acrodermatitis chronica atrophicans,** panniculitis *Rheumatologic* (~60%): joint pain, **recurrent mono- or oligoarthritis of large joints,** synovitis *Neurologic:* subacute encephalomyelitis, polyneuropathy, dementia

(*NEJM* 2001;345:115; *Lancet* 2003;362:1639)

Diagnostic studies
- In general, a *clinical* diagnosis
- **Serology** (in right clinical setting)
  - screen with **ELISA**, but
    - false ⊕ due to other spirochetal diseases, SLE, RA, EBV, HIV, etc.
    - false ⊖ due to early antibiotic therapy
  - confirm ⊕ ELISA results with **Western blot** (↑ specificity)
- CSF examination in Pts with suspected neurologic disease
  - ⊕ intrathecal Ab production if (CSF IgG/serum IgG)/(CSF albumin/serum albumin) >1

Treatment
- Prophylaxis: doxycycline 200 mg po w/in 72 hrs of finding partially-engorged, nymphal tick attached (*NEJM* 2001;345:79)
- Antibiotics: *if* clin. manifestations *and* ⊕ serology (? *and* h/o tick bite if nonendemic area)
  - local or early dissem. w/o neuro or cardiac involvement: **doxycycline** 100 mg PO bid
  - neuro (other than Bell's palsy), cardiac, chronic arthritis, preg.: **ceftriaxone** 2 g IV qd (*NEJM* 1997;337:289)
- Vaccine: 78% ↓ in occurrence of Lyme disease in Pts in endemic areas at risk for exposure (NEJM 1998;339:209); currently unavailable

• FEVER OF UNKNOWN ORIGIN (FUO) •

Definition

- **Fever >101 °F** or **>38.5 °C** on more than one occasion
- Duration ≥3 weeks
- **No diagnosis** despite 1 week of intensive evaluation

Etiologies

- Differential extensive, but following are some of the more common causes
- More likely to be *subtle manifestation of common disease* than an uncommon disease
- If known malignancy: 50% infectious (usually during neutropenia) & 50% tumor itself
- In Pts with HIV: 75% infectious, *rarely due to HIV itself*
- Up to 30% of cases undiagnosed, most spontaneously defervesce

Category	Etiologies
Infection ~30%	**Tuberculosis**: disseminated or extrapulmonary disease can have normal CXR, PPD, sputum AFB; biopsy (lung, liver, bone marrow) for granulomas has 80-90% yield in miliary disease **Endocarditis**: consider HACEK organisms, *Bartonella*, *Legionella*, and *Coxiella* **Intra-abdominal abscess**: hepatic, splenic, subphrenic, pancreatic, perinephric, pelvic, prostatic, appendicitis **Osteomyelitis,** dental abscess, sinusitis CMV, EBV, Lyme disease, malaria, babesiosis, amebiasis
Connective tissue disease ~30%	**Temporal (giant cell) arteritis**: headache, scalp pain, jaw claudication, visual disturbances, ↑ ESR **Adult onset Still's disease** (juvenile rheumatoid arthritis): fevers with evanescent, salmon-colored macular truncal rash during fevers may precede arthritis **Polyarteritis nodosa** RA, SLE, sarcoidosis
Neoplasm ~20%	**Lymphoma**: LAN, HSM, ↓ Hct or plt, ↑ LDH **Renal cell carcinoma**: microscopic hematuria, ↑ Hct **Hepatocellular carcinoma, pancreatic cancer, colon cancer** Atrial myxomas: obstruction, embolism, constitutional symptoms Leukemia, myelodysplasia
Miscellaneous ~20%	Drugs, factitious, hematoma, thyroid, adrenal insufficiency Familial Mediterranean fever: mutation in pyrin in myeloid cells *episodic* fever, peritonitis, and pleuritis ± arthritis, erythema, amyloidosis ↑ WBC & ESR during attacks

(*Lancet* 1997;350:575; *Archives* 2003;163:1033)

Workup

- History: infectious contacts, travel, pets, occupation, medications, thorough review of systems, PMHx and PSHx, TB history
- Discontinue unnecessary medications (only 20% with medication-induced FUO will have eosinophilia or rash); reassess 1-3 wks after meds d/c'd
- Careful physical exam with attention to skin findings, LAN, murmurs, HSM, arthritis
- Laboratory evaluation
  - CBC with differential, electrolytes, BUN, Cr, LFTs, ESR, ANA, RF, cryoglobulin
  - BCx × 3 sets (off antibiotics, hold for HACEK, RMSF, Q fever, Brucella), U/A, UCx, PPD, heterophile Ab, CMV antigenemia test, HIV
- Imaging studies: CXR, abdominal CT (oral and IV contrast), ? RUQ U/S, ? tagged WBC or gallium scan
- Temporal artery bx if ↑ ESR and age >60
- ? Bone marrow bx or liver bx (especially if ↑ Aϕ): even w/o localizing signs or symptoms, yield may be up to 15%

Treatment

- Empiric antibiotics *not* indicated (unless patient neutropenic)

• PITUITARY DISORDERS •

Hypopituitary Syndromes

Panhypopituitarism

- Etiologies
  - **Primary**: surgery, radiation, tumors (primary or metastatic), infection, infiltration (sarcoid, hemochromatosis), autoimmune, ischemia (including Sheehan's syndrome), carotid aneurysms, cavernous sinus thrombosis, trauma
  - **Secondary** (hypothalamic dysfunction or stalk interruption): tumors (including craniopharyngioma), infection, infiltration, radiation, surgery, trauma
- Clinical manifestations
  - **Hormonal**: weakness, easy fatigability, hypotension, bradycardia, sexual dysfunction, loss of axillary & pubic hair, hypotension, polyuria & polydipsia
  - **Mass effect**: headache, visual field Δs, cranial nerve palsies, galactorrhea
  - **Apoplexy (pituitary hemorrhage)**: sudden headache, N/V, visual field Δs, cranial nerve palsies, meningismus, Δ MS, hypoglycemia, hypotension
- Diagnostic studies
  - hormonal studies
    - *chronic:* low target gland hormone + low or normal trophic hormone
    - *acute:* hormonal studies may be *normal*
  - pituitary MRI

↓ ACTH: adrenal insufficiency similar to 1° (see "Adrenal Disorders"), *except* neither salt craving & hypokalemia (b/c aldo preserved) nor hyperpigmentation (b/c ACTH/MSH is not ↑).

↓ TSH: central hypothyroidism similar to 1° (see "Thyroid Disorders") except for absence of goiter. Full set of TFTs must be ✓'d as TSH may be low or *normal,* but *inappropriately* so in setting of low free T_4.

↓ PRL: inability to lactate (n.b., with hypothalamic hypopituitarism or stalk compression → ↓ prolactin inhibitory factor (dopamine) → ↑ PRL)

↓ GH: risk for osteoporosis, fatigue; diagnosed with failure to ↑ GH with appropriate stimulus (e.g., GHRH/arginine stimulation or insulin tolerance test)

↓ FSH & LH

- Clinical manifestations: ↓ libido, impotence, amenorrhea, oligomenorrhea, infertility
- Physical examination: loss of axillary, pubic, and body hair
- Diagnostic studies: ↓ testosterone or estradiol with low or normal FSH/LH (all levels decreased in acute illness, ∴ don't measure in hospitalized patients)
- Treatment: testosterone or estrogen replacement *vs.* correction of the underlying cause

↓ ADH (hypothalamic or stalk disease): diabetes insipidus

- Clinical manifestations: *severe* polyuria, *mild* hypernatremia (unless ↓ access to H_2O → *severe* hypernatremia)
- Diagnostic studies: see "Disorders of Sodium Homeostasis"

Hyperpituitary Syndromes

Pituitary tumors
- Pathophysiology: adenoma → excess of ≥1 trophic hormones (if tumor functional, but 30-40% are not) and potentially *deficiencies* in other trophic hormones due to compression
- Clinical manifestations
  syndromes due to oversecretion of hormones (see below)
  anatomic consequences: headache, visual Δs, diplopia, cranial neuropathies
- Workup: MRI, hormone levels, consider MEN1 (see below)

Hyperprolactinemia (↑ PRL; 50% of adenomas)
- Physiology: PRL induces lactation and inhibits GnRH → ↓ FSH & LH
- Clinical manifestations: **amenorrhea**, **galactorrhea**, **infertility**, ↓ libido, impotence
- Diagnostic studies
  ↑ **PRL**, but many false ⊕, ∴ r/o pregnancy, hypothyroidism, psychotropic medication, antiemetics, renal failure (decreased clearance), stress, high carb diet, cirrhosis
  MRI to evaluate for tumor, visual field testing if MR shows compression of optic chiasm
- Treatment
  if asymptomatic (no HA or hypogonadal sx) and microadenoma → follow with MRI
  if symptomatic or macroadenoma options include:
    medical with dopamine agonist such as bromocriptine (70-100% success rate) or cabergoline (better tolerated); side effects include N/V, orthostasis, psychosis (rare)
    surgical: trans-sphenoidal surgery (if rapidly growing tumor, visual field defect, or failed medical therapy); 10-20% recurrence rate
    radiation: if medical or surgical therapy have failed or are not tolerated

Acromegaly (↑ GH; 10% of adenomas)
- Physiology: stimulates secretion of insulin-like growth factor 1 (IGF-1)
- Clinical manifestations: ↑ soft tissue, arthralgias, jaw enlargement, headache, carpal tunnel syndrome, macroglossia, hoarseness, sleep apnea, amenorrhea, impotence, diabetes mellitus, acanthosis/skin tags, ↑ sweating, hypertension, cardiomyopathy, colonic polyps
- Diagnostic studies: *no utility in checking random GH levels because pulsatile secretion*
  ↑ **somatomedin C** (IGF-1); ± ↑ PRL; oral glucose tolerance test → GH *not* suppressed
  pituitary MRI to evaluate for tumor
- Treatment: surgery, octreotide (long and short acting preparations), dopamine agonists, pegvisomant (GH receptor antagonist), radiation
- Prognosis: w/o treatment Pts have ↑ risk of pituitary insufficiency, colon cancer, mortality

Cushing's disease (↑ ACTH; 10-15% of adenomas; see "Adrenal Disorders")

Central hyperthyroidism (↑ TSH, ↑ alpha subunit; very rare; see "Thyroid Disorders")

↑ FSH & LH (usually non-fxn, presents as *hypopituitarism* b/c of compression effects)

• DISORDERS OF MULTIPLE ENDOCRINE SYSTEMS •

Multiple Endocrine Neoplasia (MEN) Syndromes

Type	Features
1	Parathyroid hyperplasia/adenomas (→ hypercalcemia) Pancreatic islet cell neoplasia (gastrin, VIP, insulin, glucagon) Pituitary adenomas
2A	Medullary thyroid carcinoma (MTC) Pheochromocytoma (~50%) Parathyroid hyperplasia (→ hypercalcemia; 15-20%)
2B	Medullary thyroid carcinoma (MTC) Pheochromocytoma (~50%) Mucosal and gastrointestinal neuromas

Polyglandular Autoimmune (PGA) Syndromes

Type	Features
I	Mucocutaneous candidiasis Hypoparathyroidism Adrenal insufficiency
II	Adrenal insufficiency Graves' disease or hypothyroidism Type 1 diabetes mellitus

• THYROID DISORDERS •

Diagnostic Studies in Thyroid Disorders	
Test	**Comments**
Thyroid stimulating hormone (TSH)	*Most sensitive test* to detect 1° hypo- and hyperthyroidism May be inappropriately normal in central etiologies ↓ by dopamine, steroids, severe illness
T_3 and T_4 immunoassays	Measure *total* serum concentrations (∴ influenced by TBG)
Thyroxine binding globulin (TBG)	↑ TBG (∴ ↑ T_4): estrogens, OCP, pregnancy, hepatitis ↓ TBG (∴ ↓ T_4): androgens, glucocorticoids, nephrotic syndrome, cirrhosis, acromegaly, phenytoin
T_3 resin uptake (T_3RU)	Indirect measure of amount of TBG by combining Pt's serum (contains unlabeled T_4 & TBG) + labeled T_3 + thyroid hormone binding resin Amount of labeled T_3 free to bind resin (i.e., resin uptake) is *inversely proportional* to amount of TBG in Pt's serum ↑ T_3RU implies ↓ TBG; ↓ T_3RU implies ↑ TBG
Free thyroxine index (FTI)	$(T_4 \times T_3RU)/100$
Free T_4 immunoassay (FT_4)	Free T_4, not influenced by TBG
FT_4 by equilibrium dialysis	Free T_4 ("gold standard")
Reverse T_3	Inactive, ↑'d in sick euthyroid syndrome
Thyroid antibodies	Anti-thyroid peroxidase (TPO) → Hashimoto's Thyroid-stimulating Ig (TSI) → Graves' disease
Thyroglobulin	↑'d in thyroid injury, inflammation, and cancer (∴ useful marker of *recurrence* of papillary and follicular cancer).
Radioactive iodine uptake (RAIU) scan	Useful to differentiate different causes of hyperthyroidism ↑ **uptake** homogeneous = Graves' disease heterogeneous = multinodular goiter 1 focus w/ suppression of rest of gland = hot nodule **no uptake** = subacute painful or silent thyroiditis, exogenous thyroid hormone, struma ovarii, recent iodine load, or antithyroid drugs

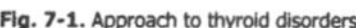

Fig. 7-1. Approach to thyroid disorders

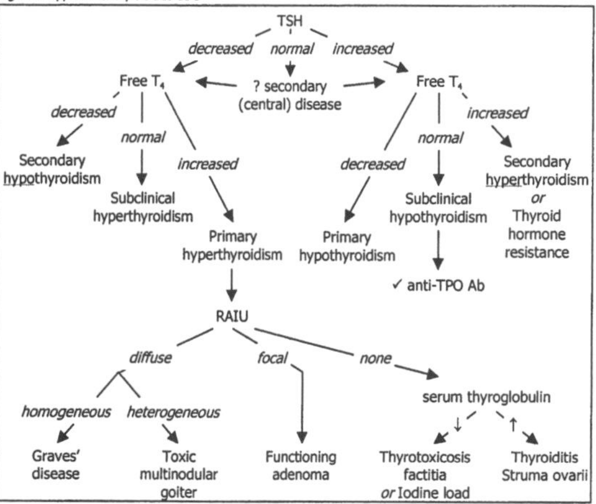

HYPOTHYROIDISM

Etiologies

- Primary (>90% of cases of hypothyroidism; ↓ free T_4, ↑ TSH)
  - Goitrous: **Hashimoto's thyroiditis**, recovery phase after thyroiditis, iodine deficiency
  - Non-goitrous: surgical destruction, s/p radioactive iodine or radiation, amiodarone
- Secondary (↓ free T_4, variable TSH): hypothalamic or pituitary failure (TSH levels may be normal although functionally inactive due to abnormal glycosylation)

Hashimoto's thyroiditis

- Autoimmune destruction with patchy lymphocytic infiltration
- Usually seen in women, 20-60 years old. May be part of polyglandular autoimmune syndrome type II (hypothyroidism, Addison's, diabetes mellitus); associated with ↑ incidence of Sjögren's syndrome, pernicious anemia, and primary biliary cirrhosis.
- ⊕ anti-thyroid peroxidase (anti-TPO) and anti-thyroglobulin (anti-Tg) Abs in >90%

Clinical manifestations (*Lancet* 2004;363:793)

- **Early**: weakness, fatigue, arthralgias, myalgias, headache, depression, cold intolerance, weight gain, constipation, menorrhagia, dry skin, coarse brittle hair, brittle nails, carpal tunnel syndrome, delayed DTRs ("hung up" reflexes), diastolic hypertension
- **Late**: slow speech, hoarseness, loss of outer third of eyebrows, **myxedema** (non-pitting skin thickening due to ↑ glycosaminoglycans), periorbital puffiness, bradycardia, pleural, pericardial or peritoneal effusions
- **Myxedema coma**: hypothermia, hypotension, hypoventilation, Δ MS
- **Subclinical hypothyroidism**: mild ↑ TSH and normal T_4 with only subtle or no sx; with high titers of antithyroid Abs, progression to overt hypothyroidism is ~4%/yr

Diagnostic studies

- ↓ **FT_4**; ↑ **TSH** in primary hypothyroidism; ⊕ antithyroid Ab in Hashimoto's thyroiditis
- Hyponatremia, hypoglycemia, anemia, ↑ cholesterol and CK

Treatment

- Levothyroxine (1.5-1.7 µg/kg/d), re✓ TSH q 5-6 wks and titrate until euthyroid; sx may take months to resolve
- Subclinical hypothyroidism: follow expectantly or treat to improve ? mild sx or abnl lipids
- Myxedema coma: 5-8 µg/kg (~500 µg) T_4 IV, then 50-100 µg IV qd; ? 5-10 µg T_3 IV q 8 hrs instead because of impaired peripheral conversion (but T_3 more arrhythmogenic); empiric *adrenal replacement therapy* as low adrenal reserves in myxedema coma

HYPERTHYROIDISM

Etiologies (*Lancet* 2003;362:459)

- **Graves' disease** (60-80% of thyrotoxicosis)
- **Thyroiditis**: thyrotoxic phase of subacute thyroiditis
- **Toxic adenomas** (single or multinodular goiter) or, rarely, functioning thyroid carcinoma
- TSH-secreting pituitary tumor or pituitary resistance to thyroid hormone (↑ TSH, ↑ free T_4)
- Miscellaneous: amiodarone, iodine-induced (Jodbasedow phenomenon when iodine is supplied to autonomous thyroid tissue), thyrotoxicosis factitia, struma ovarii (3% of ovarian dermoid tumors and teratomas), hCG-secreting tumors (e.g., choriocarcinoma)

Graves' disease

- Usually seen in women, 20-40 yrs old
- Clinical manifestations in addition to those of hyperthyroidism
  - diffuse, non-tender **goiter**, thyroid bruit
  - **ophthalmopathy** (30%; up to 90% if tested): periorbital edema, proptosis (✓ if sclera visible between lower iris and lower lid), conjunctivitis, diplopia (EOM infiltration)
  - **pretibial myxedema** (3%): infiltrative dermopathy
- ⊕ **thyroid antibodies**: TSI (⊕ in 80%), anti-microsomal, anti-thyroglobulin; ANA

Clinical manifestations

- Restlessness, insomnia, heat intolerance, sweating, moist warm skin, fine hair, ↑ HR, palpitations, AF, weight loss, ↑ freq. of bowel movements, menstrual irregularities, hyperreflexia, osteoporosis, lid lag or retraction (due sympathetic overactivity)
- **Subclinical** (↓ TSH, normal FT_4 and FT_3): ↑ risk of atrial fibrillation and osteoporosis
- **Apathetic hyperthyroidism**: seen in elderly who may present with lethargy
- **Thyroid storm** (seen with stress or thyroid surgery): delirium, fever, tachycardia, systolic hypertension, but wide pulse pressure and low MAP, GI symptoms; 20-50% mortality

Laboratory
- ↑ **FT_4** and **FT_3**; ↓ **TSH** (except in TSH-secreting tumors)
- RAIU
  - homogenous increase = Graves' disease
  - heterogeneous increase = multinodular goiter
  - single hot nodule = toxic adenoma
  - no uptake = thyroiditis, thyrotoxicosis factitia, iodine load, struma ovarii
- Rarely need to ✓ for autoantibodies except in pregnancy (to assess risk of fetal Graves')
- Hypercalcuria ± hypercalcemia, ↑ Aϕ, anemia

Treatment
- β-blockers: control tachycardia (propranolol also ↓ $T_4 \rightarrow T_3$ conversion)
- Graves' disease: either anti-thyroid drugs or radiation
  - **propylthiouracil (PTU)** or **methimazole**: 50% chance of recurrence after 1 yr; side effects include pruritus, rash, arthralgia, fever, N/V, and *agranulocytosis* in 0.5%
  - **radioactive iodine (RAI)**: preRx w/ anti-thyroid drugs to prevent ↑ thyrotoxicosis, stop >5 d before to allow RAI uptake; >75% of treated Pts will become hypothyroid
- Toxic adenoma or toxic multinodular goiter: RAI or surgery (± PTU or methimazole)
- Thyroid storm: β-blocker, PTU, iopanoic acid or iodide (for "Wolff-Chaikoff" effect) >1 hr after PTU, ± steroids (↓ $T_4 \rightarrow T_3$)

THYROIDITIS (*NEJM* 2003;348:2646)

- **Acute**: bacterial infection (fever, ↑ ESR, normal TFTs), radiation, amiodarone
- **Subacute:** transient thyrotoxicosis → transient hypothyroidism → normal
  - **painful** (= viral, granulomatous, or de Quervain's): fever, ↑ ESR; Rx = NSAIDs, steroids
  - **silent** (= post-partum, autoimmune, or lymphocytic): painless, ⊕ TPO Abs
- **Chronic**: Hashimoto's (hypothyroidism), Reidel's (idiopathic fibrosis, normal TFTs)

SICK EUTHYROID SYNDROME

- Abnormalities in TFTs due to non-thyroidal illness (∴ in acute illness, ✓ TFTs only if high concern for thyroid disease)
- Mild illness: ↓ $T_4 \rightarrow T_3$ conversion, ↑ $rT_3 \Rightarrow$ ↓ T_3
- Moderate: ↓ TBG & albumin, ↓↓ $T_4 \rightarrow T_3$ conversion, ↑↑ $rT_3 \Rightarrow$ ↓↓ T_3, ↓ T_4, normal FT_4
- Severe: same as above + ↑ degradation of T_4, central ↓ TSH ⇒ ↓↓ T_3, ↓↓ T_4, ↓ FT_4, ↓ TSH
- Recovery: ↑ TSH followed by recovery of T_4 and then T_3

AMIODARONE AND THYROID DISEASE

Hypothyroidism (occurs in ~10% of Pts on amio; more common in iodine *replete* areas)
- Pathophysiology
  - (1) "Wolff-Chaikoff" effect: iodine load ↓ I^- uptake, organification, and release of T_4 & T_3
  - (2) inhibits $T_4 \rightarrow T_3$ conversion
  - (3) ? direct/immune-mediated thyroid destruction
- Normal individuals: ↓ T_4; then escape Wolff-Chaikoff effect and have ↑ T_4, ↓ T_3, ↑ TSH; then TSH normalizes (after 1-3 mos)
- Susceptible individuals (e.g., subclinical Hashimoto's, ∴ ✓ anti-TPO) do *not* escape effects
- Treatment: thyroxine to normalize TSH

Hyperthyroidism (occurs in 3% of Pts on amio; ~20% in iodine *deficient* areas)
- Type 1 = underlying multinodular goiter or autonomous thyroid tissue
  - pathophysiology: JodBasedow effect (iodine load → ↑ synthesis of T_4 and T_3 in autonomous tissue)
  - diagnostic studies: ↑ thyroid blood flow on Doppler U/S
  - treatment: methimazole
- Type 2 = inflammatory thyroiditis
  - pathophysiology: release of pre-formed T_4 & T_3 → hyperthyroidism → hypothyroidism → recovery
  - diagnostic studies: ↑ ESR, ↓ flow on Doppler U/S
  - treatment: steroids

THYROID NODULES

- Prevalence 5-10% (>20% if screen with U/S)
- Features associated with ↑ risk of malignancy: young age, h/o neck irradiation, fixed lesion, "cold nodule" on RAIU, large size, worrisome U/S findings (hypoechoic, solid, irregular borders, microcalcifications, central blood flow)

Fig. 7-2. Approach to thyroid nodules (*NEJM* 1993;328:553)

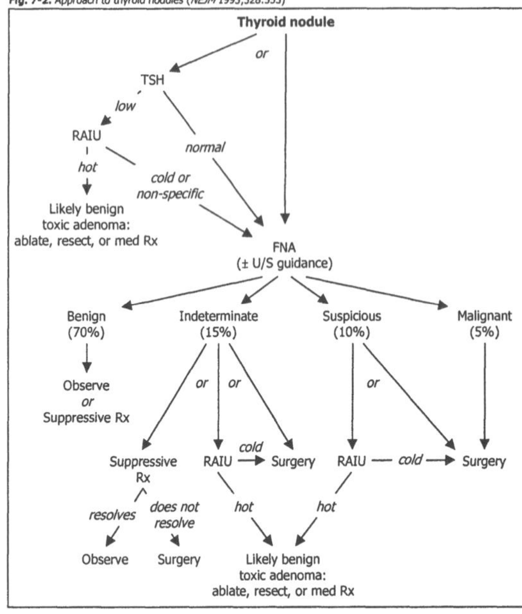

• ADRENAL DISORDERS •

CUSHING'S SYNDROME (HYPERCORTISOLISM)

Definition
- Cushing's syndrome = cortisol excess
- Cushing's disease = Cushing's syndrome 2° pituitary ACTH hypersecretion

Etiologies
- **Cushing's disease** (60-70%): pituitary adenoma or pituitary hyperplasia
- **Adrenal tumor** (15-25%): adenoma or carcinoma
- **Ectopic ACTH** (5-10%): SCLC, carcinoid, islet cell tumors, medullary thyroid cancer, pheo.

Clinical manifestations
- Glucose intolerance or DM, hypertension, obesity, and oligomenorrhea (all non-specific)
- Central obesity, buffalo hump, moon facies, wasting of the extremities, proximal myopathy, spontaneous bruising, wide striae, osteoporosis, and hypokalemia (all more specific)
- Other features: psychosis, facial plethora, acne, hirsutism, hyperpigmentation (if ↑ ACTH), fungal skin infections, nephrolithiasis, polyuria

Fig. 7-3. Approach to suspected Cushing's syndrome

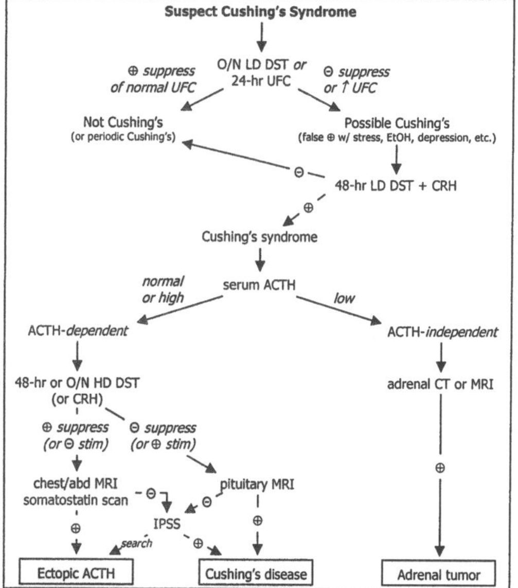

CRH = corticotropin-releasing hormone test; DST = dexamethasone suppression test; UFC = urinary free cortisol
O/N DST = 1 mg at 11 pm; ✓ 8 am serum cortisol (suppression if <5 μg/dl)
48-hr LD DST + CRH = 0.5 mg q 6 h × 2 d followed by 8 am CRH; ✓ serum cortisol 15 min later (⊕ = >1.4 μg/dl)
48-hr HD DST = 0.5 mg q 6 h × 2 d; ✓ 24-hr UFC (suppression if <10% of baseline UFC value)
O/N HD DST = 8 mg at 11 pm; ✓ 8 am serum cortisol (suppression if <32% of baseline value)
CRH test = 1 μg/kg IV; ✓ cortisol and ACTH (⊕ stim if >35% ↑ in ACTH or >20% ↑ in cortisol above baseline)
IPSS = inferior petrosal sinus vein sampling; ✓ petrosal:peripheral ACTH ratio (⊕ = >2 basal, >3 after CRH)
(*Endo & Metab Clin North Am* 1997;26:741)

Treatment

- Surgical resection of pituitary adenoma, adrenal tumor, or ectopic ACTH-secreting tumor
  if transphenoidal surgery not successful → ? pituitary XRT or bilateral adrenalectomy
- Glucocorticoid replacement therapy × 6-36 months after surgery
- Ketoconazole (± metyrapone) to ↓ cortisol production if surgery unsuccessful or contraindic

HYPERALDOSTERONISM

Etiologies

- **Primary** (adrenal disorders, ↑ aldosterone is renin-independent)
  adrenal hyperplasia (70%), adenoma (**Conn's syndrome**, 25%), carcinoma (5%)
  glucocorticoid-remediable aldosteronism (GRA; ACTH-dep. promoter rearrangement)
- **Secondary** (extra-adrenal disorders, ↑ aldosterone is renin-dependent)
  primary reninism: renin-secreting tumor
  secondary reninism
    renovascular disease: RAS, malignant hypertension
    edematous states w/ ↓ effective arterial volume: CHF, cirrhosis, nephrotic syndrome
    hypovolemia, diuretics, Bartter's (defective Na/K/2Cl transporter ≈ receiving loop diuretic), Gitelman's (defective renal Na/Cl transporter ≈ receiving thiazide diuretic)
- **Non-aldosterone mineralocorticoid** excess mimics hyperaldosteronism
  Cushing's syndrome, CAH (some enzyme defects → shunting to mineralocorticoids)
  11β-OHSD deficiency (buildup of cortisol, which binds to mineralocorticoid receptor)
  licorice (glycyrrhizinic acid inhibits 11β-OHSD)
  Liddle's syndrome (constitutively activated renal Na channel)
  exogenous mineralocorticoids

Clinical manifestations

- **Mild to moderate diastolic HTN**, headache, muscle weakness, polyuria, polydipsia
- No peripheral edema because of "escape" from Na retention
- Classically, **hypokalemia** (but can be normal), metabolic alkalosis, and mild hypernatremia

Diagnostic tests

- 5-10% of Pts w/ HTN; ∴ screen if HTN + hypokalemia, adrenal mass, or refractory HTN
- **Aldosterone** (>15-20 ng/dl) *and* **plasma aldosterone:renin ratio** (>20 if 1°; ≤10 if 2°)
  obtain 8 a.m. seated, paired values (off spironolactone for 6 wks); sens. & spec. 85-90%
- Confirm with sodium suppression test (fail to suppress aldosterone after sodium load)
  oral salt load (+ KCl) x 3d, measure 24 hr urine (⊕ if Na >200 & aldosterone >14 µg)
  or 2L NS over 4h, measure aldosterone at end of infusion (⊕ if aldosterone >10 ng/dl)
- Imaging and adrenal vein sampling to diagnose adenoma vs. hyperplasia

Fig. 7-4. Approach to suspected hyperaldosteronism

Suspect Hyperaldosteronism
↓
8 a.m. plasma renin & aldosterone

- *↓ renin, ↓ aldosterone* → **Non-aldosterone mineralocorticoid excess**: Cushing's syndrome; CAH (some forms); 11β-OHSD deficiency; licorice; Liddle's syndrome; exogenous mineralocorticoids
- *↓ renin, ↑ aldosterone, aldo:renin >20* → salt suppression test → ⊕ → **1° Hyperaldosteronism** → adrenal CT or MRI
  - *lesion* → adenoma, carcinoma
  - *no lesion* → adrenal vein sampling → *localize* → adenoma, carcinoma; *no localization* → hyperplasia or GRA
- *↑ renin, ↑ aldosterone, aldo:renin ≤10* → **2° Hyperaldosteronism**: renin-secreting tumor; renovascular disease; CHF, cirrhosis, nephrotic; hypovolemia & diuretic use; Bartter's syndrome; Gitelman's syndrome

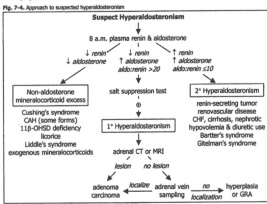

(Adapted from *Trends in Endocrine Metabolism* 1999;5:97)

Treatment
- Adenoma or carcinoma → surgery
- Hyperplasia → spironolactone; GRA → glucocorticoids ± spironolactone

ADRENAL INSUFFICIENCY

Etiologies
- **Primary** = adrenocortical disease = ***Addison's disease***
  - **autoimmune** (most common in industrialized countries):
    - isolated
    - polyglandular autoimmune syndromes (PGA)
      - PGA I = chronic mucocutaneous candidiasis + hypoparathyroidism + Addison's
      - PGA II = Addison's + thyroid disease + type 1 diabetes mellitus
  - **infection**: (most common cause worldwide): tuberculosis, CMV, histoplasmosis
  - **vascular**: hemorrhage, thrombosis, and trauma
  - **metastatic disease** (90% of the adrenals must be destroyed to cause insufficiency)
  - deposition diseases: hemochromatosis, amyloid, sarcoid
  - drugs: ketoconazole, rifampin, anticonvulsants
- **Secondary** = pituitary failure of ACTH secretion (n.b., aldosterone intact b/c RAA axis)
  - any cause of primary or secondary hypopituitarism (see "Pituitary Disorders")
  - glucocorticoid therapy (occurs after ≥2 wks of "suppressive doses", which are extremely variable: ? >20 mg/d of prednisone for >3 wks; takes 8-12 mos to recover function)
  - megestrol

Clinical manifestations (*NEJM* 1996;335:1206)
- **Primary or secondary**: **weakness and fatigability** (99%), **anorexia** (99%), **orthostatic hypotension** (90%), nausea (86%), vomiting (75%), hyponatremia (88%)
- **Primary only** (extra signs & symptoms due to lack of aldosterone and ↑ ACTH): marked orthostatic hypotension (because volume depleted), hyperpigmentation (seen in creases, mucous membranes, pressure areas, nipples), **hyperkalemia**
- **Secondary only**: ± other manifestations of hypopituitarism (see "Pituitary Disorders")

Diagnostic studies
- High dose (250 μg) **corticotropin stimulation test** (testing ability of ACTH → ↑ cortisol)
  - normal = pre- or 60 min post-ACTH cortisol ≥18 μg/dl
  - abnormal in *primary* because adrenal gland diseased and unable to give adequate output
  - abnormal in *chronic* secondary because adrenals atrophied and unable to respond
  - may be normal in *acute secondary* because adrenals still able to respond
- Low dose (1 μg) cort stim can be used to detect mild secondary (✓ cortisol 30 min post)
- Other: insulin-induced hypoglycemia; failure to ↑ 11-deoxycortisol after metyrapone
- Other laboratory abnormalities: hypoglycemia, eosinophilia, lymphocytosis, ± neutropenia
- ACTH: ↑ in primary, ↓ or low-normal in secondary
- Imaging
  - adrenal CT: small, noncalcified adrenals in autoimmune, enlarged in metastatic disease, hemorrhage, infection or deposition (although they may be normal appearing)
  - pituitary MRI: to detect pituitary abnormalities

Treatment
- *Acute* adrenal insufficiency
  - **hydrocortisone 100 mg IV q 8 hrs**
  - volume resuscitation with normal saline
- *Chronic* adrenal insufficiency
  - hydrocortisone: 20-30 mg PO qd (2/3 in am, 1/3 in pm) or prednisone 5-7.5 mg PO qd
  - fludrocortisone (not necessary in secondary adrenal insufficiency): 50 – 100 μg PO q am

Pheochromocytoma

Clinical manifestations (five P's)
- **Pressure** (hypertension, paroxysmal in 50%, severe and resistant to therapy)
- **Pain** (headache, chest pain)
- **Palpitations**, tremor, wt loss, fever
- **Perspiration** (profuse)
- **Pallor** (vasoconstrictive spell)
- "Rule of 10": 10% extra-adrenal (~15%, known as paraganglioma), 10% in children, 10% multiple or bilateral, 10% recur (↑ in paraganglioma), 10% malignant (↑ in paraganglioma), 10% (~15%) familial, 10% incidentaloma
- Associated with MEN 2A/2B, Von Hippel Lindau, neurofibromatosis type 1, familial paraganglioma (mutations in succinate dehydrogenase)

Diagnostic Studies
- Plasma free metanephrines: 99% sens., 89% spec. (*JAMA* 2002;287:1427), ∴ screening test of choice in high-risk Pts, but high rate of false ⊕ in low-prevalence population
- 24° urine for catechols, metanephrines: 90% sensitive, 98% specific (false ⊕ with severe illness, renal failure, obstructive sleep apnea, labetalol due to assay interference, TCAs, medications containing sympathomimetics)
- Adrenal CT or MRI; MIBG scan, PET to localize non-adrenal mass, but usually easy to find

Treatment
- α-blockade first ± β-blockade → surgery

Adrenal Incidentalomas

Epidemiology
- 2% of Pts undergoing abdominal CT scan have incidentally discovered adrenal mass; prevalence ↑ with age

Differential diagnosis
- **Non-functioning mass**: adenoma, cysts, abscesses, granuloma, hemorrhage, lipoma, myelolipoma, primary or metastatic malignancy
- **Functioning mass**: pheochromocytoma, adenoma (cortisol, aldosterone, sex hormones), non-classical CAH, other endocrine tumor, carcinoma
- **Non-adrenal mass**: renal, pancreatic, gastric, artifact

Workup (*NEJM* 1990;323:1401)
- **Rule-out sub-clinical Cushing's syndrome** *clinically* (lack of hypertension or obesity has NPV of 99%) and/or with dexamethasone suppression test to screen for autonomy (although only has PPV of ~3% in setting of adrenal incidentaloma)
- **Rule-out hyperaldosteronism** *if hypertensive* with plasma aldosterone & renin
- **Rule-out pheochromocytoma** *with hormonal studies:* lack of hypertension and classic symptoms has NPV of 99%, but morbidity associated with untreated pheochromocytoma warrants hormonal rule-out with urinary or plasma metanephrines
- Rule-out metastatic cancer and infection by history or CT guided biopsy if suspicious
- CT and MRI characteristics may suggest adenoma vs. carcinoma
  size <3 cm, smooth margins, homogenous and hypodense appearance, imaging *not* suggestive of malignancy → likely to be adenoma, ∴ can follow with periodic scans
  size >4 cm or ↑ size on repeat scan, h/o malignancy, imaging suggestive of malignancy (irregular margins, heterogeneous or dense appearance, or vascular), or young age (incidentaloma less common) → resection

• CALCIUM DISORDERS •

Fig. 7-5. Approach to calcium disorders based on serum calcium and PTH levels

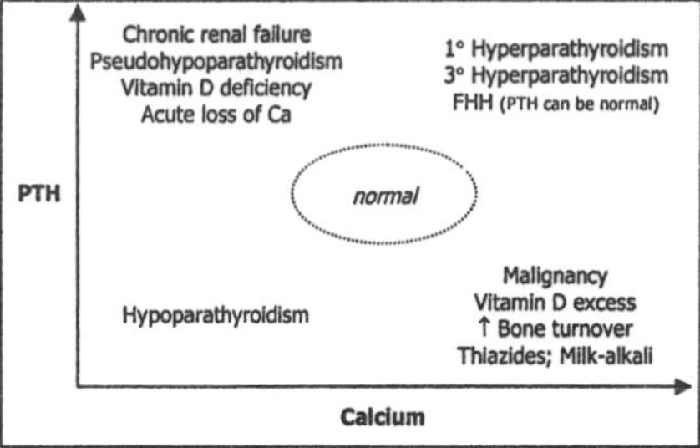

Laboratory Findings in Calcium Disorders			
Ca	**Disease state**	**PO_4**	**PTH**
↑	**Hyperparathyroidism**	↓	↑↑
	Familial hypocalciuric hypercalcemia	↓	↑ or nl
	Malignancy	var.	↓
	Vitamin D excess	↑	↓
	↑ Bone turnover	↑	↓
↓	**Hypoparathyroidism**	↑	↓
	Pseudohypoparathyroidism	↑	↑↑
	Chronic renal failure	↑	↑
	Acute calcium sequestration	var.	var.
	Vitamin D deficiency	↓	↑

Pitfalls in measuring Ca

- Physiologically active Ca is free or ionized Ca (ICa). Serum Ca reflects total calcium (bound + unbound) and ∴ influenced by albumin (main Ca binding protein).
  Corrected Ca (mg/dl) = measured Ca (mg/dl) + [0.8 × (4.0 - albumin (mg/dl))]
- Alkalosis will cause more Ca to be bound to albumin; ∴ total Ca may be normal but ↓ ICa

HYPERCALCEMIA

Etiologies of Hypercalcemia	
Category	**Etiologies**
Hyperparathyroidism	1°: adenoma (80%), hyperplasia (15-20%; spontaneous vs. MEN 1/2A, carcinoma (<1%) (n.b., 2° hyperparathyroidism = ↑ PTH in response to ↓ Ca) 3°: after long-standing 2° hyperparathyroidism (as in renal failure) → autonomous nodule develops Lithium → ↑ PTH
Familial hypocalciuric hypercalcemia (FHH)	Mutation in Ca-sensing receptor in parathyroid and kidney → ↑ Ca set point; ± ↑ PTH (and less ↑ than in 1° hyperpara.)
Malignancy	PTH related peptide (PTHrP) (e.g., squamous cell lung cancer, renal, breast, bladder) Cytokines & ↑ 1,25-$(OH)_2D_3$ (e.g., hematologic malignancies) Local osteolysis (e.g., breast cancer, myeloma)
Vitamin D excess	Granulomas (sarcoid, TB, histo) → ↑ 1-OH → ↑ 1,25-$(OH)_2D$ Vitamin D intoxication
↑ bone turnover	Hyperthyroidism, immobilization + Paget's disease, vitamin A
Miscellaneous	Thiazides; Ca-based antacids (milk-alkali syndrome); adrenal insufficiency

Clinical manifestations ("bones, stones, abdominal groans, and psychic moans")

- **Hypercalcemic crisis** (usually when Ca 13-15): polyuria, dehydration, mental status Δs
  calcium toxic to renal tubules → blocks ADH activity, causes vasoconstriction, and ↓ GFR
  → polyuria but ↑ Ca reabsorption → ↑ serum calcium → ↑ nephrotoxicity
- Osteopenia and osteitis fibrosa cystica (latter is seen in severe hyperparathyroidism only → ↑ osteoclast activity → cysts, fibrous nodules, salt & pepper appearance on X-ray)
- Nephrolithiasis, nephrocalcinosis, nephrogenic DI
- Abdominal pain, anorexia, nausea, vomiting, constipation, pancreatitis, PUD
- Fatigue, depression, confusion
- Decreased DTRs, short QT interval

Paget's disease of bone (osteitis deformans; 1-2% of population)

- Excessive bone resorption + disorganized osteoid formation with weak, vascular bone
- Clinical: asx (majority); bone pain, bowed tibias, fractures; H/A, large head, deafness; warmth over affected areas (2° ↓ SVR → ↑ CO)
- Ca *normal* (unless immob), ↑ Aϕ & urinary hydroxyproline; dense expanded bones on X-ray
- Treatment: bisphosphonates; Prognosis: ↑ risk of osteosarcoma

Diagnostic studies

- Hyperparathyroidism and malignancy account for 90% of cases of hypercalcemia
  hyperparathyroidism more likely if asx or chronic hypercalcemia
  malignancy more likely if acute or sx; malignancy usually overt or becomes so w/in mos
- Ca, alb, ICa, PTH (may be inappropriately normal in 1° hyperparathyroidism & FHH), PO_4; based on results then consider checking PTHrP, 25-(OH)D, 1,25-$(OH)_2$D, Aϕ, U_{Ca}

Acute Treatment of Hypercalcemia			
Treatment	**Onset**	**Dur.**	**Comments**
Normal saline (4-6 L/day)	hrs	during Rx	natriuresis → ↑ renal Ca excretion
Furosemide (IV q 6 hrs)	hrs	during Rx	Start only *after* Pt intravascularly replete. Promotes natriuresis and ∴ ↑ Ca excretion.
Bisphosphonates	1-2 d	10-14 d	Inhibit osteoclasts, useful in malignancy.
Calcitonin	hrs	2-3 d	Quickly develop tachyphylaxis
Glucocorticoids	days	days	? Useful in some malign. & vitamin D intox.

(*Endo & Metab Clin North Am* 1993;22:343)

HYPOCALCEMIA

Etiologies of Hypocalcemia	
Category	**Etiologies**
Hypoparathyroidism	Isolated; PGA type I (chronic mucocutaneous candidiasis + hypoparathyroid + Addison's) s/p thyroidectomy, hypomagnesemia (↓ secretion and effect)
Pseudo-hypoparathyroidism	PTH end-organ resistance (∴ ↑ serum PTH) + skeletal abnormalities, short stature, & retardation Pseudopseudohypoparathyroidism = syndrome but *normal* Ca
Vitamin D deficiency	½ of pts admitted to gen med service (*NEJM* 1998;338:777)
Chronic renal failure	↓ 1,25-$(OH)_2$D production, ↑ PO_4 from decreased clearance
Calcium sequestration	Pancreatitis, citrate excess (e.g., after blood transfusions), acute ↑↑ PO_4 (ARF, rhabdomyolysis, tumor lysis)

Clinical manifestations

- **Neuromuscular irritability**: perioral parasthesias, cramps, ⊕ **Chvostek's** (tapping facial nerve → contraction of facial muscles), ⊕ **Trousseau's** (inflation of BP cuff → carpal spasm), laryngospasm; irritability, depression, psychosis, ↑ ICP, seizures, ↑ QT
- **Renal osteodystrophy** (↓ vit D & ↑ PTH in renal failure): osteomalacia (↓ mineralization of bone due to ↓ Ca and 1,25-$(OH)_2$D) & osteitis fibrosa cystica (due to ↑ PTH)

Diagnostic studies

- Ca & alb, ICa, PTH, 25-(OH)D, 1,25-$(OH)_2$D, BUN, Cr, Mg, PO_4, Aϕ, U_{Ca}

Treatment

- Symptomatic: intravenous Ca gluconate and Vitamin D
- Asymptomatic: oral Ca and vitamin D supplementation
- In renal failure, need to give 1,25-$(OH)_2D_3$ (i.e., calcitriol) or paricalcitol (*NEJM* 2003;349:446)

• DIABETES MELLITUS •

Definition (*Diabetes Care* 2003;26:S33)

- Fasting glc >126 mg/dl *or* random glc >200 mg/dl *or* 75 g OGTT w/ 2 hr glc >200 mg/dl
- ? ↑ Hb_{A1C} (no accepted criterion as may have normal Hb_{A1C} but periodic hyperglycemia)

Categories

- **Type 1** = islet cell destruction; absolute insulin deficiency; ketosis in absence of insulin
  prevalence 0.4%; usual onset in childhood; ↑ risk if ⊕ family history; HLA associations
  anti-GAD & anti-insulin autoantibodies
- **Type 2** = insulin resistance + relative insulin deficiency (prevent ketosis but not ↑ glc)
  insulin resistance → ↑ glc → ↑ insulin secretion →→ pancreatic failure → overt diabetes
  prevalence 8%; onset in later life; ↑↑ risk if ⊕ family history; no HLA associations
  risk factors: age, race, FHx, obesity, sedentary lifestyle, metabolic abnormalities
- **Secondary causes**: exogenous or endogenous glucocorticoids, glucagonoma (3 D's = DM, DVT, diarrhea), other endocrine disease, pancreatic (pancreatitis, hemochromatosis)
- **M**ature-**O**nset **D**iabetes of the **Y**oung (MODY, *NEJM* 2001;345:971): autosomal dominant inherited form of DM due to defects in insulin secretion genes; occurs in lean young adults who do not normally require insulin

Clinical manifestations

- Polyuria, polydipsia, polyphagia with unexplained weight loss or asymptomatic

Diabetes Treatment Options	
Option	**Comments**
Diet	Type 1: ADA diet; Type 2: wt reduction diet + exercise
Oral agents	
• sulfonylureas (SU)	• ↑ insulin secretion at β cell, ↓ Hb_{A1C} 1-2%
• metformin	• ↓ hepatic gluconeogenesis, ↑ insulin sensitivity, contraindicated in renal or liver failure; ↓ Hb_{A1C} 1.5-2%
• thiazolidinediones	• ↑ insulin sensitivity at muscles, agonist at PPARγ receptor, contraindicated in liver disease, monitor LFTs; ↓ Hb_{A1C} 0.5-1%
• meglitinides	• ↑ insulin secretion, faster-acting than SU; ↓ Hb_{A1C} 0.5-1%
• α-glucosidase inhib	• ↓ intestinal CHO absorption; ↓ Hb_{A1C} 0.5%; severe gas
Insulin	Generally use a combination of long-acting (NPH or glargine) and short-acting (regular or lispro) insulin.
Other	Type 1: insulin pump, pancreatic or islet cell transplants

(*JAMA* 2002;287:360 & 373)

Complications

- Retinopathy
  non-proliferative: "dot & blot" and retinal hemorrhages, cotton wool/protein exudates
  proliferative: neovascularization, vitreous hemorrhage, retinal detachment, blindness
  treatment: photocoagulation
- **Nephropathy**: microalbuminuria → proteinuria ± nephrotic syndrome → renal failure
  diffuse glomerular basement membrane thickening/nodular pattern (Kimmelstiel-Wilson)
  usually accompanied by retinopathy; lack of retinopathy suggests another cause
  treatment: strict BP control, ACE inhibitors (*NEJM* 1993;329:1456 and *Lancet* 1997;349:1787) & ARBs (*NEJM* 2001;345:851 & 861), low protein diet, dialysis or transplant
- **Neuropathy**
  symmetric peripheral: symmetric distal sensory loss, paresthesias, ± motor loss
  autonomic: gastroparesis, neurogenic bladder, impotence, orthostatic hypotension
  mononeuropathy: sudden onset peripheral or CN deficit (footdrop, CN III > VI > IV)
- **Accelerated atherosclerosis**: coronary, cerebral, and peripheral arterial beds
- **Infections** (including mucormycosis)
- Dermatologic: necrobiosis lipoidica diabeticorum, lipodystrophy

Outpatient screening and treatment goals (*Diabetes Care* 2003;26:S33)

- Hb_{A1C} q 3-4 mos, goal <7%
  complications, especially microvascular, can be ↓ by strict glycemic control, demonstrated in Type 1 (DCCT *NEJM* 1993;329:997) and Type 2 (UKPDS *Lancet* 1998;352:837)
- Microalbuminuria yearly with spot microalbumin/Cr ratio, goal <30 mcg/mg
- BP <130/80; lipid goals LDL <100, TG <150, HDL >40 (but benefit of statins in all diabetics; HPS, *Lancet* 2003;361:2005); ASA if age >40 & other cardiac RF
- Dilated retinal exam yearly; podiatrist yearly or as needed

DIABETIC KETOACIDOSIS (DKA)

Precipitants (the 5 I's)
- **Insulin deficiency** (i.e., failure to take enough)
- **Infection** or Inflammation
- **Ischemia** or Infarction (myocardial)
- **Intra-abdominal process**: pancreatitis, cholecystitis, ischemic bowel, etc.
- **Iatrogenesis:** glucocorticoids

Pathophysiology
- Occurs in **type 1 diabetics** (and *very rarely* in severely stressed type 2 diabetics)
- ↑ glucagon and ↓ insulin
- Hyperglycemia due to: ↑ gluconeogenesis, ↑ glycogenolysis, ↓ glucose uptake into cells
- Ketosis due to: inability to utilize glucose → mobilization and oxidation of fatty acids, ↑ substrate for ketogenesis, ↑ ketogenic state of the liver, ↓ ketone clearance

Clinical manifestations (*Diabetes Care* 2003;26:S109)
- Polyuria and polydipsia
- Dehydration → ↑ HR, hypotension, dry mucous membranes, ↓ skin turgor
- Nausea, vomiting, abdominal pain (either due to intra-abdominal process or DKA), ileus
- Kussmaul's respirations (deep) to compensate for metabolic acidosis with odor of acetone
- Δ MS → somnolence, stupor, coma

Diagnostic studies
- ↑ **anion gap metabolic acidosis:** can later develop non-anion gap acidosis due to urinary loss of ketones (HCO_3 equivalents) and fluid resuscitation with chloride
- **Ketosis: ⊕ urine and serum ketones** (acetoacetate measured, but predominant ketone is β-OH-butyrate; urine ketones may be ⊕ in fasting normal individuals)
- ↑ serum glucose
- ↑ BUN and Cr (dehydration ± artifact due to ketones interfering with some Cr assays)
- Pseudohyponatremia: corrected Na = measured Na + [(2.4 × (measured glucose - 100)]
- ↓ or ↑ K (but even if serum K is elevated, usually *total body K depleted*); ↓ PO_4
- Leukocytosis, ↑ amylase (even if no pancreatitis)

Treatment of DKA

Intervention	Comments
Rule-out possible precipitants	Infection, intra-abdominal process, MI, etc.
Aggressive hydration	Initially NS 10-14 ml/kg/hr, depending on degree of dehydration & cardiovascular status
Insulin	10 U IV push → 0.1 U/kg/hr Continue insulin drip until AG normal If glucose <250 and AG still high → add dextrose to IVF and continue insulin to metabolize ketones AG normal → SC insulin (overlap IV & SC 2-3 hrs)
Electrolyte repletion	K: add 20-40 mEq/L IVF if serum K <4.5 insulin promotes K entry into cells → ↓ serum K careful K repletion in patients with renal failure HCO_3: replete if pH <7.0 or if cardiac instability PO_4: replete if <1.0

Typical DKA "Flow sheet" Setup

Time	VS	UOP	pH	HCO_3	AG	Ketones	Glc	K	PO_4	IVF	Insulin
Note: main ketone produced is β-OH-butyrate (βOHB), but ketone measured is acetoacetate (Ac-Ac). As DKA is treated, βOHB → Ac-Ac ∴ AG can decrease while measured ketones can increase											

Hyperglycemic Hyperosmolar Nonketotic Syndrome (HHNS)

Definition
- Extreme hyperglycemia (without ketoacidosis) + hyperosmolality + Δ MS

Precipitants
- Same as for DKA + dehydration and renal failure, but more likely to be *severe*

Pathophysiology (*Diabetes Care* 2003;26:S33)
- Occurs in type 2 diabetics
- Hyperglycemia → osmotic diuresis → dehydration → prerenal azotemia → ↑ glucose, etc.

Clinical manifestations
- Dehydration and Δ MS

Diagnostic studies
- ↑ **serum glucose** (usually >600 mg/dl)
- ↑ **serum osmolality** (usually >350 mOsm/L)
- No ketoacidosis
- ↑ BUN and Cr; Na may be ↑, ↓, or nl depending on degree of hyperglycemia and degree of dehydration

Treatment (always rule-out possible precipitants)
- **Aggressive hydration**: either NS or 1/2 NS depending on degrees of volume and free H_2O depletion
- **Low-dose insulin** (e.g., 0.05 U/kg/hr)

Hypoglycemia

Etiologies in diabetics
- Excessive insulin, oral agents, missed meals, renal failure (↓ insulin clearance), hypothyroidism

Etiologies in nondiabetics
- ↑ **insulin**: exogenous insulin, sulfonylureas, insulinoma, anti-insulin antibodies
- ↓ **glucose production**: hypopituitarism, adrenal insufficiency, glucagon deficiency, hepatic failure, renal failure, alcoholism, sepsis
- Postprandial, especially post-gastrectomy: excessive response to glucose load

Clinical manifestations (glucose < ~55 mg/dl)
- **CNS**: headache, visual Δs, Δ MS, weakness (neuroglycopenic sx)
- **Autonomic**: diaphoresis, palpitations, tremor

Workup (*NEJM* 1995;332:1144)
- BUN, Cr, LFTs, TFTs
- 72 hr fast with monitored blood glucoses; stop for neuroglycopenic sx
- At end of fast, give 1 mg glucagon IV and measure response of plasma glc before feeding
- *At time of hypoglycemia:* insulin, C peptide (↑ with insulinoma and sulfonylureas, ↓ with exogenous insulin), β-OH-butyrate, sulfonylurea levels, and IGF-II

• LIPID DISORDERS •

Primary Hyperlipidemias		
	Disorder	**Comments**
↑ risk of CAD	Familial hypercholesterolemia (FH)	Defective LDL receptor; autosomal co-dom; prev 1:500 Type IIa pattern (↑ LDL) → ↑↑ chol Heterozygotes develop CAD in 30-40s Familial defective apoB100 clinically identical
↑ risk of CAD	Familial combined hyperlipidemia (FCH)	Polygenic disorder; associated with obesity & diabetes Type IIb pattern (↑ VLDL & LDL) → ↑ chol and TG
↑ risk of CAD	Familial dysbetalipoproteinemia	Autosomal rec., associated w/ 2 copies of apo E2 allele Type III pattern (↑ IDL) → ↑ chol and TG
Nl risk of CAD	Familial hyperchylomicronemia	LDL deficiency Type I pattern (↑ chylomicrons) → ↑↑↑ TG ↑ risk of pancreatitis
Nl risk of CAD	Familial hypertriglyceridemia	Hepatic overproduction of VLDL; ? ↑ risk of CAD Type IV pattern (↑ VLDL) → ↑ TG ± ↑ chol
Nl risk of CAD	Type V hyperlipidemia	Multifactorial Type V pattern (↑ VLDL & chylo) → ↑↑ TG and ↑ chol

(Pattern refers to Fredrickson pattern. *Med Clin North Am* 1989;73:859)

Physical examination

- Tendon xanthomas: seen on Achilles tendon, elbows, and hands; move with flexion and extension; imply LDL >300 mg/dl (and thus most likely FH)
- Eruptive xanthomas: pimple-like lesions seen on extensor surfaces; imply TG >1000 mg/dl
- Tuberous xanthomas & palmar striated xanthomas pathognomonic of dysbetalipo.
- Xanthelasma: yellowish streaks on eyelids seen in various dyslipidemias
- Corneal arcus: common in older adults, imply hyperlipidemia in young Pts

Secondary Hyperlipidemias	
Category	**Disorders**
Endocrinopathies	Hypothyroidism (↑ LDL, ↑ TG) Diabetes (↑ TG, ↓ HDL) Cushing's syndrome & exogenous steroids (↑ LDL)
Renal diseases	Uremia (↑ TG) Nephrotic syndrome (↑ LDL)
Hepatic diseases	Acute hepatitis (↑ TG) Primary biliary cirrhosis (↑ LDL)
Lifestyle	Obesity (↑ TG, ↓ HDL); Sedentary lifestyle (↓ HDL) Alcoholism (↑ TG); Cigarette smoking (↓ HDL) OCP (↑ TG)

NCEP Guidelines			
Clinical risk	**Start lifestyle Δ's**	**Start drug Rx**	**Goal of Rx**
1 risk factor for CAD	>160 mg/dL	>190 mg/dL	<160 mg/dL
≥2 risk factors for CAD	>130 mg/dL	>130-160 mg/dL*	<130 mg/dL
⊕ CAD, DM, or PVD	>100 mg/dL	>130 mg/dL	<100 mg/dL
*Guidelines based on LDL. Risk factors: male ≥45 or female ≥55, smoking, hypertension, ⊕ FHx, HDL <40. If HDL >60 subtract 1 RF. *based on Framingham 10yr CHD risk score*			

(*JAMA* 2001;285:2486)

Treatment				
Drug	**LDL**	**HDL**	**TG**	**Side effects**
Statins	↓ 20-60%	↑ 5-10%	↓ 10-25%	Hepatitis Myopathy
Resins	↓ 20%	↑ 5%	? ↑	GI distress
Ezetimibe	↓ 20%	↑ 5%	-	Well tolerated
Fibrates	↓ 5-15% may ↑	↑ 10-20%	↓ 30%	GI distress, gallstones Myopathy risk w/ statin
Nicotinic acid	↓ 10-25%	↑ 15-30%	↓ 40%	Flushing (Rx w/ ASA), pruritis, ↑ glc, gout, GI distress, hepatitis

• ARTHRITIS – OVERVIEW •

Fig. 8-1. Approach to arthritis

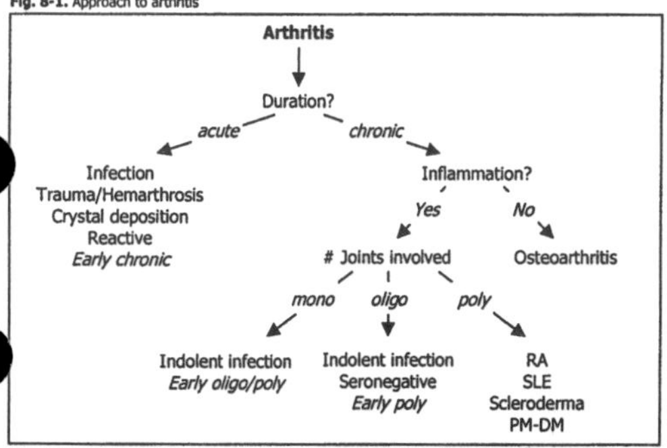

(Adapted from Braunwald E, et al., eds. *Harrison's Principles of Internal Medicine*, 15th ed., 2001)

Comparison of Major Arthritides

Feature	OA	RA	Crystal	Seronegative
Onset	gradual	gradual	acute	variable
Inflammation	⊖	⊕	⊕	⊕
Pathology	degeneration	pannus	microtophi	enthesitis
# of joints	poly	poly	mono	oligo or poly
Type of joints	large	small	small or large	large
Location	DIP weight-bearing	MCP wrists	MTP feet, ankles	sacroiliac spine peripheral
Special articular Δs	Bouchard's nodes Heberden's nodes	ulnar dev. swan neck boutonnière	crystals	en bloc spine enthesopathy
Bone changes	osteophytes	osteoporosis erosions	erosions	erosions ankylosis
Extra-articular features		SC nodules pulmonary cardiac splenomegaly	tophi olec. bursitis	uveitis conjunctivitis aortic pulmonary psoriasis IBD
Lab data	normal	⊕ RF, ↑ ESR	↑ UA	HLA-B27

Analysis of Joint Fluid

Test	Normal	Noninflammatory	Inflammatory	Septic
Appearance	clear	clear, yellow	clear to opaque yellow-white	opaque
WBC/mm^3	<200	<2,000	>2,000	>2,000 often ↑↑↑
Polys	<25%	<25%	≥50%	≥75%
Culture	⊖	⊖	⊖	⊕
Glucose	≈ serum	≈ serum	25 < glc < serum	glc < 25
Conditions		OA, trauma	RA, crystal CTD seronegative	infection

(Adapted from *Current Medical Diagnosis and Treatment*, 41st ed., 2002)

• RHEUMATOID ARTHRITIS (RA) •

Definition and epidemiology

- Chronic debilitating destructive polyarthritis
- Genetic factors affect susceptibility. ↑ incidence in those with Class II MHC DRB1 and DR4.
- Prevalence = 1% of adults; female:male = 3:1; onset 35-50 yrs

Clinical manifestations (*Lancet* 2001;358:903)

- Chronic, symmetric, sterile, erosive **synovitis of joints** (typically PIPs, MCPs, wrists, knees, ankles, MTPs, and cervical spine) with **morning stiffness** for ≥1 hr
- Joint immobilization, muscle shortening, bone & cartilage destruction, joint deformities:
  - **ulnar deviation**
  - **swan neck deformity** (MCP flexion, PIP hyperextension, DIP flexion)
  - **boutonnière deformity** (PIP flexion, DIP hyperextension)
  - **cock-up deformities** and subluxations of the MTP heads.
- **C1-C2 instability** → myelopathy, ∴ ✓ C-spine flex/ext films prior to elective intubation
- **Rheumatoid nodules** (20-30%; usually in RF ⊕ patients): SC nodules on extensor surfaces along tendon sheaths and in bursae; also occur in lung, pericardium and sclera
- Ocular: keratoconjunctivitis sicca (associated Sjögren's), scleritis, corneal melt
- Malaise, mild fever, weight loss
- Pulmonary
  - ILD: COP, fibrosis, nodules, Caplan's syndrome (pneumoconiosis + rheumatoid nodules)
  - pleural disease: pleuritis, pleural effusions (low or no glucose)
  - airway disease: obstruction (cricoarytenoid arthritis), bronchiolitis, bronchiectasis
- Cardiac: pericarditis, pericardial effusion, aortitis
- Heme: anemia of chronic disease, leukemia, lymphoma
- Carpal tunnel syndrome
- Long-standing seropositive, erosive RA:
  - Raynaud's phenomenon
  - small nail fold infarcts, palpable purpura, leukocytoclastic vasculitis
  - secondary amyloidosis (AA)
  - *Felty's syndrome* (1%): active RA, splenomegaly and neutropenia; ↑ risk of NHL
- Remember that rheumatoid joints can become *superinfected*

Laboratory and radiologic studies

- ⊕ **RF** (IgM anti-IgG Ab) in 85% of Pts; levels correlate only loosely with disease activity
  - *non*-specific as also seen in other rheumatic diseases (SLE, Sjögren's), chronic inflammation (SBE, hepatitis, TB), type II cryoglobulinemia, 5% of healthy population
- Anti-CCP (cyclic citrullinated peptides): less sens. (~60%) but more spec. (~90%) for RA
- ↑ ESR and CRP; ⊕ ANA in ~15%; ↑ globulin during periods of active disease
- Radiographs of hands and wrists: erosions, deformities and periarticular decalcification

Classification criteria (4 of 7; ~90% sens. and spec.; *Arthritis Rheum* 1988;31:315)

- **Morning stiffness** ≥1 hr × 6 wks
- **Arthritis** ≥3 joints simultaneously × 6 wks
- **Hand joint arthritis** × 6 wks
- **Symmetric joint involvement** × 6 wks
- **Rheumatoid nodules**
- ⊕ **Rheumatoid factor**
- **Radiographic changes** consistent with RA (i.e., erosions and periarticular decalcification)

Treatment (*Arthritis Rheum* 2002;46:328)

- Symptomatic relief & ↓ inflammation
  - 1st line: **NSAIDs/COX-2 inhibitors**
  - 2nd line: **glucocorticoids** (joint injection and/or low-dose oral)
- **DMARDs** for any Pt w/ established disease and ongoing inflammation
  - 1st line: hydroxychloroquine or sulfasalazine, methotrexate (MTX) for very active disease
  - 2nd line: leflunomide, anti-TNF Rx (etanercept, infliximab, or adalimumab), anakinra (IL-1 receptor antagonist); MTX + etanercept superior to either alone (*Lancet* 2004;363:675)
  - Other agents: azathioprine, penicillamine, gold, minocycline, cyclosporine

Prognosis

- Typical disease course variable with exacerbations & remissions
- 15% of patients will have a complete remission
- 10% of patients will have severe, progressive arthritis despite Rx
- Poor prognostic signs: ↑↑ RF, ⊕ ANA, persistently ↑ ESR & CRP, nodules, erosions

• CRYSTAL DEPOSITION ARTHRITIDES •

Gout

Definition
- Urate crystal deposition in joints and other tissues → acute and chronic inflammation

Epidemiology
- More common in men than in women; peak incidence 5th decade
- Most common cause of inflammatory arthritis in men over 30
- *Rare* in premenopausal women (estrogens promote renal urate excretion), ∴ if confirm diagnosis of gout, search for cause of secondary hyperuricemia (see below)
- Predisposing factors: obesity, hypertriglyceridemia, diabetes mellitus

Etiologies
- Uric acid (UA) is end-product of purine catabolism and is renally excreted. Serum level reflects balance between production and excretion.

	Overproduction	Underexcretion
Primary hyperuricemia (inherited)	**Idiopathic** Rare enzyme (HGPRT, PRPP) deficiencies	**Idiopathic**
Secondary hyperuricemia (acquired)	**Excessive dietary purine or alcohol** **Myelo- & lymphoproliferative dis.** Chronic hemolytic anemia Cytotoxic drugs, psoriasis Severe muscle exertion	**Dehydration** ↓ renal function Drugs: **diuretics**, PZA, EMB, salicylates, CsA Keto- or lactic acidosis

Clinical manifestations
- **Acute arthritis**: sudden onset, frequently nocturnal, of **painful monoarticular arthritis**
  location: **MTP of great toe** ("podagra"), feet, ankles, knees
  occasionally polyarticular (in women more than in men)
  overlying skin is warm, tense, dusky red; patient may be febrile
  precipitants: rapid Δ UA; ↑ purine or alcohol; surgery; infection; diuretics, dehydration
  recovery: subsides over 3-10 d with desquamation and pruritis overlying affected area
- **Tophi**: deposits of urate crystals leading to foreign body reaction, found in Heberden's nodes, synovium, subchondral bone, or Achilles tendons; more rarely in aortic walls, cardiac valves, eyelids, nasal cartilage and pinna of the ear.
- **Bursitis**: olecranon, patellar (must be differentiated from intra-articular knee effusion)
- **Chronic arthritis**: gross deformities, functional loss, disability
- **Renal**: uric acid stones; gouty nephritis (interstitial deposits)

Diagnostic studies
- ↑ UA, but can be misleading and does *not* make the diagnosis of acute attack
- Arthrocentesis
  take care not to tap through an infected area thus introducing infections into joint space
  polarized microscopy → **needle-shaped, *negatively* birefringent crystals** (yellow *parallel* and blue perpendicular to axis marked on polarizer), intra- or extracellular
  WBC 20,000-100,000/mm^3, >50% polys
  infection can co-exist with acute attacks, ∴ always check gram stain and culture
- Radiographs
  early → show soft tissue swelling; useful to exclude chondrocalcinosis or septic changes
  late → bony erosions with sclerotic margins, calcifications

Acute Treatment for Gout		
Drug	**Mechanism**	**Comments**
NSAIDs	↓ inflammation	Gastritis; ↓ dose in renal insufficiency
Colchicine (PO or IV)	Inhibits polymerization of microtubules → prevention of chemotaxis and phagocytosis	Nausea, vomiting and diarrhea IV and high PO doses → bone marrow suppression, myopathy, neuropathy ↓ dose in renal insufficiency
Corticosteroids (PO or intra-artic)	↓ inflammation	Highly effective for recalcitrant cases Rule-out joint infection first

(*NEJM* 2003;349:1647)

Chronic treatment

- ↓ urate production by avoiding foods high in purine (e.g., meats, beans, peas, spinach, beer); ↓ alcohol; avoid dehydration; avoid hyperuricemic drugs (e.g., diuretics, low-dose ASA)
- Prophylaxis: colchicine or NSAIDs if frequent attacks
- **Hypouricemic therapy** for tophi, frequent attacks, nephrolithiasis; goal is UA <5 mg/dl
  however, do not start until 2-4 wks after acute attack as Δ in serum UA concentration can precipitate an attack
  allopurinol (xanthine oxidase inhibitor); side effects: hypersensitivity, rash, diarrhea, dyspepsia, headache, renal failure, BM suppression, and hepatitis
  probenecid or **sulfinpyrazone** (uricosuric agents) for underexcreters (urine UA <600 mg/24 hrs)

CALCIUM PYROPHOSPHATE DIHYDRATE (CPPD) DEPOSITION DISEASE

Definition

- Deposition of CPPD crystals w/in tendons, ligaments, articular capsules, synovium, cartilage
- **Chondrocalcinosis**: calcified cartilage secondary to CPPD deposition

Pathogenesis

- ↑ synovial & joint fluid levels of inorganic pyrophosphate, produced by articular chondrocytes from ATP hydrolysis in response to a variety of insults or inherited defects

Epidemiology

- More common in the elderly: 4% of adult population at age 72 has CPPD crystal deposition

Etiologies

- Most cases ***idiopathic***, but consider search for underlying cause, especially in the young
- **Metabolic**: hypomagnesemia, alkaline phosphatase deficiency, hyperparathyroidism, hypothyroidism, familial hypocalciuric hypercalcemia, gout, Gitelman's syndrome, X-linked hypophosphatemic rickets, hemochromatosis
- Trauma
- Joint injections with hyaluronate can precipitate attacks
- Familial chondrocalcinosis (autosomal dominant disorder)

Clinical manifestations

- "Pseudogout": acute, usually symmetric, mono- or oligoarticular arthritis
  location: knees, wrists and MCP joints; precipitants: surgery or severe illness
- "PseudoRA": chronic polyarticular arthritis with morning stiffness; ± RF
- Premature OA: destruction of articular cartilage and bony overgrowths → degen. of joints

Diagnostic studies

- Arthrocentesis
  take care not to tap through an infected area thus introducing infections into joint space
  polarized microscopy → **rhomboid-shaped, weakly *positively* birefringent crystals** (yellow *perpendicular* and blue parallel to axis marked on polarizer)
  WBC 2000-100,000/mm^3, > 50% polys
  infection can co-exist with acute attacks, ∴ always check gram stain and culture
- Screen for metabolic diseases when dx a new case: ✓ Ca, Mg, TSH, Fe, glc, UA
- **Radiographs**: punctate and linear densities in articular hyaline, chondrocalcinosis, especially in menisci, small joints of fingers, and symphysis pubis

Treatment

- Acute therapy: same as for gout
- Chronic therapy: treat underlying disease

• SERONEGATIVE SPONDYLOARTHROPATHIES •

General

Definition (*Annals* 2002;136:896)
- Multisystem inflammatory arthritides affecting spine, peripheral joints, and periarticular structures
- Includes: ankylosing spondylitis, reactive arthritis, psoriatic arthritis, enteropathic arthritis, and undifferentiated spondyloarthropathies
- Notable for *absence* of rheumatoid factor or autoantibodies; ± ↑ ESR
- ↑ prevalence of HLA-B27 (⊕ in 50-90% vs. 6-8% of general pop.), but *not* used for dx
- Synovial fluid of affected joints shows an inflammatory, non-septic picture

Ankylosing Spondylitis

Epidemiology
- Onset in teens or mid-20's; onset after age 40 very unusual; male:female ratio = 3:1; HLA-B27 ⊕ in 90%

Clinical manifestations
- Gradual onset of chronic, intermittent bouts of lower back pain and stiffness
- **Morning stiffness** that improves with hot shower and exercise
- Mild constitutional symptoms in early stages
- Slow cephalad progression of **limitation of back motion** and chest expansion
  ⊕ modified **Wright-Schober test** (<4 cm ↑ in distance between a point at lumbosacral junction and one 10 cm above, when going from standing to maximum forward flexion)
- **Enthesitis** (inflammation at site of ligament insertion into bone) causes tenderness at costochondral junctions, spinous processes, scapulae, iliac crests, heels
- **Transient arthritis in peripheral joints** (hips, shoulders, knees), occasionally permanent
- Acute anterior **uveitis** (25% at some time during disease): presents with unilateral blurred vision, lacrimation and photophobia. Resolves in 4-8 wks
- Cardiovascular disease (5%): ascending aortitis, AI, conduction system abnormalities
- Neurologic symptoms: due to spinal fracture or dislocation even with minor trauma

Radiographs
- **Sacroiliac joint disease** with erosions and sclerosis
- Calcification of spinal ligaments with bridging syndesmophytes ("bamboo spine")
- Squaring and generalized demineralization of vertebral bodies, "shiny corners"

Treatment
- Physical therapy, NSAIDs, steroid injection, short course systemic steroids, sulfasalazine, methotrexate

Reactive Arthritis

Epidemiology
- Worldwide distribution, but rare in African-Americans, male:female ratio = 5:1

Pathogenesis
- Response in genetically susceptible host to genitourinary or gastrointestinal infection
- Thought to be secondary to infection with *Chlamydia* and *Ureaplasma urealyticum* as well as *Shigella, Salmonella, Yersinia, Campylobacter, Klebsiella, C. difficile, Trophyrema whippelii*, HIV

Clinical Presentation
- Originally described as *Reiter's Syndrome* = triad of **seronegative arthritis, nongonococcal urethritis** and **non-infectious conjunctivitis**
- **Arthritis**: 10-30 d post inciting infection → mild constitutional sx, low back pain, asymmetric, mono- or oligoarticular arthritis of primarily large joints (knees, ankles, feet, wrists), enthesopathy, and sacroiliitis. Can develop *sausage digits* of extremities.
- **Urethritis**: usually chlamydial infection preceding arthritis, but also can see sterile urethritis in post-dysenteric reactive arthritis
- **Conjunctivitis**: non-infectious, unilateral or bilateral and ± uveitis, iritis and keratitis

- Cutaneous manifestations (may go unnoticed by patient)
  - **balantitis circinata**: shallow, painless ulcers of glans penis and urethral meatus
  - **keratoderma blenorrhagica**: hyperkeratotic skin lesions on soles of feet, scrotum, palms, trunk, scalp
  - stomatitis and superficial oral ulcers
- Gastrointestinal tract: diarrhea and abdominal pain either with or without infectious agent
- Cardiovascular: AI from inflammation and scarring of aorta and AoV; conduction defects

Imaging
- **Sacroiliitis** eventually in 70% patients
- **Soft tissue swelling** around affected joints
- Joint space narrowing in small joints

Diagnostic studies
- PCR of urine or genital swab for *Chlamydia*, stool cultures, C. difficile toxin, HIV, etc., but ⊖ studies do not rule out

Treatment and prognosis
- NSAIDs, steroids for keratoderma blenorrhagica, sulfasalazine
- Antibiotics if evidence of infection
- Arthritis may persist for months to years and recurrences are common

Psoriatic Arthritis

Epidemiology
- 15% of Pts with psoriasis develop arthritis; not necessarily those with severe skin disease
- Arthritis may precede onset of skin disease, even by years
- 40% of patients with psoriatic arthritis have an associated spondyloarthropathy
- Men and women are affected equally and most patients in 30's and 40's

Clinical manifestations
- Several clinical patterns of arthritis:
  - **monoarticular/oligoarticular** (e.g., large joint, DIP joint, dactylitic digit) most common initial manifestation
  - **polyarthritis** (small joints of the hands and feet, wrists, ankles, knees, elbows); indistinguishable from RA
  - **arthritis mutilans**: severe destructive resorptive arthritis
  - **axial disease**: similar to ankylosing spondylitis ± peripheral arthritis
- Enthesopathies
- Fingernails: pitting, transverse depressions, onycholysis, subungal hyperkeratosis
- Eye inflammation (30%): conjunctivitis, iritis, episcleritis and keratoconjunctivitis sicca
- Psoriatic skin lesions

Radiographs
- **"Pencil-in-cup"** deformity seen at DIP joints
- Spinal involvement, sacroiliitis

Treatment
- 1st line: NSAIDs/COX-2 inhibitors
- 2nd line (failure of NSAIDs or aggressive disease)
  - methotrexate, PUVA to improve skin and peripheral joint disease
  - sulfasalazine for peripheral joint disease without skin disease
- Other: etanercept, infliximab, retinoic acid, CsA, antimalarials, gold, penicillamine, AZA

Enteropathic (IBD-Associated)

Epidemiology
- 20% of patients with IBD develop arthritis; more frequently seen in Crohn's than UC

Clinical manifestations
- **Peripheral, asymmetric, non-deforming oligoarthritis**: abrupt onset, large joints, course *parallels* GI disease
- **Spondylitis:** associated more strongly with HLA-B27, course does *not* parallel GI disease
- Erythema nodosum, pyoderma gangrenosum, anterior uveitis

Treatment
- 5-ASA compounds, etc. for underlying IBD (see "IBD")

• INFECTIOUS ARTHRITIS •

NONGONOCOCCAL

Epidemiology
- **Abnormal or immunosuppressed host** (e.g., diabetics, HIV, elderly)
- **Bacteremia** secondary to IVDA, endocarditis, or skin infection; also can occur due to direct inoculation or spread from a contiguous focus (e.g., cellulitis, septic bursitis, osteomyelitis)
- **Damaged joints**: RA, OA, gout, trauma, prosthetic, prior arthrocentesis

Microbiology
- GPC: ***S. aureus*** (most frequent), *S. epidermidis* (post-procedure, prostheses), streptococci
- GNR (especially in IVDA): *E. coli*, *Pseudomonas* and *Serratia*

Clinical manifestations
- Acute onset of **monoarticular arthritis** (>80%) with pain, swelling, and warmth
- Location: **knee** (most common), hip, wrist, shoulder, ankle. In IVDA, tends to involve other areas such as sacroiliac joint, symphysis pubis, sternoclavicular and manubrial joints.
- In knee, septic pre-patellar bursitis (no intra-articular effusion, preserved range of motion) must be differentiated from septic intra-articular knee effusion
- **Constitutional symptoms**: fevers, chills, sweats, malaise, myalgias, pain
- Infection can track from initial site to form fistulae, abscesses, or osteomyelitis

Diagnostic studies
- **Leukocytosis** with left shift
- **Arthrocentesis** should be performed as soon as suspected
  take care not to tap through an infected area thus introducing infections into joint space
  synovial fluid: **WBC usually >100,000** (but can be as low as 1000), **>90% polys**
  (crystals do *not* rule out septic arthritis!)
  gram stain ⊕ in ~75% of staphylococcal infections, ~50% of GNR infections
  culture ⊕ in >90% of cases
- **Blood cultures**: ⊕ in >50% of cases
- Conventional radiographs rarely helpful as normal until after ~2 wks of infection when can then see bony erosions, joint space narrowing, osteomyelitis, periostitis
- **CT and MRI** useful especially for suspected hip infection or epidural abscess

DISSEMINATED GONOCOCCAL INFECTION (DGI)

Epidemiology
- Most frequent type of infectious arthritis in young adults.
- **Normal host** as well as patients with deficiencies of terminal components of complement
- Female:male ratio = 4:1. ↑ incidence during menses, pregnancy and postpartum period. ↑ incidence in homosexual males. Rare after age 40.

Clinical manifestations
- Preceded by **mucosal infection** (e.g., endocervix, urethra or pharynx) that is often asx
- **Prodrome**: fever, malaise, **migratory polyarthralgias** (wrist, knees, ankles, elbows)
- Acute onset of **tenosynovitis** (60%) in wrists, fingers, ankles, toes
- **Purulent monoarthritis** (40%) usually of the knees, wrists, hands, or ankles
- **Rash** (>50%): gunmetal gray pustules on an erythematous base on extremities & trunk
- Rarely: pericarditis, meningitis, aortitis, endocarditis, myocarditis, osteomyelitis, hepatitis

Diagnostic studies
- **Leukocytosis** with left shift; ↑ ESR
- **Arthrocentesis** should be performed as soon as suspected
  take care not to tap through an infected area thus introducing infections into joint space
  synovial fluid: **WBC > 50,000** (but can be as low as 1000), **poly-predominant**
  (crystals do *not* rule out septic arthritis!)
  gram stain ⊕ in ~25% of cases
  culture ⊕ in up to 50% of cases if culture anaerobically on Thayer-Martin media
  PCR for gonococcal DNA can improve sensitivity (not yet widely available)
- Blood culture: more likely ⊕ in tenosynovitis; rarely in monoarthritis
- Gram stain and culture of skin lesions occasionally ⊕
- Cervical, urethral, pharyngeal, rectal cultures should be submitted on Thayer-Martin media

TREATMENT

Therapy
- Prompt antibiotics guided by gram stain

Gram stain	Antibiotic regimen
GPC	Nafcillin *or* Vancomycin if suspect MRSA (e.g., hospitalized Pt)
Gram-negative cocci	Ceftriaxone
GNR	Ceftriaxone + anti-pseudomonal aminoglycoside if suspect IVDA
No organism seen	Nafcillin *or* Vancomycin + Ceftriaxone + anti-pseudomonal aminoglycoside if suspect IVDA

- Antibiotic regimen then tailored based on culture and sensitivity data and clinical response
- Local aspiration or surgical drainage/lavage if not improving
- Prognosis: if polyarticular non-gonococcal sepsis, mortality ≈ 30%

• CONNECTIVE TISSUE DISEASES •

Fig. 8-2. Venn diagram of connective tissue diseases

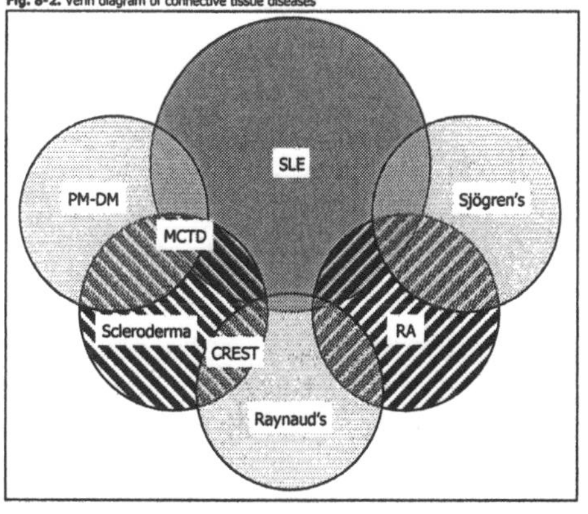

Autoantibodies in Connective Tissue Diseases (%)										
Disease	**ANA & Pattern**	**RF**	**dsDNA**	**Sm**	**Ro**	**La**	**Scl-70**	**Cent**	**Jo**	**RNP**
SLE	95-99 D, S, N	20	50-70	30	35	15	0	0	0	30-50
RA	15-35 D	85	<5	0	10	5	0	0	0	10
Sjögren's	>90 D, S	75	<5	0	55	40	0	0	0	15
Diffuse sclero.	>90 S, N, D	30	0	0	5	1	40	<5	0	30
Limited sclero.	>90 S, N, D	30	0	0	5	1	<15	70	0	30
PM-DM	75-95	33	0	0	0	0	10	0	25	0
MCTD	95-99 S, D	50	0	0	<5	<5	0	0	0	100

(D = diffuse or homogeneous, S = speckled, N = nucleolar; *Primer on the Rheumatic Diseases*, 12th ed., 2001)

see "Systemic Lupus Erythematosus" and "Rheumatoid Arthritis" for those diseases

SCLERODERMA (SYSTEMIC SCLEROSIS)

Definition and epidemiology

- Patients present in their 20's-40's; more common in women than in men
- **Subtypes**
  - **Systemic:** multiorgan involvement
    - systemic sclerosis with *diffuse cutaneous disease* (incl. proximal extremities & trunk)
    - systemic sclerosis with *limited cutaneous disease* (CREST syndrome)
    - systemic sclerosis *sine scleroderma* (visceral disease w/o skin involvement)
  - **Localized:** *morphea* (plaques of fibrotic skin), *linear* (fibrotic bands), "*en coup de saber*" (linear scleroderma involving one side of scalp and forehead ≈ saber scar)

Classification criteria (1 major or 2 minor; 97% sens, 98% spec; *Arthritis Rheum* 1980;23:581)

- *Major*: **skin findings *proximal* to MCP or MTP joints**
- *Minor*: **sclerodactyly** (skin findings limited to the fingers)
  - **digital pitting scars** of loss of substance from the finger pad
  - bibasilar **pulmonary fibrosis**

Clinical Manifestations of Scleroderma	
Organ	**Involvement**
Skin	Tightening and thickening of extremities, face, and trunk "Puffy" hands, carpal tunnel syndrome, sclerodactyly Nail fold capillary dilatation & dropout Immobile, pinched, "mouse-like" facies and "purse-string" mouth Calcinosis cutis (subcutaneous calcification) Telangiectasias
Arteries	Raynaud's phenomenon (80%); digital or visceral ischemia
Renal	Scleroderma renal crisis = sudden onset severe HTN, RPGN, MAHA
GI	GERD and erosive esophagitis Esophageal dysmotility → dysphagia and odynophagia Gastric dysmotility → early satiety and gastric outlet obstruction Small intestinal dysmotility → bloating, diarrhea, malabsorption
Musculoskel	Polyarthralgias & joint stiffness; muscle weakness, tendon friction rubs
Cardiac	Myocardial fibrosis, pericarditis; conduction abnormalities
Pulmonary	Pulmonary fibrosis; pulmonary hypertension
Endocrine	Amenorrhea and infertility common; thyroid fibrosis ± hypothyroidism

Systemic Sclerosis		
	Limited	**Diffuse**
Skin	Thickening of distal extremities and face only	Thickening of extremities, face, *and trunk*
Nails	Capillary dropout ± dilatation	Capillary dropout & *dilatation*
Pulmonary	Pulmonary fibrosis (67%) *PHT* (10%)	Pulmonary fibrosis (67%)
GI	GERD, hypomotility *Biliary cirrhosis*	GERD, hypomotility
Renal		Renovascular HTN
Cardiac		Restrictive cardiomyopathy
Other	**CREST syndrome =** **C**alcinosis **R**aynaud's **E**sophageal dysmotility **S**clerodactyly **T**elangiectasias	
Antibodies	Anti-centromere (70%)	Anti-Scl 70 (40%)
Prognosis	Survival >70% at 10 yrs	Survival 40-60% at 10 yrs

Diagnostic studies

- Autoantibodies
  - ⊕ **anti-Scl-70** (anti-topoisomerase 1): 40% of diffuse, 15% of limited
  - ⊕ **anti-centromere**: <5% of diffuse, 60-80% of limited
  - ⊕ ANA (>90%), ⊕ RF (30%)
- ↑ ESR, ↑ globulin
- If renal involvement → ↑ BUN and Cr, proteinuria
- If pulmonary involvement → interstitial pattern on CXR, restriction on PFTs, ± PHT

Treatment

- DMARDs: MTX, CsA, cyclophosphamide, AZA
- Raynaud's: CCB (but may worsen GERD), avoid cold & cigarettes, IV prostaglandins
- GI: PPI (GERD); abx (malabsorption); metoclopramide/erythromycin (hypomotility)
- Hypertensive crises: ACE inhibitors (not ARB), poor prognosis with 50% mortality
- Pulmonary: steroids, cyclophosphamide, AZA (fibrosis); IV epoprostenol or bosentan (PHT)

POLYMYOSITIS (PM) – DERMATOMYOSITIS (DM)

Definition and epidemiology (*Lancet* 2003;362:971)

- **Polymyositis**: *T cell-mediated muscle injury* → skeletal muscle inflammation & weakness
- **Dermatomyositis**: *immune complex deposition in blood vessels* → skeletal muscle inflammation & weakness *+ skin manifestations*
- Patients typically in 40's and 50's; more common in women than in men
- ↑ incidence of cancer (especially ovarian) in ~10% of Pts with DM (lower incidence in PM)

Clinical manifestations
- **Muscle weakness**: gradual, progressive, bilateral, and *proximal* with tenderness of affected areas; typically with difficulty climbing stairs and arising from chairs.
- **Dermatologic**
  - **erythematous rash** on sun-exposed areas, butterfly area of face, neck, shoulders
  - **heliotrope rash** (purplish discoloration) over upper eyelids
  - **Gottron's papules** (*pathognomonic*): lacy, pink or violaceous areas symmetrically over dorsum of PIP, MCP, elbows, patellae, medial malleoli
  - subungal erythema, cuticular telangiectasias, **"mechanic's hands"** (cracking of skin of distal fingertips)
- Polyarthralgias or polyarthritis
- Vasculitis of skin, muscle, GI tract and eyes, and Raynaud's phenomenon (30%)
- Visceral involvement
  - pulmonary: acute alveolitis, chronic ILD, weakness of respiratory muscles
  - cardiac (33%): myocarditis, pericarditis and arrhythmias
  - GI: dysphagia and delayed gastric emptying

Diagnostic studies
- ↑ **CK**, aldolase, SGOT, and LDH
- Autoantibodies
  - ⊕ **anti-Jo-1** (25%), associated with PM + deforming polyarthritis, Raynaud's, ILD
  - ⊕ **anti-Mi-2** (5-10%), associated with dermatomyositis
  - ⊕ ANA (>75%), ⊕ RF (33%)
- ± ↑ ESR
- **EMG**: ↑ spontaneous activity, ↓ amplitude, polyphasic potentials with contraction
- Muscle biopsy
  - PM: cellular infiltrate within the muscle fascicle
  - DM: perifascicular, often perivascular cellular infiltrate, complement in vessel walls

Classification criteria (DM = 3 criteria + derm features; PM = 4 criteria; *NEJM* 1975;292:344)
1. Symmetrical weakness
2. Muscle biopsy evidence
3. Elevation of muscle enzymes
4. EMG evidence
5. Dermatologic features

Treatment
- 1st line: **high-dose steroids**
- 2nd line: DMARDs (e.g., MTX, AZA, cyclophosphamide)
- ✓ for occult malignancy
- Monitor respiratory muscle weakness (e.g., negative inspiratory force)

Myositides, Myopathies, and Myalgias					
Disease	**Weakness**	**Pain**	**↑ CK**	**↑ ESR**	**Biopsy**
DM/PM	⊕	⊖	⊕	±	as above
Inclusion body	⊕	⊖	⊕	⊖	eosinophilic inclusions
Hypothyroidism	⊕	±	⊕	⊖	mild necrosis inflammation atrophy
Steroid-induced	⊕	⊖	⊖	⊖	atrophy
PMR	⊖ (limited by pain)	⊕	⊖	⊕	normal
Fibromyalgia	⊖ (limited by pain)	⊕ (tender points)	⊖	⊖	normal

SJÖGREN'S SYNDROME (SICCA SYNDROME)

Definition and epidemiology
- Chronic dysfunction of **exocrine glands** due to lymphoplasmacytic infiltration
- Can be primary or secondary (associated with RA, scleroderma, SLE, PM, HIV)
- More prevalent in women than in men; typically presents between 40-60 yrs of age

Clinical manifestations
- **Dry eyes** → keratoconjunctivitis
- **Dry mouth** (xerostomia) → difficulty speaking and swallowing; dental caries

- Parotid gland enlargement
- Systemic manifestations: chronic arthritis; interstitial nephritis (40%), type I RTA (20%); vasculitis (25%); pleuritis; pancreatitis; neuropsychiatric disorders
- ↑ risk of lymphoproliferative disorders (~50x ↑ risk of lymphoma and Waldenström's macroglobulinemia in primary Sjögren's)

Diagnostic studies
- Autoantibodies
  Sjögren's alone: ⊕ **anti-Ro** (anti-SS-A, 55%) and ⊕ **anti-La** (anti-SS-B, 40%)
  ⊕ ANA (95%), ⊕ RF (75%)
- **Schirmer test**: filter paper in palpebral fissures to assess tear production
- **Rose-Bengal** staining: dye which reveals devitalized epithelium of cornea/conjunctiva
- **Biopsy** (minor salivary, labial, lacrimal, or parotid gland): lymphoplasmacytic infiltration

Classification criteria (4 of 6 has 94% sens. and 94% spec.; *Arthritis Rheum* 1993;36:340)
1. Dry eyes
2. Dry mouth
3. Positive Schirmer test or Rose-Bengal staining
4. Salivary gland involvement
5. Antibodies to Ro/SS-A or La/SS-B

Treatment
- Supportive: artificial tears, sugarfree gum, lemondrops, cholinergic Rx for xerostomia
- Systemic manifestations: NSAIDs, steroids, DMARDs

Mixed Connective Tissue Disease (MCTD)

Definition
- Patients with MCTD tend to have features of **SLE**, **scleroderma**, and/or **polymyositis**.

Clinical manifestations
- **Raynaud's phenomenon** typical presenting symptom; hand edema → sclerodactyly
- RA-like **arthritis** without erosions
- Pulmonary involvement (85%) with **pulmonary hypertension**, fibrosis
- GI dysmotility (70%)
- Renal disease (25%) typically with membranous nephropathy

Diagnostic studies
- **Anti-U1-RNP** present by definition in MCTD, but *not* specific (seen in up to 50% SLE Pts)
- RF (50%)

Treatment
- As per specific rheumatic diseases detailed above

Raynaud's Phenomenon

Clinical manifestations
- Episodic digital ischemia, classically with triphasic color response: **blanching** (ischemia) → **cyanosis** (venule dilatation) → **rubor** (resolution with reactive hyperemia); changes usually well-demarcated and confined to fingers & toes
- Associated sx include cold, numbness, & paresthesias → throbbing & pain
- Precipitated by cold, emotional stress

Primary = Raynaud's disease (50%; excluded all secondary causes)
- Onset age 20-40 yrs, female:male = 5:1
- Clinical: mild, symmetric episodic attacks; no evidence of peripheral vascular disease, no tissue injury, normal nailfold capillary examination, ⊖ ANA, normal ESR

Secondary = Raynaud's phenomenon (50%)
- Etiologies
  collagen vascular disease: scleroderma, SLE, RA, PM-DM (*abnormal nailfold exam*)
  arterial disease: peripheral atherosclerosis, thromboangiitis obliterans (*abnormal pulses*)
  hematologic disorders: cryoglobulinemia, Waldenström's macroglobulinemia
  trauma (vibration or repetitive motion injury) & drugs (ergot alkaloids)

Treatment
- Avoid cold, cigarettes, trauma
- Long-acting CCB, α-blockers, topical nitrates, ASA; IV prostaglandins if severe

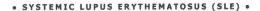

• SYSTEMIC LUPUS ERYTHEMATOSUS (SLE) •

Definition

- Multisystem inflammatory autoimmune disease with a broad spectrum of clinical manifestations in association with antinuclear antibody (ANA) production

Epidemiology

- Prevalence 15-50/100,000; predominantly affects women 2nd to 4th decade
- Female:Male ratio = 8:1; African-American:Caucasian ratio = 4:1
- HLA-linked (DR3)
- **Drug-induced lupus (DLE)**
  drugs: procainamide, hydralazine, INH, methyldopa, quinidine, chlorpromazine
  clinical: milder disease with predominantly arthritis and serositis
  laboratory: ⊕ anti-histone (95%); ⊖ anti-ds-DNA & anti-Sm; normal complement levels
  course: usually reversible within 4-6 wks

Classification Criteria and Other Clinical Manifestations of SLE		
Organ System	**Am. Coll. Rheum. Criteria**	**Other Features**
Constitutional (84%)		Fever, malaise, anorexia, weight loss
Cutaneous (81%)	**1. Malar rash** **2. Discoid rash** (erythematous papules w/ keratosis & plugging) **3. Photosensitivity** **4. Oral/nasopharyngeal ulcers**	Alopecia Vasculitis Subacute cutaneous lupus Panniculitis (lupus profundus) Urticaria
Musculoskeletal (85%)	**5. Non-erosive arthritis**: episodic, oligoarticular, symmetrical, migratory	Arthralgias and myalgias Avascular necrosis of bone
Cardiopulmonary (33%)	**6. Serositis**: pleuritis (37%) or pleural effusion, pericarditis (29%) or pericardial effusion	Pneumonitis, IPF, PHT Myocarditis Libman-Sacks endocarditis
Renal (77%)	**7. Proteinuria** (>500 mg/dl or 3+ on dipstick) or **urinary cellular casts**	Nephrotic syndrome Lupus nephritis (WHO class.): I = normal; II = mesangial; III = focal & seg. prolif.; IV = diffuse proliferative; V = membranous; VI = sclerotic
Neurologic (54%)	**8. Seizures or psychosis** without other cause	Organic brain syndrome Cranial or periph. neuropathies
Gastrointestinal (~30%)		Serositis (peritonitis, ascites) Vasculitis (bleeding, perf.) Abdominal pain Hepatitis, pancreatitis
Hematologic	**9. Hemolytic anemia** (DAT ⊕) *or* **leukopenia** (<4000/mm^3), *or* **lymphopenia** (<1500/mm^3), *or* **thrombocytopenia** (<100,000/mm^3)	Anemia of chronic disease Lupus anticoagulant ± thrombosis Splenomegaly Lymphadenopathy
Other		Sicca syndrome Conjunctivitis or episcleritis Raynaud's (20%) Nail fold capillary changes
Serologies	**10. ⊕ ANA** **11. ⊕ anti-ds-DNA, anti-SM, or anti-phospholipid Abs**	⊕ RF, ↑ ESR, ↑ CRP ↓ complement (during flare)

If ≥4 of 11 criteria met, sens. & spec. for SLE >95%. However, Pt may have SLE but not have 4 criteria at a given point in time. (*Arthritis Rheum* 1982;25:1271 & 1997;40:1725; *NEJM* 1994;330:1871; *Annals* 1995;122:940 & 123:42)

Autoantibodies in SLE		
Autoantibody	**Frequency**	**Clinical Associations**
ANA	95-99% if active disease ~90% if in remission Usually high titer Homogeneous or speckled pattern Sensitive but not specific May appear yrs before disease overt (*NEJM* 2003;349:1526)	Any or all of the broad spectrum of clinical manifestations
anti-ds-DNA	70%; very specific for SLE Titers parallel disease activity, especially renal disease	Lupus nephritis Vasculitis
anti-Sm	30%; very specific for SLE	Lupus nephritis
anti-Ro **anti-La**	15-35% ⊕ anti-Ro in ANA ⊖ SLE	Sjögren's/SLE overlap Neonatal lupus Photosensitivity Subacute cutaneous lupus
anti-U1-RNP	40%	MCTD; Raynaud's Tend *not* to have nephritis
anti-histone	drug-induced lupus (DLE), SLE	Mild arthritis and serositis

Workup

- Autoantibodies: ANA, if ⊕ → ✓ anti-ds-DNA, anti-Sm, anti-Ro, anti-La, anti-U1-RNP
- Complement levels
- Electrolytes, BUN, Cr
- U/A, urine sediment, 24-hr urine for creatinine clearance and protein
- CBC, Coombs' test, PTT, anti-cardiolipin and lupus anticoagulant

Treatment of SLE		
Drug	**Indication**	**Adverse Effects**
NSAIDs **COX-2 inhibitors**	Arthralgias/arthritis, myalgias Mild serositis	Gastritis, UGIB Renal failure
Hydroxychloroquine	Mild disease complicated by serositis, arthritis, skin Δs	Macular damage Stevens-Johnson syndrome Myopathy
Corticosteroids	Low doses for mild disease unresponsive to hydroxychloroquine High doses for major manifestations including renal and hematologic	Adrenal suppression Immunosuppression Infection Osteopenia Avascular necrosis of bone Myopathy
Azathioprine (AZA)	Mild nephritis Steroid-sparing agent	Myelosuppression Hepatotoxicity Lymphoproliferative disorders
Methotrexate (MTX)	Skin and joint disease Serositis	Myelosuppression Hepatotoxicity Pneumonitis ± fibrosis Alopecia, stomatitis
Cyclophosphamide	Severe nephritis, vasculitis or CNS disease	Myelosuppression Myeloproliferative disorders Immunosuppression Hemorrhagic cystitis, bladder cancer Infertility, teratogen
Cyclosporine (CsA)	Renal disease	Hyperplastic gums, HTN Hirsutism Renal impairment, anemia
Mycophenolate	Renal disease	Myelosuppression

Prognosis

- 5-yr survival rate >90%, 10-yr survival rate >80%
- Leading causes of morbidity and mortality: **infection, renal failure**, neurologic and cardiac events

• VASCULITIS •

LARGE-VESSEL VASCULITIS

Takayasu's arteritis ("pulseless disease")

- Definition: systemic granulomatous vasculitis involving aorta and its branches
- Epidemiology: most common in **Asia** and in **young women** of reproductive age
- Clinical manifestations
  - Phase I: inflammatory period with **fever**, **arthralgias**, weight loss
  - Phase II: vessel pain and tenderness, ↓ **and unequal pulses in extremities**, **bruits** subclavian (93%), carotid (58%), Ao (50%), renal (38%), pulm (20%), coronary (10%) pyoderma gangrenosum and erythema nodosum of skin
  - Phase III: burnt out, fibrotic period
- Diagnostic studies: ↑ ESR (75%), CRP; **arteriography** → occlusion, stenosis, irregularity and aneurysms; carotid Doppler studies; MRI/MRA; pathology → focal panarteritis, cellular infiltrate with granulomas and giant cells
- Classification criteria (3 of 6 is 90.5% sens. & 97.8% spec.; *Arthritis Rheum* 1990;33:1129)
  1. age ≤40 yrs
  2. claudication of the extremities
  3. decreased brachial artery pulse
  4. systolic BP difference >10 mm Hg
  5. bruit over subclavian arteries or aorta
  6. arteriogram abnormality (Ao, primary branches, or prox. large arteries in extremities)
- Treatment: steroids, methotrexate, anti-platelet therapy

Giant cell arteritis (Temporal arteritis) (*NEJM* 2003;349:160)

- Definition: vasculitis affecting cranial branches of arch of aorta, especially the temporal artery, but can be more generalized
- Epidemiology: Pts **older than 50** (90% older than 60); female:male ratio = 2:1
- Clinical manifestations
  - constitutional symptoms: **low grade fevers**, **fatigue**, weight loss, myalgias, anorexia
  - ophthalmic artery → optic neuritis, amaurosis fugax and blindness
  - headache; tender temporal arteries and scalp and absent temporal artery pulsation
  - facial arteries → **jaw claudication**
  - Raynaud's phenomenon; intermittent claudication of the extremities
- **Polymyalgia rheumatica** (50%): symmetrical aching proximal muscle pain & stiffness especially of shoulder girdle; morning stiffness with gelling after inactivity
- Diagnostic studies: ↑ ESR, CRP, **temporal artery biopsy** (vasculitis, granulomas)
- Classification criteria (3 of 5 is 93.5% sens. & 91.2% spec.; *Arthritis Rheum* 1990;33:1122)
  1. age ≥50 yrs
  2. new headache
  3. temporal artery tenderness or decreased pulsation
  4. ↑ ESR
  5. biopsy → vasculitis & granulomas
- Treatment: **steroids** (if vision threatened *do not await path results* before starting Rx); follow ESR and clinical status

MEDIUM-VESSEL VASCULITIS

Polyarteritis nodosa (PAN) (*JAMA* 2002;288:1632)

- Definition: acute or chronic systemic necrotizing vasculitis, typically of renal and other visceral arteries, *without granuloma formation*
- Epidemiology: more common in *men* than women; average age of onset ~50 yrs; strongly **associated with HBV**
- Clinical manifestations (Cupps & Fauci. *The Vasculitides*. Philadelphia: Saunders, 1981)
  - constitutional symptoms: **weight loss**, fevers, fatigue
  - musculoskeletal (64%): **myalgias**, arthralgias, arthritis
  - renal involvement (60%) with **active urinary sediment**, **hypertension**, **renal failure**
  - nervous system (51%): **peripheral neuropathies**, mononeuritis multiplex, stroke
  - gastrointestinal (44%): **abdominal pain**, GI bleeding/infarction, cholecystitis
  - cutaneous lesions (43%): **livedo reticularis**, **purpura**, Raynaud's
  - cardiac (36%): coronary arteritis, cardiomyopathy, pericarditis
  - GU (25%): testicular or ovarian pain

- Diagnostic studies
  angiogram (mesenteric vessels) → aneurysms and focal vessel narrowings
  MRA may not be adequate to make the diagnosis
  biopsy (sural nerve or skin) → vasculitis with fibrinoid necrosis *without granulomas*
  ↑ ESR, ↑ WBC, rare eosinophilia, ⊕ HBsAg (30%), p-ANCA (<20%)
- Classification criteria (3 of 10 criteria is 82% sens. & 87% spec.; *Arthritis Rheum* 1990;33:1088)
  1. weight loss ≥4 kg
  2. **livedo reticularis**
  3. testicular pain/tenderness
  4. myalgias, weakness, leg tenderness
  5. mononeuropathy or polyneuropathy
  6. diastolic BP >90 mm Hg
  7. elevated BUN >40 mg/dL or Cr >1.5 mg/dL
  8. Hepatitis B virus
  9. Arteriographic abnormality (aneurysms, occlusion of visceral arteries)
  10. Biopsy → vasculitis of small or medium-sized vessel
- Treatment: **steroids**, cyclophosphamide; antiviral therapy for HBV-related PAN

ANCA-ASSOCIATED SMALL-VESSEL VASCULITIS

Disease	Gran.	Renal	Pulm.	Asthma	ANCA Type*	ANCA ⊕
Wegener's granulomatosis	⊕	80%	90%	–	c-ANCA (anti-PR3)	90%
Microscopic polyangiitis	–	90%	50%	–	p-ANCA (anti-MPO)	70%
Churg-Strauss syndrome	⊕	45%	70%	⊕	p-ANCA (anti-MPO)	50%

*Predominant ANCA type; either p- or c-ANCA can be seen in all three disease. (*NEJM* 1997;337:1512)

Differential Diagnosis of ANCA

- **c-ANCA (anti-PR3)**: Wegener's granulomatosis, Churg-Strauss, microscopic polyangiitis
- **p-ANCA (anti-MPO)**: microscopic polyangiitis, Churg-Strauss, PAN, Wegener's granulomatosis, drug-induced vasculitis, nonvasculitic rheumatic diseases
- **atypical ANCA patterns**: drug-induced vasculitis, nonvasculitic rheumatic diseases, ulcerative colitis, primary sclerosing cholangitis, endocarditis, cystic fibrosis

Wegener's granulomatosis

- Definition: necrotizing systemic vasculitis, particularly involving respiratory tract and kidney
- Epidemiology: can occur at any age, but ↑ incidence in young and middle-aged adults
- Clinical manifestations
  pulmonary (90%)
    upper: sinusitis, otitis, rhinitis, nasal mucosal ulceration, saddle-nose deformity
    lower: pleurisy, pulmonary infiltrate, nodules, hemorrhage, hemoptysis
  renal (80%): hematuria, RPGN
  ocular (50%): episcleritis, uveitis and proptosis from orbital granulomas
  neurologic: cranial and peripheral neuropathies, mononeuritis multiplex
- Diagnostic studies: **90% ⊕ ANCA** (80-95% c-ANCA, remainder p-ANCA)
  biopsy → necrotizing granulomatous inflammation of arterioles, capillaries, veins
  ↑ BUN and Cr, **hematuria, active urine sediment** with RBC casts & dysmorphic RBCs
- Classification criteria (2 of 4 criteria is 88% sens. & 92% spec.; *Arthritis Rheum* 1990;33:1101)
  1. nasal or oral inflammation- oral ulcers, purulent or bloody nasal discharge
  2. CXR showing nodules, fixed infiltrates, or cavities
  3. microscopic hematuria or urinary red cell casts
  4. granulomatous inflammation on biopsy
- Treatment (*Annals* 1992;116:488; *NEJM* 2003;349:36)
  cyclophosphamide (2 mg/kd/d × ≥1 yr) & **methylprednisolone** (1 mg/kg/d, taper over 6 mos)
  MTX for mild disease/long-term maintenance; AZA for maintenance
  TMP-SMX may prevent relapse incited by respiratory infections
  consider plasmapheresis for dialysis-dependent renal disease

Microscopic polyangiitis (MPA)

- Definition: necrotizing small-vessel vasculitis → glomerulonephritis, dermal leukocytoclastic venulitis, and pulmonary capillary alveolitis. Similar to Wegener's *but without granulomas.*
- Epidemiology: *not* associated with HBV (unlike classic polyarteritis nodosa)
- Clinical manifestations
  constitutional symptoms: weight loss, fevers, fatigue, myalgias
  renal: hematuria, RPGN (vs. microaneurysms in classic PAN)
  pulmonary: cough and/or hemoptysis
- Diagnostic studies: **70% ⊕ ANCA** (almost all p-ANCA), **biopsy → necrotizing inflammation** of arterioles, capillaries, & venules *w/o granulomas or eosin. infiltrates*
  urine sediment and CXR findings similar to those seen in Wegener's
- Treatment: **cyclophosphamide**; **methylprednisolone**; AZA for maintenance; plasmapheresis in some cases

Churg-Strauss syndrome

- Definition: granulomatous inflammation, involving skin, peripheral nerves, lungs & kidneys
- Epidemiology: rare condition that can present at any age, but typically 30-40
- Clinical manifestations
  asthma and allergic rhinitis (new asthma in an adult raises suspicion)
  eosinophilic infiltrative disease or eosinophilic pneumonia
  systemic small-vessel vasculitis with *granulomas* (within 3 yrs onset of asthma)
    neuropathy, coronary arteritis, and myocarditis frequent and severe
    glomerulonephritis and serositis less frequent and less severe
- Diagnostic studies: **50% ⊕ ANCA** (c-ANCA or p-ANCA), **eosinophilia** (80%), **biopsy → microgranulomas**, fibrinoid necrosis and thrombosis of small arteries and veins with **eosinophilic infiltrates**; CXR may show shifting pulmonary infiltrates
- Classification criteria (4 of 6 criteria is 85% sens. & 99.7% spec.; *Arthritis Rheum* 1990;33:1094)
  1. asthma
  2. eosinophilia >10%
  3. mononeuropathy or polyneuropathy
  4. migratory or transitory pulmonary infiltrates
  5. paranasal sinus abnormality
  6. extravascular eosinophils on biopsy
- Treatment: high dose **corticosteroids** (+ cyclophosphamide or other DMARDs if nec.)

Immune Complex-Associated Small-Vessel Vasculitis

Henoch-Schönlein purpura (HSP)

- Epidemiology: most common systemic vasculitis in children. Peak incidence age 5. Rare in adults (1.2 cases/million/year, *Semin Arthritis Rheum* 1994;37:187)
  begins after an upper respiratory tract infection or drug exposure; IgA-mediated
- Clinical manifestations: **purpura** on extensor surfaces & buttocks; **fever**; non-deforming **polyarthralgias** especially involving hips, knees and ankles; colicky **abdominal pain** ± GIB or intussusception; nephritis ranging from **microscopic hematuria** and proteinuria to ESRD
- Diagnostic studies: normal plt count, ↑ serum IgA (<50%), hematuria and proteinuria
  skin biopsy → leukocytoclastic vasculitis with IgA and C3 deposition in vessel wall
- Criteria for classification (2 of 4 is 87% sens. and 88% spec.; *Arthritis Rheum* 1990;33:1114)
  1. palpable purpura
  2. age ≤20 yrs at disease onset
  3. bowel angina
  4. biopsy showing granulocytes in the walls of arterioles or venules
- Treatment: supportive; steroids for renal or severe disease

Cryoglobulinemic vasculitis: see "Cryoglobulinemia"

Connective tissue disease-associated vasculitis

- Definition: vasculitis associated with RA, SLE, or Sjögren's syndrome
- Clinical manifestations
  distal arteritis: Raynaud's phenomenon, livedo reticularis, palpable purpura, cutaneous ulceration
  visceral arteritis: pericarditis and mesenteric ischemia
  peripheral neuropathy
- Diagnostic studies: skin and sural nerve biopsies, angiography, EMG
- Treatment: steroids, cyclophosphamide, MTX (other DMARDs)

Cutaneous leukocytoclastic angiitis (Hypersensitivity vasculitis)

- Definition: heterogeneous group of clinical syndromes due to immune complex deposition in capillaries, venules, and arterioles
- Epidemiology: overall the most common type of vasculitis
- Etiologies
  drugs: penicillin, aspirin, amphetamines, thiazides, chemicals, immunizations
  infections: strep throat, bacterial endocarditis, TB, hepatitis, staphylococcal infections
  tumor antigens
  foreign proteins (serum sickness)
- Clinical manifestations: abrupt onset after exposure to the offending agent of **palpable purpura**, **cutaneous ulceration** and **transient arthralgias**; peripheral neuropathy
- Diagnostic studies: ↑ ESR, ↓ **complement levels**, eosinophilia, **skin biopsy → leukocytoclastic vasculitis with neutrophils**, nuclear fragments secondary to karyorrhexis, perivascular hemorrhage and fibrinoid deposits
- Classification criteria (3 of 5 criteria is 71% sens. & 84% spec.; *Arthritis Rheum* 1990;33:1108)
  1. age >16 years
  2. medication taken at disease onset
  3. palpable purpura
  4. maculopapular rash
  5. biopsy showing granulocytes in a perivascular or extravascular location
- Treatment: withdrawal of offending agent ± rapid prednisone taper

Behcet's syndrome

- Definition: systemic leukocytoclastic vasculitis primarily affecting venules
- Classification criteria (#1 + ≥2 others is 91% sens. & 96% spec.; *Lancet* 1990;335:1078)
  1. recurrent oral aphthous ulceration (at least 3 times in one year)
  2. recurrent genital ulceration
  3. eye lesions: uveitis (with hypopyon), scleritis, retinal vasculitis, optic neuritis
  4. skin lesions: pustules, papules, folliculitis, erythema nodosum
  5. ⊕ pathergy test (prick forearm with sterile needle → pustule)
- Other clinical manifestations
  arthritis: mild, chronic and non-destructive, involving knees and ankles
  neurologic: focal deficits and pleocytosis accompanying cerebral vasculitis
  superficial or deep vein thrombosis (25%)
- Diagnostic studies: ulcer biopsy, cerebral angiography (rarely necessary); slit lamp exam and funduscopy
- Treatment (*Arthritis Rheum* 1997;40:769)
  superficial ulcers: topical steroids, dapsone, thalidomide (in males), MTX
  uveitis or CNS involvement: **oral steroids** + **azathioprine** or CsA
    azathioprine early improves prognosis and helps prevent ocular disease, ulcerations
  arthritis: colchicine, IFN

• CRYOGLOBULINEMIA •

Definition (*Arthritis & Rheum* 1999;42:2507)
- **Proteins that precipitate on exposure to the cold**
- **Type 1**: *monoclonal* Ig (usually IgM or IgG)
- **Type 2** (mixed): *monoclonal* IgM w/ activity against *polyclonal* IgG (i.e. rheumatoid factor)
- **Type 3** (mixed): *polyclonal* IgM w/ activity against *polyclonal* IgG

Epidemiology
- Female predominance
- Age of onset ~50 years

Etiologies
- **Lymphoproliferative disorders**: multiple myeloma, Waldenström's macroglobulinemia, CLL, B cell NHL. Usually associated with *Type 1* cryoglobulinemia.
- **HCV infection**: >80% of Pts with mixed cryoglobulinemia are HCV RNA ⊕ (*NEJM* 1992;327:1490); usually associated with *Type 2* cryoglobulinemia
- **Autoimmune syndromes**: usually associated with *Type 3* cryoglobulinemia
- Infections: viral (EBV, CMV), bacterial (endocarditis), and parasitic infections
- Essential (idiopathic)

Pathophysiology
- Immune complex deposition, complement activation
- Platelet aggregation, small vessel thromboses, vasculitis

Clinical manifestations
- General: **weakness**, low-grade fever
- Dermatologic: lower extremity **purpura**, **livedo reticularis**, leg ulcers, Raynaud's phenomenon, leukocytoclastic vasculitis
- Rheumatologic: symmetric, migratory **arthralgias** of small or medium joints
- Renal (50%): **glomerulonephritis** (proteinuria, hematuria, ARF, hypertension, edema)
- Hematologic: anemia, thrombocytopenia
- GI: abdominal pain, hepatosplenomegaly, abnormal LFTs
- Neurologic: peripheral neuropathy and mononeuritis multiplex

Diagnostic studies
- ⊕ **cryocrit** (amount not necessarily associated with disease activity), **cryoglobulin electrophoresis**
- ⊕ rheumatoid factor (RF)
- ↓ **C4 levels**, variable C3 levels, ↑ ESR
- If blood sample not kept at 37° C → cryoprecipitation → loss of RF and ↓↓ complement
- In Type 2 cryoglobulinemia: ⊕ HCV RNA, ⊖ anti-HCV Ab
- Biopsy of affected area (skin, kidney)

Treatment
- Treat underlying disorder
- NSAIDs for mild disease
- Prednisone + other immunosuppressants (e.g., cyclophosphamide) for major organ involvement
- Plasmapheresis in severe disease
- IFN-α for HCV RNA ⊕ (*NEJM* 1994;330:751); avoid steroids if possible

• AMYLOIDOSIS •

Accumulation of insoluble fibrillar proteins that form β-pleated sheets

Classification of Amyloidosis			
Type	**Precursor**	**Causative diseases**	**Organ systems**
AL ("Primary")	Ig light chain (monoclonal)	MM Light chain disease (λ>κ) MGUS, WM	**Renal, cardiac, GI, neuro, cutaneous,** hepatic, pulmonary, musculoskel, heme
AA ("Secondary")	Serum amyloid (SAA)	Chronic infections: osteo, TB, empyema, leprosy Inflam: RA, IBD, FMF Neoplasms: renal, HD	**Renal, GI, hepatic,** neuro, cutaneous
Hereditary	Transthyretin (TTR), et al.	Mutant proteins	**Neurologic**, cardiac
Senile	TTR, ANP	*Normal* proteins; 2° aging	**Cardiac**, aorta, GI
Aβ_2M	β_2-microglobulin	Dialysis-associated (β2m normally renally excreted)	Musculoskeletal
Organ-specific	β-amyloid protein Peptide hormones et al.	Localized production and processing	Neurologic Endocrine et al.

(Adapted from *NEJM* 1997;337:898 and 2003;349:583)

Clinical Manifestations of Amyloidosis		
System	**Manifestations**	**Amyloid**
Renal	Proteinuria or nephrotic syndrome	AL, AA
Cardiac	Cardiomyopathy (restrictive & dilated) ↓ QRS amplitude, conduction abnormalities, AF Orthostatic hypotension	AL, hereditary, senile, organ-specific
GI	Diarrhea, malabsorption, protein loss Ulceration, hemorrhage, obstruction Macroglossia → dysphonia and dysphagia	all systemic
Neurologic	Peripheral neuropathy with painful paresthesias Autonomic neuro → impotence, dysmotility, ↓ BP Carpal tunnel syndrome	hereditary, AL, organ-specific, Aβ_2m
Cutaneous	Waxy, non-pruritic papules; periorbital ecchymoses "Pinch purpura" = skin bleeds with minimal trauma	AL
Hepatic & Splenic	Hepatomegaly, usually *without* dysfunction Splenomegaly, usually *without* leukopenia or anemia	all systemic
Endocrine	Deposition with rare hormonal insufficiency	organ-specific
Musculoskel	Arthralgias and arthritis	AL, Aβ_2m
Pulmonary	Airway obstruction	AL, AA
Hematologic	Factor X deficiency	AL

Diagnostic studies

- Abdominal SC fat pad or rectal biopsy → apple-green birefringence on Congo red stain
- If suspect AL → ✓ SPEP, SIEP, UPEP, ± BM bx
- If suspect renal involvement: ✓ U/A (proteinuria)
- If suspect cardiac involvement: ✓ ECG (↓ voltage, conduction abnormalities) & echocardiogram (biventricular thickening with "*granular sparkling*" appearance)
- Genetic testing for hereditary forms

Treatment

- AL: melphalan + prednisone (*NEJM* 1997;336:1202), ? iododoxorubicin, ? stem cell transplant
- AA: treatment of underlying disease
  Familial Mediterranean Fever: colchicine (*NEJM* 1986;314:1001)
- For hereditary amyloidoses in which amyloid precursor protein is produced by the liver (e.g. TTR), liver transplantation may prevent further deposition
- Heart, kidney and liver transplantation may be considered in those with advanced disease

Prognosis

- AL amyloid: median survival ~12-18 mos; if cardiac involvement, median survival ~6 mos

• CHANGE IN MENTAL STATUS •

Definitions

- **Confusion** (encephalopathy): unable to maintain coherent thought process
- **Delirium**: confusional state with additional sympathetic signs
- **Drowsiness**: ↓ level of consciousness, but rapid arousal to verbal or noxious stimuli
- **Stupor**: impaired arousal to noxious stimuli, but preserved purposeful movements
- **Coma**: sleep-like state of unresponsiveness, with no purposeful response to stimuli

Etiologies	
Primary Neurologic	**Systemic** *(especially in elderly)*
Stroke	Cardiac: severe CHF, HTN encephalopathy
Seizure (post-ictal, status, subclinical)	Pulmonary: ↓ P_aO_2, ↑ P_aCO_2
Infection: meningoencephalitis, abscess	GI: liver failure, constipation, Wilson's
Epidural/subdural hematoma	Renal: uremia, hypo- and hypernatremia
Concussion	Endocrine: ↓ glc, DKA, HHNS, ↑ Ca, hypo- or hyperthyroidism, Addisonian crisis
Hydrocephalus	
Venous occlusion	ID: pneumonia, UTI, sepsis
Cholesterol or fat emboli	Hypo- and hyperthermia
CNS vasculitis	Medications (espec. opiates & sedatives)
TTP	Alcohol & toxins

Initial evaluation

- **History** (typically from others): previous or recent illnesses, including psychiatric disorders; head trauma; medications, drug or alcohol use
- **General physical examination** including signs of trauma, stigmata of liver disease, embolic phenomena, signs of drug use, nuchal rigidity (may be present in meningitis or subarachnoid hemorrhage, but *do not test* if question of trauma/cervical spine fracture)
- **Neurologic examination**
  - Observation for spontaneous movements, response to stimuli, papilledema
  - Cranial nerves: eye position at rest, response to visual threat, corneal reflex, facial grimace to nasal tickle, cough/gag (with ET tube manipulation if necessary)
  - Pupil size & reactivity: pinpoint → opiates; midposition & fixed → midbrain lesion; fix & dilated → severe anoxic encephalopathy
  - Intact oculocephalic ("doll's eyes", eyes move opposite head movement) or oculovestibular ("cold calorics", eyes move towards lavaged ear) imply brainstem intact
  - Look for signs of ↑ ICP: H/A, vomiting, HTN, ↓ HR, papilledema, unilateral dilated pupil
  - Motor response in the extremities to noxious stimuli – noting purposeful *vs.* posturing
  - Deep tendon reflexes, Babinski response

Glasgow Coma Scale			
Eye opening	**Best verbal response**	**Best motor response**	**Points**
		Follows commands	6
	Oriented	Localizes pain	5
Spontaneous	Confused	Withdraws from pain	4
To voice	Inappropriate words	Flexor response	3
To painful stimuli	Unintelligible sounds	Extensor response	2
None	None	None	1
Sum points from each of the 3 categories to calculate the score			

Initial treatment

- Control airway, monitor vital signs, IV access
- Immobilization of C-spine if concern for cervical trauma
- Thiamine (100 mg IV) *prior to dextrose* to prevent exacerb. of Wernicke's encephalopathy
- Dextrose (50 g IV push)
- Naloxone 0.01 mg/kg if opiates suspected; flumazenil 0.2 mg IV if benzos suspected
- If concern for ↑ ICP and herniation: ↑ head of bed; osmotherapy with mannitol; hyperventilation; dexamethasone; consider emergent surgical decompression

Diagnostic studies

- Head CT; radiographs to rule-out C-spine fracture
- Laboratory: electrolytes, BUN, Cr, ABG, LFTs, CBC, PT, PTT, tox screen, TSH, U/A
- Lumbar puncture to r/o meningitis
- EEG to r/o subclinical seizures

• SEIZURES •

Definitions

- **Seizure** = abnormal, paroxysmal, excessive discharge of CNS neurons; occurs in 5-10% of the population; clinical manifestations can range from dramatic to subtle
- **Epilepsy** = recurrent seizures due to an underlying cause; 0.5-1.0% of population
- **Generalized seizures** (involves brain diffusely)
  - *Tonic-clonic* (grand mal): tonic phase (10-20 sec) with contraction of muscles (causing expiratory moan, cyanosis, pooling of secretions, tongue biting) → clonic phase (~30 sec) with intermittent relaxing and tensing of muscles
  - *Absence* (petit mal): transient lapse of consciousness w/o loss of postural tone
  - *Myoclonic* (infantile spasms & juvenile myoclonic epilepsy): sudden, brief contraction
- **Partial or focal seizures** (involves discrete areas, implies a focal, structural lesion)
  - *Simple:* without impairment of consciousness; may be motor, sensory, or autonomic
  - *Complex:* with impairment of consciousness; may be temporal or frontal lobe, with automatisms or psychogenic features
  - *Partial with secondary generalization:* starts focal, becomes diffuse

Ddx

- **Syncope**: lacks true aura (although Pt may describe feeling unwell with diaphoresis, nausea, and tunneling of vision), motor manifestations <30 sec (convulsive activity for <10 sec may occur with transient cerebral hypoperfusion), and w/o post-ictal disorientation, muscle soreness, or sleepiness
- **Psychogenic seizure**: may see side-to-side head turning, asymmetric large amplitude limb movements, diffuse twitching w/o LOC, and crying/talking during event
- Other: metabolic disorders (e.g., alcoholic blackouts, hypoglycemia); migraines; TIAs; narcolepsy; non-epileptic myoclonus

Etiologies

- **A**lcohol withdrawal, illicit drugs, medications (e.g., β-lactams, meperidine, cyclosporine)
- **B**rain tumor or penetrating trauma
- **C**erebrovascular disease, including subdural hematomas
- **D**egenerative disorders of the CNS (e.g., Alzheimer's)
- **E**lectrolyte (hyponatremia) & other metabolic (e.g., uremia, liver failure, hypoglycemia)

Clinical manifestations

- **Aura** (sec to mins): premonition consisting of abnormal smells/tastes, unusual behavior, oral or appendicular automatisms.
- **Ictal period** (sec to mins): tonic and/or clonic movements of head, eyes, trunk or extrem.
- **Post-ictal period** (mins to hrs): slowly resolving period of confusion, disorientation and lethargy. May be accompanied by focal neurological deficits ("Todd's paralysis").
- **Status epilepticus***:* continuous tonic-clonic seizure ≥30 mins, or repeated seizures such that there is no resolution of post-ictal periods. Complications include neuronal death, rhabdomyolysis, and lactic acidosis.

Clinical evaluation

- Seizure: patient usually w/o recollection, must talk to witnesses
  - unusual behavior before seizure (i.e., an aura)
  - type and pattern of abnormal movements, including head turning and eye deviation (gaze preference *away* from seizure focus)
  - loss of responsiveness
- HPI: recent illnesses/fevers, head trauma
- PMH: prior seizures or ⊕ FHx, prior meningitis/encephalitis, prior stroke or head trauma
- Medications, alcohol, and illicit drug use
- General physical exam should include the skin, looking for neuro-ectodermal disorders (e.g., neurofibromatosis, tuberous sclerosis) that are associated with seizures
- Neurological exam should look for focal abnormalities → underlying structural abnormality

Diagnostic studies

- Laboratory: full electrolytes, BUN, Cr, glc, LFTs, tox screen, medication levels
- EEG
  - frequent seizures: can confirm by demonstrating repetitive rhythmic activity (n.b., generalized seizures will always have abnormal EEG; partial seizures may not)
  - infrequent seizures: may show inter-ictal epileptiform activity (e.g., spikes or sharp waves), but such patterns seen in up to 2% of normal population
  - sleep-deprivation ↑ dx yield of EEG; video-monitoring may help with psychogenic seizures

- MRI to r/o structural abnormalities; ↑ sens. w/ fine coronal cuts of frontal & temporal lobes
- Lumbar puncture (after ruling-out space-occupying lesion): if suspect meningitis or encephalitis and in *all* HIV ⊕ patients

Treatment
- Treat any underlying causes, including CNS infections, alcohol or drug intoxication or withdrawal, hyponatremia, etc.
- Antiepileptic drug therapy is usually reserved for Pts with an underlying structural abnormality or an idiopathic seizure *plus* (1) status epilepticus on presentation, (2) focal neurologic exam, (3) post-ictal Todd's paralysis, or (4) abnormal EEG
- Generalized tonic-clonic seizures: valproic acid, phenytoin, carbamazepine, phenobarbital
- Partial seizures: carbamazepine, phenytoin, valproic acid
- Absence seizures: ethosuximide, valproic acid
- Secondary agents: gabapentin, lamotrigine, topiramate, clonazepam, leviteracitam
- Introduce gradually, monitor carefully
- May consider withdrawal if seizure-free (typically for at least 1 year) and normal EEG
- Individual state laws mandate different durations of Pt being seizure-free before being allowed to drive

Antiepileptic Drugs and Side Effects			
Medication	**Avg daily dose**	**Side effects**	
		Neurologic	*Systemic*
Phenytoin	300-400 mg	Dizziness Ataxia Diplopia Confusion	Gum hyperplasia, ↓ Ca, ↑ K
Carbamazepine	600-1800 mg		Aplastic anemia Leukopenia Hepatotoxicity Hyponatremia
Valproic acid	750-2000 mg		Hepatotoxicity Thrombocytopenia
Phenobarbital	60-180 mg		Rash
Ethosuximide	750-1250 mg		Rash Bone marrow suppression
Gabapentin	900-2400 mg		GI upset

(*JAMA* 2004;291:605 & 615)

Status epilepticus (consult neurology)
- Place Pt in semi-prone position to ↓ risk of aspiration
- Oral airway or, if prolonged, endotracheal intubation
- IV access, start normal saline infusion
- STAT labs including glc, Na, Ca, serum & urine toxicology screen, anticonvulsant levels
- Thiamine (100 mg IV) *prior to dextrose* to prevent exacerbation of Wernicke's encephalopathy
- Dextrose (50 g IV push)
- Na or Ca repletion as needed

Treatment of Status Epilepticus *(proceed to next step if seizures continue)*			
Step	**Antiepileptic**	**Dosing regimen**	**Typical adult dose**
1	**Lorazepam** or **Diazepam**	0.1 mg/kg at 2 mg/min 0.2 mg/kg at 5 mg/min	Successive 2-4 mg IV pushes Successive 5-10 mg IV pushes
	Lorazepam marginally slower onset of action (3 vs. 2 min) but at least as efficacious (success 65%) & longer duration of effect (12-24 hrs vs. 15-30 min) (*JAMA* 1983;249:1452; *NEJM* 1998;339:792)		
2	**Phenytoin** or **Fosphenytoin**	20 mg/kg at 50 mg/min 20 mg PE/kg at 150 mg/min + 5-10 mg/kg if still seizing	1.0-1.5 g IV over 20 mins 1.0-1.5 g PE IV over 5-10 mins + 500 mg IV if still seizing
Subsequent steps typically mandate intubation, EEG monitoring, and ICU admission			
3	Phenobarbital	20 mg/kg at 50-75 mg/min + 5-10 mg/kg if still seizing	1.0-1.5 g IV over 30 mins + 500 g IV if still seizing
4	General anesthesia with midazolam, pentobarbital, or propofol		

(*NEJM* 1998;338:970)

• STROKE •

ISCHEMIC (~70%)

Etiologies
- Embolic (~75%): artery → artery, cardioembolic, or cryptogenic
- Thrombotic (~25%): lacunar (arteriolar, seen in HTN & DM) or large vessel
- Other: dissection, vasculitis, hyperviscosity

Clinical Manifestations	
Embolic: rapid onset at maximum severity, usually during activity *Thrombotic: progression of sx over hrs to days with stuttering course*	
Artery	**Deficits**
ICA/Ophth	Amaurosis fugax (transient monocular blindness)
ACA	Hemiplegia (leg > arm) Confusion, urinary incontinence, primitive reflexes
MCA	Hemiplegia (arm & face > leg); hemianesthesia; homonymous hemianopia Aphasia if dom. hemisphere: ant. div. → expressive; post. → expressive Apraxia and neglect if nondominant hemisphere Drowsiness & stupor seen later (due to brain swelling)
PCA	Thalamic syndromes with contralateral hemisensory disturbance, aphasia Macular-sparing homonymous hemianopia
Vertebral	Wallenberg's syndrome = numbness of ipsilateral face and contralateral limbs, diplopia, dysarthria, ipsilateral Horner's
Basilar	Pinpoint pupils, long tract signs (quadriplegia and sensory loss), cranial nerve abnormalities, cerebellar dysfunction
Cerebellar	Vertigo, nausea/vomiting, nystagmus, ipsilateral limb ataxia
Lacunar	Pure hemiplegia, pure hemianesthesia, ataxic hemiparesis, or dysarthria + clumsy hand
Transient ischemia attacks (TIAs) are sudden neurologic deficits caused by cerebral ischemia that resolve within 24 hrs (usually within 1 hr) and are a harbinger of stroke.	

Physical examination
- General including rhythm, murmurs, carotid & subclavian bruits, signs of peripheral embol.
- Neurologic including NIH stroke scale (NIHSS)

Diagnostic studies
- Laboratory: electrolytes, Cr, glc, CBC, PT, PTT, LFTs, tox screen;
  hypercoagulable w/u (consider in young Pts; send once stable & ideally before anticoag)
- ECG
- **Urgent CT** is usually the initial imaging study because of its rapidity and availability
  first, non-contrast CT to r/o hemorrhage (sens. for ischemic Δs is only 50% w/in 6 hrs)
  then, CT angio to evaluate cerebrovascular anatomy & patency and cerebral perfusion
- MRI offers superior imaging but may not identify acute hemorrhage and should be avoided if Pt is unstable or will delay therapy
- Carotid Doppler U/S, transcranial Doppler (TCD), echocardiography w/ bubble study to r/o PFO, Holter monitoring

Treatment of TIA
- **Heparin IV → warfarin** for known or presumptive cardioembolic TIAs; consider for large vessel atherothrombotic
- **Antiplatelet therapy** with ASA, clopidogrel, or ASA + dipyridamole
- Carotid revascularization if >70% ipsilateral stenosis (NASCET, *NEJM* 1991;325:445)

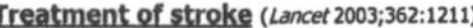

Treatment of stroke (*Lancet* 2003;362:1211)

- **Thrombolysis** (IV): 0.9 mg/kg (max 90 mg), w/ 10% as bolus over 1 min, rest over 1 hr
  consider if onset w/in 3 hrs, large deficit, ∅ hemorrhage, and ∅ contraindication to lysis
  12% absolute ↑ in excellent functional outcome, 5.8% absolute ↑ ICH, 4% absolute ↓ mortality (p=NS) (NINDS rt-PA Stroke Study, *NEJM* 1995;333:1381)
- Intra-arterial therapy with thrombolysis (PROACT II, *JAMA* 1999;282:2003) or catheter-based techniques promising (66% rate of recanalization) but still experimental
  currently reserved for occlusion of a major vessel (ICA, MCA, basilar)
- Anticoagulation with UFH of no proven benefit with ↑ risk of hemorrhagic transformation
  consider infusion w/o bolus if not Pt thrombolysed and having progressive sx
  long-term warfarin if embolic stroke; no role in non-embolic stroke (*NEJM* 2001;345: 1444)
- **Aspirin** reduces the rate of death and recurrent stroke (*Stroke* 2000;31:1240)
- BP should *not* be lowered unless severe SBP >200 or evidence of MI or CHF
  if considering thrombolysis, then lower to <180/110 with nitrates or labetalol
- DVT prophylaxis
- Cerebral edema → ↑ ICP requiring
  elevated head of bed >30°
  intubation and hyperventilation to P_aCO_2 ~30 (transient benefit)
  osmotherapy with mannitol IV 1 gm/kg → 0.25 gm/kg q 6 hrs; ± hypertonic saline
  surgical decompression

HEMORRHAGIC (~30%)

Etiologies

- Intracerebral (ICH, ~90%): HTN, AVM, amyloid angiopathy, anticoagulation/thrombolysis
- Subarachnoid (SAH, ~10%): ruptured aneurysm, trauma

Clinical manifestations

- ICH
  sudden impairment in level of consciousness
  vomiting ± headache
  progressive focal neurologic deficit depending on site of hemorrhage
- SAH
  severe headache, nausea & vomiting
  nuchal rigidity and other signs of meningeal irritation
  impairment in level of consciousness

Diagnostic studies

- CT
- Cerebral angiography to determine the source of bleeding (aneurysm, AVM)
- LP to ✓ for xanthochromia if no evidence on CT of hemorrhage and suspicious for SAH

Treatment

- Reversal of any coagulopathies
- Strict BP control with goal SBP <140, unless risk for hypoperfusion because critical carotid stenosis
- ICH: surgical decompression for large hemorrhage with clinical deterioration
- SAH: nimodipine to ↓ risk of vasospasm, phenytoin for seizure prophylaxis, endovascular or surgical correction of aneurysm/AVM to prevent rebleeding

• WEAKNESS & NEUROMUSCULAR DYSFUNCTION •

Feature	Upper Motor Neuron	Lower Motor Neuron	Myopathy
Distribution of weakness	Regional	Distal, segmental	Proximal
Atrophy	None	Severe	Mild
Fasciculations	None	Common	None
Tone	↑	↓	Normal or ↓
DTRs	++++	0/+	+/++
Babinski	Present	Absent	Absent

PERIPHERAL NEUROPATHIES

Etiologies
- **Mononeuropathy** (one nerve): entrapment, compression, trauma, DM, Lyme
- **Mononeuropathy multiplex** (multiple, noncontiguous, separate nerves)
  Axonal: vasculitis, sarcoidosis, diabetes, hereditary neuropathy with pressure palsies
- **Polyneuropathy** (multiple symmetric nerves)
  Demyelinating
    acute: acute idiopathic demyelinating polyneuropathy (AIDP) = Guillain-Barré
    subacute: CIDP, meds (taxol)
    chronic: diabetes, hypothyroidism, toxins, paraneoplastic, paraproteinemia, hereditary
  Axonal
    acute: porphyria
    subacute: meds (cisplatin, taxol, vincristine, INH, ddI), alcohol, B_{12} defic., sepsis
    chronic: diabetes, uremia, lead, arsenic, Lyme, HIV, paraneoplastic, paraproteinemia

Clinical manifestations
- Motor and/or sensory dysfunction with weakness and/or dysesthesias
- Depressed or absent DTRs

Diagnostic studies
- Electrolytes, BUN, Cr, Glc, Hb_{A1C}, CBC, TSH, LFTs, ANA, ESR, SPEP
- HIV, Lyme titers, heavy metal screening as indicated by clinical history
- EMG, NCS, nerve biopsy

GUILLAIN-BARRÉ SYNDROME (GBS)

Definition and epidemiology
- Acute idiopathic demyelinating polyneuropathy (AIDP)
- Incidence 1-2 per 100,000
- Precipitants: viral illness (EBV, CMV, HSV), URI (*Mycoplasma*), gastroenteritis (*Campylobacter*), surgery, older immunizations

Clinical manifestations
- Ascending paralysis over hours to days
- *Hypoactive or absent reflexes*
- Sensory dysesthesias
- Respiratory compromise requiring ventilatory assistance occurs in 30%; autonomic instability and arrhythmias also may occur

Diagnostic studies
- Lumbar puncture: albuminocytologic dissociation = ↑ protein w/o pleocytosis (<20 lymphs)
- EMG & NCS: ↓ nerve conduction velocity and conduction block

Treatment
- Plasma exchange (*Neurology* 1985;35:1096) or IVIg (*NEJM* 1992, 326:1123)
  no additional benefit with both (*Lancet* 1997;349:225)
- Supportive care with monitoring in ICU setting
- Watch for autonomic dysfunction: labile BP, dysrhythmias

Myasthenia Gravis

Definition and epidemiology
- Autoimmune disorder with Ab directed against acetylcholine receptor (AChR) in NMJ
- Prevalence 1 in 7500
- Occurs at all ages; peak for women in 20s-30s; peak for men in 60s-70s

Clinical manifestations
- Weakness and *fatigability* with weakness worse with repetitive use, relieved by rest
- Cranial muscles involved early → ptosis, diplopia, difficulty chewing, dysarthria, dysphagia
- Limb weakness proximal > distal; DTRs preserved
- Exacerbations triggered by stressors such as URI, surgery, meds (e.g., aminoglycosides, procainamide)
- Myasthenic crisis = exacerbation → need for respiratory assistance
- Cholinergic crisis = weakness due to *overtreatment* with anticholinesterase medications; may have excessive salivation, abdominal cramping and diarrhea

Diagnostic studies
- Bedside tests: timing of sustained upgaze, forced mouth closure on tongue blade, etc.
- Edrophonium (Tensilon) test: temporary ↑ strength; false ⊕ & ⊖ occur; atropine at bedside
- EMG: ↓ response with repetitive nerve stimulation (vs. ↑ response in Lambert-Eaton)
- Anti-AChR Ab: sens. 80%, 50% if ocular disease only; spec. >90%
- CT or MRI of thorax to evaluate thymus (65% hyperplasia, 10% thymoma)

Treatment
- Anticholinesterase medications (e.g., pyridostigmine)
- Thymectomy: mandatory if thymoma; also leads to improvement in 85% Pts w/o thymoma
- Immunosuppression: prednisone, azathioprine, cyclophosphamide
- Myasthenic crisis: treat precipitant, d/c anticholinesterase medications (to r/o cholinergic crisis), aggressive immunosuppression with glucocorticoids, IVIg, plasmapheresis

Myopathies (also see Rheumatology)

Etiologies
- Hereditary: Duchenne, Becker, limb-girdle, myotonic
- Endocrine: hypothyroidism, hyperparathyroidism, Cushing's syndrome
- Toxic: statins, fibrates, glucocorticoids, zidovudine, alcohol
- Polymyositis and dermatomyositis

Clinical manifestations
- Progressive weakness, proximal > distal
- ± Myalgias
- Eventually muscle atrophy

Diagnostic studies
- CK (↑ in inflammatory myopathies)
- EMG/NCS
- Muscle biopsy

• HEADACHE •

Primary headache syndromes
- Tension: associated with muscle contraction in neck or lower head
- Migraine: *see below*
- Cluster: periodic, paroxysmal, brief, sharp, orbital headache that may awaken from sleep ± lacrimation, rhinorrhea, conjunctival injection, or unilateral Horner's syndrome

Secondary causes of headaches
- Vascular: stroke, intracerebral hemorrhage, SAH, subdural hematoma AVM, unruptured aneurysm, arterial hypertension, venous thrombosis
- Infection: meningitis, encephalitis, abscess
- Brain tumor
- CSF disorder: ↑ (hydrocephalus) or ↓ (s/p LP)
- Trigeminal neuralgia
- Extracranial: sinusitis, TMJ syndrome, temporal arteritis

Clinical evaluation
- History: quality, severity, location, duration, time of onset, precipitants/relieving factors
- Associated symptoms (visual Δs, nausea, vomiting, photophobia)
- Focal neurologic symptoms
- Head or neck trauma, constitutional symptoms
- Medications, substance abuse
- General and neurologic examination
- *Warning signs: worst headache ever, worsening over days, vomiting precedes headache, precipitated by bending or cough, wakes from sleep, fever, abnormal neurologic exam → neuroimaging*

MIGRAINE

Epidemiology
- Affects 15% of women and 6% of men; onset usually by 30 yrs

Clinical manifestations (*Lancet* 2004;363:381)
- Unilateral or bilateral, retro-orbital throbbing headache; lasts 4-72 hrs
- Often accompanied by nausea, vomiting, photophobia
- Classic = visual aura (scotomata with jagged or colored edge) precede headache
- Common = headache without aura
- Complicated = accompanied by transient neurologic deficit
- Precipitants: stress, hunger, foods (cheese, chocolate) and food additives (MSG), fatigue, alcohol, menstruation, exercise

Treatment
- Eliminate precipitants
- Prophylaxis: TCA, βB, CCB, valproic acid, topiramate (*JAMA* 2004;291:965)
- Abortive therapy
  - ASA, acetaminophen, caffeine, high-dose NSAIDs
  - metoclopramide IV, prochlorperazine IM or IV
  - 5-HT_1 agonists ("triptans"); contraindicated in Pts with CAD
  - ergotamine, dihydroergotamine; use with caution in Pts with CAD

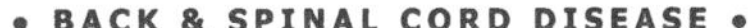

• BACK & SPINAL CORD DISEASE •

Ddx of back pain

- **Musculoskeletal**
  strain (experienced by up to 80% of the population at some time)
  osteoarthritis, vertebral compression fracture
  ankylosing spondylitis
- **Disk herniation syndromes** (see below)
- **Metastatic**: lung, breast, prostate, multiple myeloma, lymphoma
- **Infectious**: vertebral osteomyelitis or epidural abscess (see ID section)
- **Visceral disease with referred pain**
  PUD, cholelithiasis
  pancreatitis, pancreatic cancer
  pyelonephritis, nephrolithiasis
  uterine or ovarian cancer, salpingitis
  leaking aortic aneurysm

Initial evaluation

- **History**: location, radiation, neurologic symptoms, infection, malignancy
- **General physical examination**: local tenderness, ROM, signs of infection or malignancy
  straight leg raise (⊕ = radicular pain at <60°)
  ipsilateral: 95% sens., 40% spec.; crossed (contralateral): 25% sens., 90% spec.
- **Neurologic examination**: full motor (including sphincter tone), sensory (including perineal region), and reflexes (including anal and cremasteric)
- **Laboratory** (depending on suspicions): CBC, ESR, Ca, PO_4, Aϕ
- **Neuroimaging** (depending on suspicions): X-rays, CT or CT myelography, MRI, bone scan
- EMG/NCS may be useful to distinguish root/plexopathies from peripheral neuropathies

Disk Herniation Syndromes

Clinical manifestations

- Back pain aggravated by activity (especially bending, straining, and coughing), relieved by resting on unaffected side with affected leg in flexed posture
- "Sciata" = aching pain that radiates from the buttocks down the lateral aspect of the leg, often to the knee or lateral calf ± numbness and paresthesias radiating to lateral foot

Cervical and Lumbar Disk Herniation Patterns

Disk	Root	Pain / Paresthesias	Sensory loss	Motor loss	Reflex loss
C4-C5	C5	Neck, shoulder upper arm	Shoulder	Deltoid, biceps	Biceps
C5-C6	C6	Neck, shoulder, lateral arm, radial forearm, thumb & index finger	Lateral arm, radial forearm, thumb & index finger	Biceps	Biceps, supinator
C6-C7	C7	Neck, lateral arm, ring & index fingers	Radial forearm, index & middle fingers	Triceps, extensor carpi ulnaris	Triceps, supinator
C7-T1	C8	Ulnar forearm and hand	Ulnar half of ring finger, little finger	Intrinsic hand muscles, wrist extensors	None
L3-L4	L4	Anterior thigh, inner shin	Antero-medial thigh and shin, inner foot	Quadriceps	Patella
L4-L5	L5	Lateral thigh and calf, dorsum of foot, great toe	Lateral calf and great toe	Extensor hallicus longus, ± foot dorsiflexion and eversion	None
L5-S1	S1	Back of thigh, lateral posterior calf, lateral foot	Lateral calf, lateral foot, smaller toes	Gastrocnemius ± foot eversion	Achilles

Treatment
- Conservative: avoid bending/lifting; NSAIDs
- Surgery: cord compression or cauda equina syndrome (see below); progressive loss of motor function; bowel or bladder dysfunction; failure to respond to conservative therapy

Cord Compression

Clinical manifestations
- Spastic paraparesis
- Hyperactive reflexes
- Posterior column dysfunction in legs (loss of vibratory sense or proprioception)
- Bilateral Babinski responses
- *Conus medullaris syndrome*: saddle anesthesia, bladder & bowel dysfunction (urinary retention, ↓ anal tone), absent bulbocavernosus and anal reflexes
- *Cauda equina syndrome*: severe back pain, leg weakness and/or sensory loss, ± ↓ reflexes in lower extremities, relative sparing of bowel & bladder function (but occurs)

Evaluation & Treatment
- STAT MRI and neurology consultation
- Empiric dexamethasone 10 mg IV or methylprednisolone 30 mg/kg IVB over 15 mins → 5.4 mg/kg/hr starting 45 min after bolus and continuing for 23 hrs
- Emergent radiation therapy for compression due to metastatic disease
- Emergent neurosurgical consultation

Spinal Stenosis

Clinical manifestations
- Neurogenic claudication = back or buttocks pain induced by walking or prolonged standing, relieved by rest
- ± Focal weakness, sensory loss, diminished reflexes
- Unlike claudication: max discomfort in anterior thighs, preserved lower extremity pulses
- Unlike disk herniation: pain relieved by sitting

Evaluation & Treatment
- MRI

Treatment
- Conservative: avoid bending/lifting; NSAIDs
- Surgical decompression if failure to respond to conservative therapy

• ACLS ALGORITHMS •

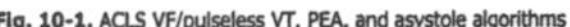

Fig. 10-1. ACLS VF/pulseless VT, PEA, and asystole algorithms

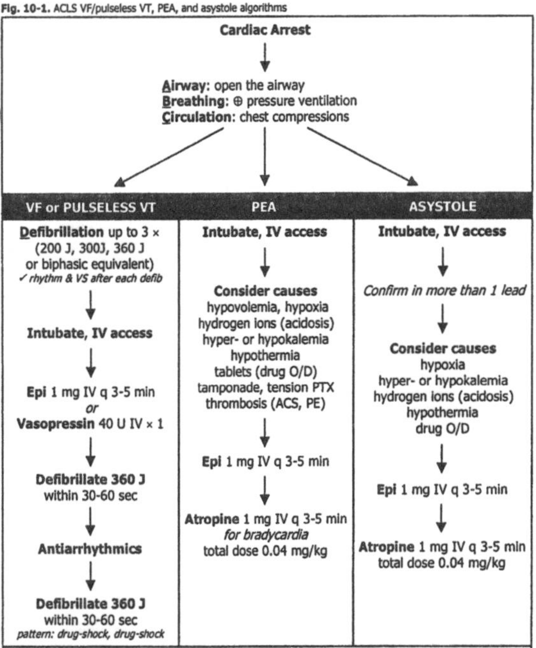

Cardiac Arrest

↓

Airway: open the airway
Breathing: ⊕ pressure ventilation
Circulation: chest compressions

↓

VF or PULSELESS VT	PEA	ASYSTOLE
Defibrillation up to 3 × (200 J, 300J, 360 J or biphasic equivalent) ✓ *rhythm & VS after each defib*	**Intubate, IV access**	**Intubate, IV access**
↓	↓	↓
Intubate, IV access	**Consider causes** hypovolemia, hypoxia hydrogen ions (acidosis) hyper- or hypokalemia hypothermia tablets (drug O/D) tamponade, tension PTX thrombosis (ACS, PE)	*Confirm in more than 1 lead*
↓	↓	↓
Epi 1 mg IV q 3-5 min *or* **Vasopressin** 40 U IV × 1	**Epi** 1 mg IV q 3-5 min	**Consider causes** hypoxia hyper- or hypokalemia hydrogen ions (acidosis) hypothermia drug O/D
↓	↓	↓
Defibrillate 360 J within 30-60 sec	**Atropine** 1 mg IV q 3-5 min *for bradycardia* total dose 0.04 mg/kg	**Epi** 1 mg IV q 3-5 min
↓		↓
Antiarrhythmics		**Atropine** 1 mg IV q 3-5 min total dose 0.04 mg/kg
↓		
Defibrillate 360 J within 30-60 sec *pattern: drug-shock, drug-shock*		

Antiarrhythmics

Amiodarone: 300 mg IVP ± 150 mg IVP in 3-5 mins
Lidocaine: 1.0-1.5 mg/kg IVP (avg dose 100 mg), repeat in 5-10 min
Procainamide: 17 mg/kg at 50 mg/min (avg dose 1 gm over 20 mins)

Treatment of reversible causes of PEA & asystole

Hypovolemia: volume infusion
Hypoxia: oxygenate
Hydrogen ions (acidosis): $NaHCO_3$
Hyperkalemia: Ca, $NaHCO_3$, insulin
Hypokalemia: KCl
Hypothermia: warming
Tablets: med-specific
Tamponade: pericardiocentesis
Tension PTX: needle decompression
Thrombosis (ACS): lysis or PCI, IABP
Thrombosis (PE): lysis, thrombectomy

(Adapted from *ACLS Provider Manual*, 2002. For out-of-hospital cardiac arrest, vasopressin 40 U IV × 2 followed by epinephrine may be superior to epinephrine alone. *NEJM* 2004;350:105.)

Fig. 10-2. ACLS tachycardia algorithms

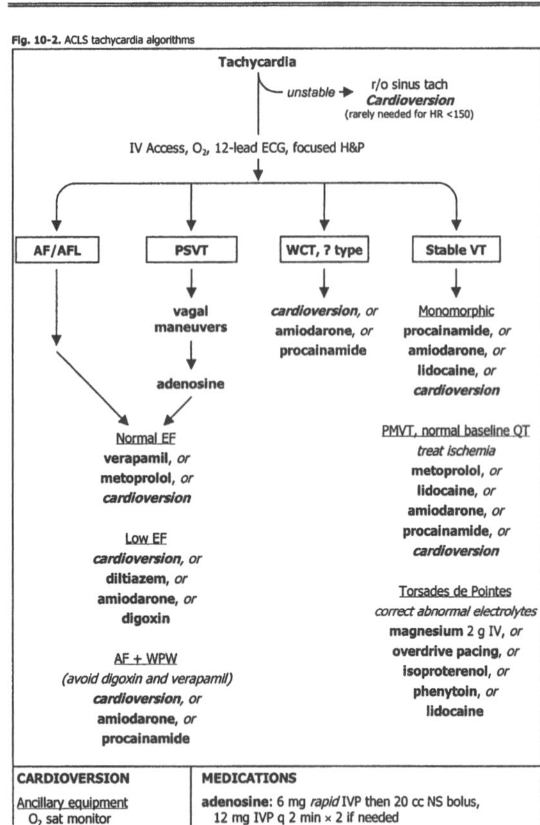

CARDIOVERSION	MEDICATIONS
Ancillary equipment O_2 sat monitor suction device IV line intubation equipment	**adenosine**: 6 mg *rapid* IVP then 20 cc NS bolus, 12 mg IVP q 2 min × 2 if needed **amiodarone** 150 mg IV over 10 mins **digoxin**: 0.5 mg IV, 0.25 mg IV q 6hrs × 2
Premedicate *call anesthesia service* midazolam 1-5 mg fentanyl 100-300 mcg titrate to effect	**diltiazem**: 15-20 mg IV over 2 mins, 20-25 mg 15 mins later if needed **lidocaine** 1.0-1.5 mg/kg IVP, repeat in 5-10 min **metoprolol** 5 mg IV q 5 min × 3
Synchronized cardioversion **100, 200, 300, 360 J** or biphasic equivalent	**procainamide** 17 mg/kg at 50 mg/min *(avoid if EF ↓)* **verapamil** 2.5-5 mg IV over 2 mins, 5-10 mg 15-30 mins later if needed

(Adapted from *ACLS Provider Manual*, 2002)

Fig. 10-3. ACLS bradycardia algorithms

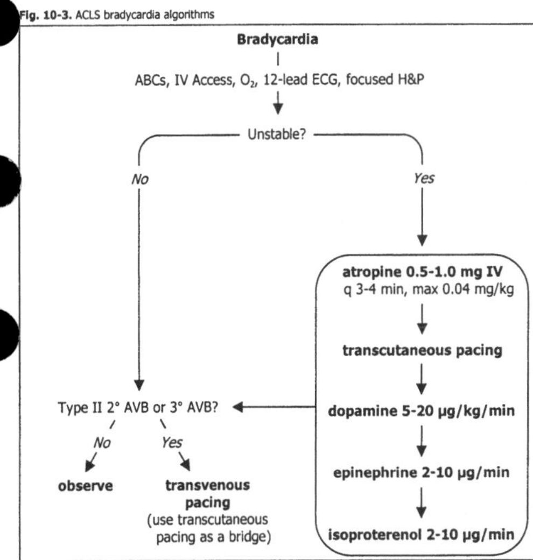

(Adapted from *ACLS Provider Manual*, 2002)

Fig. 10-4. ACLS pulmonary edema, hypotension, or shock algorithm

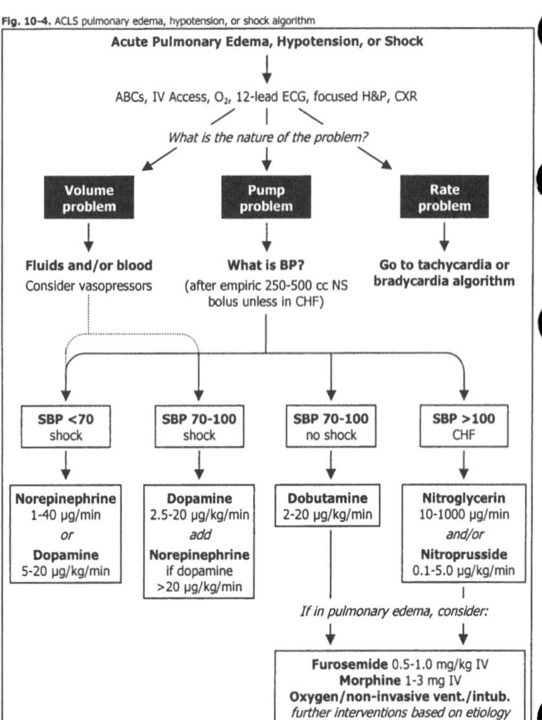

(Adapted from Emergency Cardiac Care Committee and Subcommittee, American Heart Association. Guidelines for Cardiopulmonary Resuscitation and Emergency Cardiac Care. *JAMA* 1992;268:2171.)

• ICU MEDICATIONS •

Drug	Class	Dose	
		per kg	average
Pressors, Inotropes, and Chronotropes			
Phenylephrine	α_1	10-300 μg/min	
Norepinephrine	$\alpha_1 > \beta_1$	1-40 μg/min	
Epinephrine	$\alpha_1, \alpha_2, \beta_1, \beta_2$	2-20 μg/min	
Isoproterenol	β_1, β_2	0.1-10 μg/min	
Dopamine	D β, D α, β, D	0.5–2 μg/kg/min 2–10 μg/kg/min >10 μg/kg/min	50-200 μg/min 200-500 μg/min 500-1000 μg/min
Dobutamine	$\beta_1 > \beta_2$	2–20 μg/kg/min	50-1000 μg/min
Amrinone	PDE	0.75 mg/kg over 3 min then 5-10 μg/kg/min	40-50 mg over 3 min then 250-900 μg/min
Milrinone	PDE	50 μg/kg over 10 min then 0.375-0.75 μg/kg/min	3-4 mg over 10 min then 20-50 μg/min
Vasopressin	V_1	0.1-0.6 U/hr	
Vasodilators			
Nitroglycerin	NO	10-1000 μg/min	
Nitroprusside	NO	0.1–10 μg/kg/min	5-800 μg/min
Nesiritide	BNP	2 μg/kg IVB then 0.01 μg/kg/min	
Labetalol	α_1, β_1, and β_2 blocker	20 mg over 2 min then 20-80 mg q 10 min or 10-120 mg/hr	
Fenoldopam	D	0.1-1.6 μg/kg/min	10-120 μg/min
Epoprostenol	vasodilator	2-20 ng/kg/min	
Enalaprilat	ACE	0.625–2.5 mg over 5 min then 0.625–5 mg q 6 hrs	
Hydralazine	vasodilator	5-20 mg q 20-30 min	
Anti-arrhythmics			
Amiodarone	K *et al.* (Class III)	150 mg over 10 min, then 1 mg/min × 6 hrs, then 0.5 mg/min × 18 hrs	
Lidocaine	Na channel (Class IB)	1-1.5 mg/kg then 1-4 mg/min	100 mg then 1-4 mg/min
Procainamide	Na channel (Class IA)	17 mg/kg over 60 min then 1-4 mg/min	1 g over 60 min then 1-4 mg/min
Ibutilide	K channel (Class III)	1 mg over 10 min, may repeat × 1	
Propranolol	β blocker	0.5-1.0 mg q 5 min then 1-10 mg/hr	
Esmolol	$\beta_1 > \beta_2$ blocker	500 μg/kg then 25–300 μg/kg/min	20-40 mg over 1 min then 2-20 mg/min
Verapamil	CCB	2.5–5 mg over 1-2 min repeat 5-10 mg in 15-30 min prn 5-20 mg/hr	
Diltiazem	CCB	0.25 mg/kg over 2 min reload 0.35 mg/kg × 1 prn then 5-15 mg/hr	20 mg over 2 min reload 25 mg × 1 prn then 5-15 mg/hr
Adenosine	purinergic	6 mg rapid push if no response: 12 mg → 12-18 mg	

Drug	Class	Dose	
		per kg	average
		Sedation	
Morphine	opioid	1-unlimited mg/hr	
Fentanyl	opioid	50-100 µg then 50–unlimited µg/hr	
Thiopental	barbiturate	3-5 mg/kg over 2 min	200-400 mg over 2 min
Etomidate	anesthetic	0.2-0.5 mg/kg	100-300 mg
Propofol	anesthetic	1-3 mg/kg then 0.3-5 mg/kg/hr	50-200 mg then 20-400 mg/hr
Diazepam	BDZ	1-5 mg q 1-2 hrs then q 6 hrs prn	
Midazolam	BDZ	0.5–2 mg q 5 min prn or 0.5-4.0 mg then 1-10 mg/hr	
Ketamine	anesthetic	1-2 mg/kg	60-150 mg
Haloperidol	antipsychotic	2-5 mg q 20-30 min	
Naloxone	opioid antag.	0.4-2 mg q 2-3 min to total of 10 mg	
Flumazenil	BDZ antag.	0.2 mg over 30 sec then 0.3 mg over 30 sec if still lethargic may repeat 0.5 mg over 30 sec to total of 3 mg	
		Paralysis	
Succinylcholine	depolar. paralytic	0.6-1.1 mg/kg	70-100 mg
Tubocurare	nACh	10 mg then 6-20 mg/hr	
Pancuronium	nACh	0.08 mg/kg	2-4 mg q30-90′
Vecuronium	nACh	0.08 mg/kg then 0.05-0.1 mg/kg/hr	5-10 mg over 1-3 min then 2-8 mg/hr
Cisatracurium	nACh	5-10 µg/kg/min	
		Miscellaneous	
Aminophylline	PDE	5.5 mg/kg over 20 min then 0.5-1 mg/kg/hr	250-500 mg then 10-80 mg/hr
Insulin		10 U then 0.1 U/kg/hr	
Glucagon		5-10 mg then 1-5 mg/hr	
Octreotide	somatostatin analog	50 µg then 50 µg/hr	
Phenytoin	antiepileptic	20 mg/kg at 50 mg/min	1-1.5 g over 20-30 min
Fosphenytoin	antiepileptic	20 mg/kg at 150 mg/min	1-1.5 g over 10 min
Phenobarbital	barbiturate	20 mg/kg at 50-75 mg/min	1-1.5 g over 20 min
Mannitol	osmole	1.5-2 g/kg over 30-60 min repeat q 6-12 hrs to keep osm 310-320	

• ANTIBIOTICS •

The following tables of spectra of activity for different antibiotics are generalizations. Sensitivity data at your own institution should be used to guide therapy.

Spectrum of Penicillins						
Class	***Strep***	***Staph***	***H. flu M. cat***	**Enterics**	***Pseud.***	**Anaerobes**
Natural	⊕					±
PCNase-resist.	⊕	⊕				
Amino	⊕		±	±		±
Extended	⊕		⊕	⊕	⊕	⊕
Carbapenem	⊕	⊕	⊕	⊕	⊕	⊕
Aztreonam			⊕	⊕	⊕	
β-lact. inhib.		⊕	⊕	⊕		⊕

[*Staph* refers to methicillin-sensitive *Staph. aureus*; methicillin-resistant *Staph. aureus* (MRSA) are resistant to all penicillins.]

Spectrum of Cephalosporins			
Gen.	**GPC**	**GNR**	**Anaerobes**
1st	⊕⊕⊕	⊕	
2nd	⊕⊕	⊕⊕	⊕⊕
3rd	⊕⊕	⊕⊕⊕	⊕
4th	⊕⊕⊕	⊕⊕⊕	⊕

(The multiple ⊕ symbols are used to show *relative* differences within the family of cephalosporins and do not imply that cephalosporins are superior to antibiotics in other charts where only single ⊕ symbols are used.)

Spectrum of Fluoroquinolones					
Gen.	**GPC**	**GNR**	***Pseudomonas***	**Atypicals**	**Anaerobes**
1st		⊕ (UTI)			
2nd	±	⊕	⊕	±	
3rd	⊕	⊕	⊕	⊕	
4th	⊕	⊕	⊕	⊕	⊕

Spectrum of Other Antibiotics						
Antibiotic	**GPC**	**MRSA**	**VRE**	**GNR**	**Atypicals**	**Anaerobes**
Vancomycin	⊕	⊕				
Linezolid	⊕	⊕	⊕			
Quinopristin/ Dalfopristin	⊕	⊕	⊕			
Chloramphenicol	±		±	±		
Doxycycline	±	±	±	±	⊕	
Macrolides	⊕			±	⊕	
Nitrofurantoin	±			±		
TMP-SMZ	⊕	±		⊕		
Aminoglycosides	±			⊕		
Clindamycin	⊕					⊕
Metronidazole						⊕

(For MRSA and VRE, antibiotics with ± activity have only limited efficacy and are only rarely used for those pathogens.)

Penicillins				
Antibiotic	**Normal dose**	**Dose in renal failure** (by GFR)		
		>50	10-50	<10
Natural penicillins				
Penicillin G	0.4-4 MU IM/IV q 4 hrs	NC	NC	1-2 MU q 4 hrs
Penicillin V	250-500 mg PO q 6 hrs	NC	NC	NC
Penicillinase-resistant penicillins				
Cloxacillin	0.5-1.0 g PO q 6 hrs	NC	NC	NC
Dicloxacillin	250-500 mg PO q 6 hrs	NC	NC	NC
Nafcillin	1-2 g IM/IV q 4 hrs	NC	NC	NC
Oxacillin	1-2 g IM/IV q 4 hrs	NC	NC	NC
Aminopenicillins				
Amoxicillin	250-500 mg PO q 8 hrs	NC	250-500 mg q 8-12 hrs	250 mg q 12 hrs
Amox-clav	250-500 mg PO q 8 hrs	NC	250-500 mg q 8-12 hrs	250 mg q 12 hrs
Ampicillin	1-2 g IM/IV q 4 hrs	NC	1-2 g q 8 hrs	1-2 g q 12 hrs
Amp-sulbact	1.5-3.0 g IM/IV q 6 hrs	NC	1.5-3.0 g q 12 hrs	1.5-3.0 g q 24 hrs
Extended-spectrum penicillins				
Azlocillin	2-4 g IM/IV q 4-6 hrs	NC	2-3 g q 6 hrs	2-3 g q 12 hrs
Mezlocillin	2-4 g IV q 4-6 hrs	NC	2-3 g q 6 hrs	2-3 g q 12 hrs
Piperacillin	2-4 g IM/IV q 4-6 hrs	NC	2-4 g q 8 hrs	2-4 g q 12 hrs
Pip-tazo	3.375 g IV q 6 hrs	NC	2.25 g q 6 hrs	2.25 g q 8 hrs
Ticarcillin	2-4 g IM/IV q 4 hrs	NC	2-3 g q 6 hrs	2 g q 12 hrs
Ticar-clav	3.1 g IV q 4 hrs	NC	3.1 g q 6 hrs	2 g q 12 hrs
Other β-lactams				
Aztreonam	1-2 g IM/IV q 8 hrs	NC	1 g q 8 hrs	0.5 g q 8 hrs
Imipenem	250-500 mg IV q 6 hrs	NC	250-500 mg q 8-12 hrs	250-500 mg q 12 hrs
Meropenem	1 g IV q 8 hrs	NC	0.5-1 g IV q 12 hrs	0.5 g IV q 24 hrs

Cephalosporins				
Antibiotic	**Normal dose**	**Dose in renal failure** (by GFR)		
		>50	10-50	<10
1st generation				
Cefadroxil	0.5-1 g PO q 12 hrs	NC	0.5 g q 12-24 hrs	0.5 g q 36 hrs
Cefazolin	1 g IM/IV q 8 hrs	NC	1 g q 12 hrs	1 g q 24 hrs
Cephalexin	250-500 mg PO q 6 hrs	NC	NC	NC
2nd generation				
Cefaclor	250-500 mg PO q 8 hrs	NC	NC	NC
Cefotetan	1-2 g IM/IV q 12 hrs	NC	1-2 g q 24 hrs	1 g q 24 hrs
Cefoxitin	1-2 g IM/IV q 4 hrs	1-2 g q 6 hrs	1-2 g q 8 hrs	1 g q 12 hrs
Cefprozil	250-500 mg PO q 12-24 hrs	NC	NC	250 mg q 12 hrs
Cefuroxime	750-1500 mg IM/IV q 6 hrs	NC	750-1500 mg q 8 hrs	750 mg q 24 hrs
Loracarbef	200-400 mg PO q 12 hrs	NC	200 mg q 12 hrs	200 mg q 3-5 days
3rd generation				
Cefdinir	600 mg PO qd	NC	NC	300 mg qd
Cefixime	400 mg PO q 24 hrs	NC	300 mg q 24 hrs	200 mg q 24 hrs
Cefoperazone	1-3 g IV q 8 hrs	NC	NC	NC
Cefotaxime	1-2 g IM/IV q 6 hrs	NC	NC	1-2 g q 12 hrs
Cefpodoxime	100-400 mg PO q 12 hrs	NC	NC	400 mg q 24 hrs
Ceftazidime	1-2 g IV q 8 hrs	NC	1-2 g q 12 hrs	1 g q 24 hrs
Ceftibuten	400 mg PO qd	NC	200 mg qd	100 mg qd
Ceftizoxime	1-2 g IV q 6 hrs	NC	1 g q 12 hrs	0.5 g q 12 hrs
Ceftriaxone	1-2 g IM/IV q 12-24 hrs	NC	NC	NC
4th generation				
Cefepime	1-2 g IM/IV q 12 hrs	NC	1-2 g q 16-24 hrs	1-2 g q 24-48 hrs

Fluoroquinolones				
Antibiotic	**Normal dose**	**Dose in renal failure** (by GFR)		
		>50	10-50	<10
		1st generation		
Nalidixic acid	1 g PO qid	n/a	n/a	n/a
		2nd generation		
Ciprofloxacin	500-750 mg PO q 12 hrs 200-400 mg IV q 12 hrs	NC	250-500 mg q 12 hrs	250-500 mg q 24 hrs
Lomefloxacin	400 mg PO qd	NC	200-400 mg qd	200 mg qd
Norfloxacin	400 mg PO q 12 hrs	NC	400 mg q 12-24 hrs	400 mg q 24 hrs
Ofloxacin	200-400 mg PO/IV q 12	NC	400 mg q 24 hrs	200 mg q 24 hrs
		3rd generation		
Levofloxacin	250-500 mg PO/IV q 24	NC	250 mg q 24 hrs	250 mg q 48 hrs
Sparfloxacin	400 mg PO on day 1, then 200 mg PO q 24 hrs	NC	200 mg q 48 hrs	? 200 mg q 48 hrs
		4th generation		
Gatifloxacin	400 mg PO/IV qd	NC	200 mg qd	200 mg qd
Moxifloxacin	400 mg PO qd	NC	NC	NC
Trovafloxacin	100-200 mg PO q 24 hrs 200-300 mg IV q 24 hrs	NC	NC	NC

Other Antibiotics				
Antibiotic	**Normal dose**	**Dose in renal failure** (by GFR)		
		>50	10-50	<10
		Aminoglycosides		
Gentamicin Tobramycin	1.0-1.7 mg/kg q 8 hrs	60-90% q 8-12 hrs	30-70% q 12-18 hrs	20-30% q 24-48 hrs
		or ~ 1.0-1.7 mg/kg q (8 × serum Cr) hrs		
Amikacin	5 mg/kg q 8 hrs	60-90% q 8-12 hrs	30-70% q 12-18 hrs	20-30% q 24-48 hrs
		or ~ 5.0 mg/kg q (8 × serum Cr) hrs		
		Macrolides		
Azithromycin	500 mg IV qd 500 mg PO on d 1, then 250 mg PO qd	NC	NC	NC
Clarithromycin	250-500 mg PO bid	? ↓	? ↓	? ↓
Erythromycin	0.5-1 g IV q 6 hrs 250-500 mg PO qid	NC	NC	250-500 mg IV or 250 mg PO q 6 hrs
		Others		
Chloramphenicol	0.5-1 g IV/PO q 6	NC	NC	NC
Clindamycin	600 mg IV q 8 hrs 150-300 mg PO qid	NC	NC	NC
Doxycycline	100 mg PO/IV q 12-24 hrs	NC	NC	NC
Linezolid	400-600 mg IV/PO q 12 hrs	NC	NC	NC
Metronidazole	1000 mg load then 500 mg IV/PO q 6	NC	NC	NC
Nitrofurantoin	50-100 mg PO qid	NC	avoid	avoid
Quinopristin/ Dalfopristin	7.5 mg/kg IV q 8-12 hrs	NC	NC	NC
TMP-SMX*	2-5 mg TMP/kg PO/IV q 6 hrs	NC	2-5 mg TMP/kg q 12 hrs	avoid
Vancomycin	500 mg IV q 6 hrs 1 g IV q 12 hrs	1 g q 24-72 hrs	follow random levels, redose with 1 g when level <10	

(* single strength table = 1 ampule = 80 mg of TMP + 400 mg SMX)

• FORMULAE & QUICK REFERENCE •

CARDIOLOGY

Hemodynamic parameters	Normal value
Mean arterial pressure (MAP) $= \frac{(SBP \times 2) + DBP}{3}$	70-100 mm Hg
Heart rate (HR)	60-100 bpm
Right atrial pressure (RA)	≤6 mm Hg
Right ventricular (RV)	systolic 15-30 mm Hg diastolic 1-8 mm Hg
Pulmonary artery (PA)	systolic 15-30 mm Hg mean 9-18 mm Hg diastolic 6-12 mm Hg
Pulmonary capillary wedge pressure (PCWP)	≤12 mm Hg
Cardiac output (CO)	4-8 L/min
Cardiac index (CI) $= \frac{CO}{BSA}$	2.6-4.2 L/min/m²
Stroke volume (SV) $= \frac{CO}{HR}$	60-120 ml/contraction
Stroke volume index (SVI) $= \frac{CI}{HR}$	40-50 ml/contraction/m²
Systemic vascular resistance (SVR) $= \frac{\text{MAP - mean RA}}{\text{CO}} \times 80$	800-1200 dynes × sec/cm⁵
Pulmonary vascular resistance (PVR) $= \frac{\text{mean PA - mean PCWP}}{\text{CO}} \times 80$	120-250 dynes × sec/cm⁵

("Rule of 6's" for PA catheter measured pressures: RA ≤6, RV ≤30/6, PA ≤30/12, WP ≤12)
(1 mmHg = 1.36 cm water or blood)

Fick cardiac output

Oxygen consumption (L/min) = CO (L/min) × arteriovenous (AV) oxygen difference

CO = oxygen consumption / AV oxygen difference

Oxygen consumption must be measured (can estimate w/ 125 ml/min/m², but inaccurate)

AV oxygen difference = Hb (g/dl) × 10 (dl/L) × 1.36 (ml O_2/g of Hb) × (S_aO_2-S_vO_2)

S_aO_2 is measured in any arterial sample (usually 93-98%)

S_vO_2 (mixed venous O_2) is measured in RA, RV, or PA (assuming no shunt) (normal ~75%)

∴ **Cardiac output** (L/min) $= \frac{\text{Oxygen consumption}}{\text{Hb (g/dl)} \times 13.6 \times (S_aO_2 - S_vO_2)}$

Shunts

$Q_p = \frac{\text{Oxygen consumption}}{\text{pulm. vein } O_2 \text{ sat - pulm. artery } O_2 \text{ sat}}$ (if no R → L shunt, PV O_2 sat ≈ S_aO_2)

$Q_s = \frac{\text{Oxygen consumption}}{S_aO_2 \text{ - mixed venous } O_2 \text{ sat}}$ (MVO_2 drawn proximal to potential L → R shunt)

$\frac{Q_p}{Q_s} = \frac{S_aO_2 \text{ - MV } O_2 \text{ sat}}{\text{PV } O_2 \text{ sat - PA } O_2 \text{ sat}} \approx \frac{S_aO_2 \text{ - MV } O_2 \text{ sat}}{S_aO_2 \text{ sat - PA } O_2 \text{ sat}}$ (if only L → R and no R → L shunt)

Valve area

Gorlin equation: Valve area $= \dfrac{CO/(\text{DFP or SEP}) \times HR}{44.3 \times \text{constant} \times \sqrt{\Delta P}}$ (constant = 1.0 for AS, 0.85 for MS)

Hakki equation: Valve area $\approx \dfrac{CO}{\sqrt{\Delta P}}$

Coronary artery anatomy

Fig. 10-5. Coronary arteries

LEFT CORONARY ARTERY

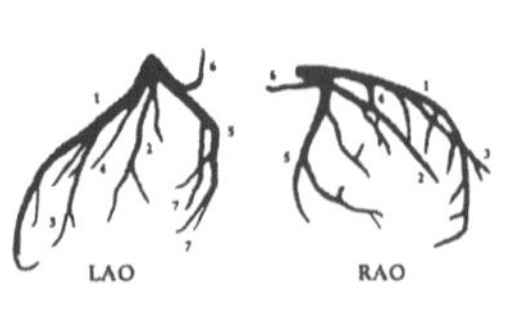

RIGHT CORONARY ARTERY

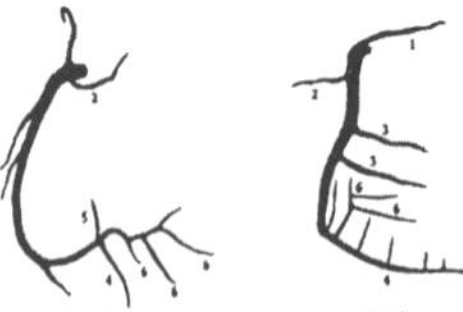

Left coronary artery:

1. **Left anterior descending artery (LAD)**
2. Ramus medianus artery
3. Diagonal branches
4. Septal branches
5. **Left circumflex artery (LCx)**
6. Left atrial circumflex artery
7. Obtuse marginal branches

Right coronary artery:

1. Conus artery
2. SA node artery
3. Acute marginal branches
4. Posterior descending artery (PDA)
5. AV node artery
6. Posterior left ventricular artery (PLV)

(From Grossman WG. *Cardiac Catheterization and Angiography*, 4th ed. Philadelphia: Lea & Febiger, 1991, with permission).

PULMONARY

Dead space = lung units that are ventilated but not perfused
Intrapulmonary shunt = lung units that are perfused but not ventilated

Alveolar gas equation: $P_AO_2 = [F_IO_2 \times (760 - 47)] - \dfrac{P_aCO_2}{R}$ (where R ≈ 0.8)

$$P_AO_2 = 150 - \frac{P_aCO_2}{0.8} \quad \text{(on room air)}$$

A-a gradient = $P_AO_2 - P_aO_2$ (normal A-a gradient ≈ age × 0.4)

Minute ventilation ($\dot{V}_E$) = tidal volume (V_T) × respiratory rate (RR) (normal 4-6 L/min)

Tidal volume (V_T) = alveolar space (V_A) + dead space (V_D)

Fraction of tidal volume that is dead space $\left(\dfrac{V_D}{V_T}\right) = \dfrac{P_aCO_2 - P_{expired}CO_2}{P_aCO_2}$

$$\mathbf{P_aCO_2} = k \times \frac{CO_2 \text{ production}}{\text{alveolar ventilation}} = k \times \frac{\dot{V}_{CO_2}}{RR \times V_T \times \left(1 - \dfrac{V_D}{V_T}\right)}$$

RENAL

Compensation for Acid/Base Disorders	
Primary disorder	**Expected compensation**
Metabolic acidosis	↓ P_aCO_2 = 1.25 × ΔHCO_3 (also, $PaCO_2$ = last two digits of pH)
Metabolic alkalosis	↑ P_aCO_2 = 0.75 × ΔHCO_3
Acute respiratory acidosis	↑ HCO_3 = 0.1 × ΔP_aCO_2 (also, ↓ pH = .008 × ΔP_aCO_2)
Chronic respiratory acidosis	↑ HCO_3 = 0.4 × ΔP_aCO_2 (also, ↓ pH = .003 × ΔP_aCO_2)
Acute respiratory alkalosis	↓ HCO_3 = 0.2 × ΔP_aCO_2
Chronic respiratory alkalosis	↓ HCO_3 = 0.4 × ΔP_aCO_2

Fig. 10-6. Acid-Base nomogram

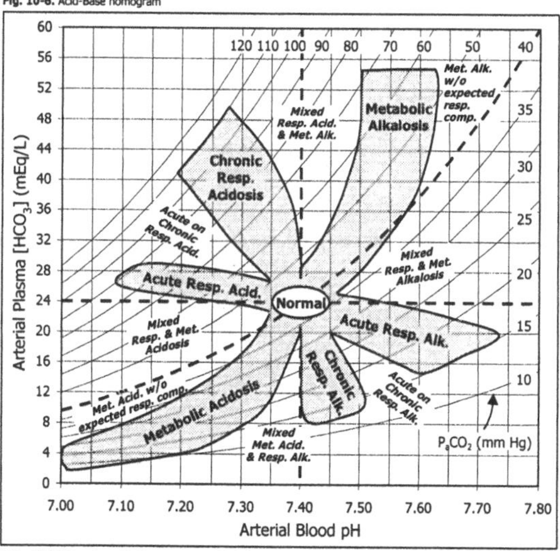

N.B., If ABG not available, can use VBG, but note that pH ~0.04 ↓, $PaCO_2$ ~8 mm Hg ↑, and HCO_3 ~2 mEq ↑. (Adapted from Brenner BM, ed. *Brenner & Rector's The Kidney*, 5th ed., 1996 and Ferri F, ed. *Practical Guide to The Care of the Medical Patient*, 5th ed., 2001)

Anion gap (AG) = Na - (Cl + HCO_3) (normal 12 ± 2 mEq)

Delta-delta ($\Delta\Delta$) = Δ AG (calculated AG -12) vs. Δ HCO_3 (24 - measured HCO_3)

Urine anion gap (UAG) = $(U_{Na} + U_K) - U_{Cl}$

Calculated osmoles = $(2 \times Na) + \left(\frac{glc}{18}\right) + \left(\frac{BUN}{2.8}\right) + \left(\frac{EtOH}{4.6}\right)$

Osmolal gap (OG) = measured osmoles - calculated osmoles (normal <10)

Estimated creatinine clearance = $\frac{[140 - \text{age (yrs)}] \times \text{wt (kg)}}{\text{serum Cr (mg/dl)} \times 72}$ (× 0.85 in women)

Calculated creatinine clearance (CrCl) based on 24-hour urine collection

$$P_{Cr}\ (^{mg}/_{dl}) \times 0.01\ (^{dl}/_{ml}) \times \text{CrCl}\ (^{ml}/_{min}) \times 1400\ (^{min}/_{24\ hrs}) = U_{Cr}\ (^{mg}/_{ml}) \times U_{vol}\ (^{ml}/_{24\ hrs})$$

$$\text{CrCl} = \frac{[U_{Cr}\ (\text{mg/ml}) \times U_{vol}\ (\text{ml/24 hrs})]}{[P_{Cr}\ (\text{mg/dl}) \times 14.4]}$$

Fractional excretion of Na (FE_{Na}, %) = $\left[\frac{\frac{U_{Na}\ (\text{mEq/L})}{P_{Na}\ (\text{mEq/L})} \times 100\%}{\frac{U_{Cr}\ (\text{mg/ml})}{P_{Cr}\ (\text{mg/dl})} \times 100\ (\text{ml/dl})}\right] = \frac{U_{Na}}{P_{Na}} \Big/ \frac{U_{Cr}}{P_{Cr}}$

Total body water (TBW) = 0.60 × IBW (× 0.85 if female and × 0.85 if elderly)

Corrected Na in hyperglycemia

estimate in all Pts: corrected Na = measured Na + $\left[2.4 \times \frac{(\text{measured glc} - 100)}{100}\right]$

however, Δ in Na depends on glc (*Am J Med* 1999;106:399)
Δ is 1.6 mEq per each 100 mg/dl ↑ in glc ranging from 100-440
Δ is 4.0 mEq per each 100 mg/dl ↑ in glc beyond 440

Total body water (TBW) = 0.60 × IBW (× 0.85 if female and × 0.85 if elderly)

Δ $[Na]_{serum}$ per L infusate = $\frac{[Na]_{infusate} - [Na]_{serum}}{TBW + 1}$ *(assuming no Na excretion)*

Δ TBW (⊕ → excretion; ⊖ → retention) = $\left[\frac{osm_{infusate}}{U_{osm}} - 1\right]$ *(assuming all Na excreted)*

Free H_2O deficit = $TBW \times \left(\frac{[Na]_{serum} - 140}{140}\right) \approx \left(\frac{[Na]_{serum} - 140}{3}\right)$ (in 70 kg patient)

Trans-tubular potassium gradient (TTKG) = $\frac{U_K}{P_K} \Big/ \frac{U_{Osm}}{P_{Osm}}$

Treatment of Hyperkalemia			
Intervention	**Dose**	**Onset**	**Comment**
Calcium gluconate **Calcium chloride***	1-2 amps IV	few min	transient effect stabilizes cell membrane
Insulin	reg. insulin 10 U IV + 1-2 amps $D_{50}W$	15-30 min	transient effect drives K into cells
Bicarbonate	1-3 amps IV	15-30 min	transient effect drives K into cells in exchange for H
β2 agonists	albuterol 10-20 mg inh. or 0.5 mg IV	30-90 min	transient effect drives K into cells
Kayexalate	30-90 g PO/PR	1-2 hrs	↓ total body K exchanges Na for K in gut
Diuretics	furosemide ≥40 mg IV	30 min	↓ total body K
Hemodialysis			↓ total body K

*calcium chloride contains more calcium and is typically reserved for use in codes

HEMATOLOGY

Heparin for Thromboembolism	
80 U/kg bolus 18 U/kg/hr	
PTT	**Adjustment**
<40	bolus 5000 U, ↑ rate 300 U/hr
40-49	bolus 3000 U, ↑ rate 200 U/hr
50-59	↑ rate 100 U/hr
60-85	no Δ
86-95	↓ rate 100 U/hr
96-120	hold 30 min, ↓ rate 150 U/hr
>120	hold 60 min, ↓ rate 200 U/hr

(*Circ* 2001;103:2994)

Heparin for ACS	
STEMI w/ fibrinolysis 60 U/kg bolus (max 4000 U) 12 U/kg/hr (max 1000 U/hr)	
UA/NSTEMI 60-75 U/kg bolus (max 5000 U) 12-15 U/kg/hr (max 1000 U/hr)	
PTT	**Adjustment**
<40	bolus 3000 U, ↑ rate 100 U/hr
40-49	↑ rate 50 U/hr
50-70	no Δ
71-85	↓ rate 50 U/hr
86-100	hold 30 min, ↓ rate 100 U/hr
101-150	hold 60 min, ↓ rate 150 U/hr
>150	hold 60 min, ↓ rate 300 U/hr

(ACC/AHA 1999 Guideline Update for STEMI)

✓ PTT q 6 hrs after every change (half-life of heparin is ~90 min)

✓ PTT qd or bid once PTT is therapeutic

✓ CBC qd (to ensure Hct and plt counts are stable)

Reversal with protamine sulfate IV

after bolus: protamine 1 mg / 100 U heparin (not to exceed 50 mg)
after infusion: dose to reverse 2× the amount of heparin given per hour

LMWH reversal by protamine is **incomplete**; direct thrombin inhibitors have **no antidote**

Warfarin Loading Nomogram					
	INR				
Day	**<1.5**	**1.5-1.9**	**2.0-2.5**	**2.6-3.0**	**>3.0**
1-3	5 mg (7.5 mg if >80 kg)		2.5-5.0 mg	0-2.5 mg	0 mg
4-5	10 mg	5-10 mg	0-5 mg		0-2.5 mg
6	Dose based on requirements over preceding 5 days				

(*Annals* 1997;126:133 & *Archives* 1999;159:46)

Warfarin-Heparin overlap therapy

- Indications: when failure to anticoagulate carries ↑ risk of morbidity or mortality (e.g., DVT/PE, intracardiac thrombus)
- Rationale: (1) Half-life of factor VII (3-6 hrs) is shorter than half-life of factor II (60-72 hrs); ∴ warfarin can elevate PT *before achieving a true antithrombotic state*
  (2) Protein C also has half-life less than that of factor II; ∴ theoretical concern of *hypercoagulable state* before antithrombotic state
- Method: (1) Therapeutic PTT is achieved using heparin
  (2) Warfarin therapy is initiated
  (3) Heparin continued until INR therapeutic for ≥2 d and ≥4-5 d of warfarin (roughly corresponds to ~2 half-lives of factor II or a reduction to ~25%)

Reversal of warfarin *(in addition to holding warfarin)*

- INR >5.0, but no bleeding: **vitamin K** 1-5 mg PO (superior to SC, *Annals* 2002;137:251)
- Bleeding: **vitamin K** 10 mg IV **+ FFP** 2-4 units IV q 6-8 hrs

Other

Ideal body weight (IBW) = [50.0 kg (men) or 45.5 kg (women)] + 2.3 kg/inch over 5 feet

Body surface area (BSA, m^2) = $\sqrt{\frac{\text{height (cm)} \times \text{weight (kg)}}{3600}}$

		Disease	
		present	absent
Test	⊕	a (true ⊕)	b (false ⊕)
	⊖	c (false ⊖)	d (true ⊖)

Prevalence $= \frac{\text{all diseased}}{\text{all patients}} = \frac{a+c}{a+b+c+d}$

Sensitivity $= \frac{\text{true positives}}{\text{all diseased}} = \frac{a}{a+c}$

Specificity $= \frac{\text{true negatives}}{\text{all healthy}} = \frac{d}{b+d}$

⊕ predictive value $= \frac{\text{true positives}}{\text{all positives}} = \frac{a}{a+b}$

⊖ predictive value $= \frac{\text{true negatives}}{\text{all negatives}} = \frac{d}{c+d}$

Accuracy $= \frac{\text{true positives + true negatives}}{\text{all patients}} = \frac{a+d}{a+b+c+d}$

• ABBREVIATIONS •

AAA abdominal aortic aneurysm
Ab antibody
ABE acute bacterial endocarditis
ABG arterial blood gas
abnl abnormal
ABPA allergic bronchopulmonary aspergillosis
AC assist control
ACD anemia of chronic disease
ACE angiotensin converting enzyme
ACEI ACE inhibitor
ACL anticardiolipin antibody
ACTH adrenocorticotrophic hormone
ADH antidiuretic hormone
ADL activities of daily living
AF atrial fibrillation
AFB acid-fast bacilli
AFL atrial flutter
AFTP ascites fluid total protein
AG aminoglycoside
anion gap
Ag antigen
AGN acute glomerulonephritis
AI aortic insufficiency
AIDS acquired immunodeficiency syndrome
AIHA autoimmune hemolytic anemia
AIN acute interstitial nephritis
ALL acute lymphocytic leukemia
ALT alanine aminotransferase
AML acute myelogenous leukemia
AMM/MF agnogenic myeloid metaplasia/myelofibrosis
ANA antinuclear antibody
ANCA antineutrophilic cytoplasmic antibody
angio angiogram
AoV aortic valve
Aϕ alkaline phosphatase
APC activated protein C
APS antiphospholipid antibody syndrome
ARDS adult respiratory distress syndrome
ARF acute renal failure
ARVD arrhythmogenic RV dysplasia
AS aortic stenosis
ASD atrial septal defect
AST aspartate aminotransferase
asx asymptomatic
AT atrial tachycardia
ATII angiotensin II
ATIII antithrombin III
ATN acute tubular necrosis
ATRA all-*trans*-retinoic acid
AV atrioventricular
AVA aortic valve area
AVNRT AV nodal reentrant tachycardia
AVR aortic valve replacement
AVRT AV reciprocating tachycardia
AZA azathioprine
b/c because
BAL bronchoalveolar lavage
βB beta-blocker
BBB bundle branch block
BCx blood culture
BDZ benzodiazepines
bili. bilirubin
BiPAP Bilevel positive airway pressure
BM bone marrow
BMT bone marrow transplantation
BP blood pressure
BPH benign prostatic hypertrophy
BRBPR bright red blood per rectum
BT bleeding time
BUN blood urea nitrogen
bx biopsy
C′ complement
CAD coronary artery disease
CALLA common ALL antigen
CAPD chronic ambulatory peritoneal dialysis
CBC complete blood count
CBD common bile duct
CCB calcium channel blocker
CCl_4 carbon tetrachloride
CD Crohn's disease
ceph. cephalosporin
CFU colony forming units
CHB complete heart block
CHD congenital heart disease
CHF congestive heart failure
CI cardiac index
CIARF contrast-induced acute renal failure
CLL chronic lymphocytic leukemia
CML chronic myelogenous leukemia
CMML chronic myelomonocytic leukemia
CMP cardiomyopathy
CMV cytomegalovirus
CO cardiac output
COX cyclooxygenase
CPAP continuous positive airway pressure
CPPD calcium pyrophosphate dihydrate
Cr creatinine
CsA cyclosporine A
CSM carotid sinus massage
CT computed tomogram
CV cardiovascular
CVA cerebrovascular accident
CVD cerebrovascular disease
CVVH continuous veno-venous hemofiltration

c/w	compared with consistent with
CXR	chest radiograph
d	day
Δ MS	change in mental status
DAT	direct antiglobulin test
DBP	diastolic blood pressure
d/c	discharge discontinue
DCIS	ductal carcinoma *in situ*
DCMP	dilated cardiomyopathy
Ddx	differential diagnosis
DFA	direct fluorescent antigen detection
DI	diabetes insipidus
DIC	disseminated intravascular coagulation
diff.	differential
DIP	desquamative interstitial pneumonitis
DIP	distal interphalangeal
DL_{CO}	diffusion capacity of the lung
DM	diabetes mellitus
DMARD	disease-modifying anti-rheumatic drug
DRE	digital rectal exam
DTRs	deep tendon reflexes
DVT	deep vein thrombosis
dx	diagnosis
EAD	extreme axis deviation
EAV	effective arterial volume
ECG	electrocardiogram
echo	echocardiogram
ECMO	extracorporeal membrane oxygenation
EDP	end-diastolic pressure
EDV	end-diastolic volume
EF	ejection fraction
EGD	esophagogastroduodenoscopy
EIA	enzyme-linked immunoassay
ELISA	enzyme linked immunosorbent assay
EP	electrophysiology
Epo	erythropoietin
EPS	electrophysiology study
ERCP	endoscopic retrograde cholangiopancreatography
ERV	expiratory reserve volume
ESP	end-systolic pressure
ESR	erythrocyte sedimentation rate
ESRD	end-stage renal disease
ESV	end-systolic volume
ET	essential thrombocytosis
ETT	endotracheal tube
FDP	fibrin degradation product
FEV_1	forced expiratory volume in 1 second
FFP	fresh frozen plasma
FHx	family history
FMF	familial Mediterranean fever
FOBT	fecal occult blood testing
FQ	fluoroquinolone
FRC	functional residual capacity
FSGS	focal segmental glomerulosclerosis
FSH	follicle stimulating hormone
FTI	free thyroxine index
FVC	forced vital capacity
G-CSF	granulocyte colony stimulating factor
G6PD	glucose-6-phosphate dehydrogenase
GBM	glomerular basement membrane
gen.	generation
GERD	gastroesophageal reflux disease
GGT	γ-glutamyl transpeptidase
GH	growth hormone
GIB	gastrointestinal bleed
glc	glucose
GNR	gram negative rods
GnRH	gonadotropin releasing hormone
GPC	gram positive cocci
GVHD	graft-versus-host disease
HA	headache
HAV	hepatitis A virus
Hb	hemoglobin
HBIG	hepatitis B immune globulin
HBV	hepatitis B virus
HCC	hepatocellular carcinoma
HCMP	hypertrophic cardiomyopathy
Hct	hematocrit
HCV	hepatitis C virus
HD	hemodialysis
HD	Hodgkin's disease
HDL	high-density lipoprotein
HDV	hepatitis D virus
HELLP	hemolysis, abnormal LFTs, low plts
HEV	hepatitis E virus
HGPRT	hypoxanthine-guanine phosphoribosyl transferase
HHNS	hyperglycemic hyperosmolar nonketotic coma
HIT	heparin-induced thrombocytopenia
HK	hypokinesis
h/o	history of
hpf	high power field
HR	heart rate
hr	hour
HRT	hormone replacement therapy
HS	hereditary spherocytosis
HSCT	human stem cell transplantation
HSP	Henoch-Schönlein purpura
HTN	hypertension
HUS	hemolytic uremic syndrome
IABP	intraaortic balloon pump
IBD	inflammatory bowel disease
IC	inspiratory capacity
ICa	ionized calcium
ICD	implantable cardiac defibrillator
ICH	intracranial hemorrhage

ICP	intracranial pressure
ICU	intensive care unit
IDDM	insulin-dependent diabetes mellitus
IE	infective endocarditis
IGF	insulin-like growth factor
ILD	interstitial lung disease
ITP	idiopathic thrombocytopenic purpura
IVDA	intravenous drug abuser
IVF	intravenous fluids
IVIg	intravenous immunoglobulin
JVD	jugular venous distention
JVP	jugular venous pulse
LA	left atrium
LA	lupus anticoagulant
LAD	left anterior descending coronary artery
LAD	left axis deviation
LAE	left atrial enlargement
LAN	lymphadenopathy
LAP	leukocyte alkaline phosphatase
LBBB	left bundle branch block
LCIS	lobular carcinoma *in situ*
LCx	left circumflex coronary artery
LDH	lactate dehydrogenase
LDL	low-density lipoprotein
LES	lower esophageal sphincter
LFTs	liver function tests
LGIB	lower gastrointestinal bleed
LH	luteinizing hormone
LM	left main coronary artery
LN	lymph node
LOC	loss of consciousness
LP	lumbar puncture
lpf	low power field
LUSB	left upper sternal border
LV	left ventricle
LVAD	LV assist device
LVEDP	LV end-diastolic pressure
LVEDV	LV end-diastolic volume
LVH	left ventricular hypertrophy
LVSD	LV systolic dimension
MAC	mitral annular calcification
MAC	*Mycobacterium avium* complex
MAHA	microangiopathic hemolytic anemia
MAT	multifocal atrial tachycardia
MCD	minimal change disease
MCP	metacarpal phalangeal
MCTD	mixed connective tissue disease
MCV	mean corpuscular volume
MDI	metered dose inhaler
MEN	multiple endocrine neoplasia
MGUS	monoclonal gammopathy of uncertain significance
MI	myocardial infarction
min	minute
min.	minimal
MM	multiple myeloma
MMEFR	maximal mid-expiratory flow rate
MN	membranous nephropathy
mos	months
mod.	moderate
Mϕ	macrophage
MPGN	membranoproliferative glomerulonephritis
MPD	myeloproliferative disorder
MR	mitral regurgitation
MRA	magnetic resonance angiography
MRI	magnetic resonance imaging
MRSA	methicillin-resistant *S. aureus*
MS	mitral stenosis
MTb	*Mycobacterium tuberculosis*
MTP	metatarsal phalangeal
MTX	methotrexate
MV	mitral valve
MVP	mitral valve prolapse
MVR	mitral valve replacement
NAFLD	non-alcoholic fatty liver disease
NGT	nasogastric tube
NHL	Non-Hodgkin's lymphoma
NIDDM	non-insulin dependent diabetes mellitus
nl	normal
NM	neuromuscular
NMJ	neuromuscular junction
NPJT	non-paroxysmal junctional tachycardia
NPO	nothing by mouth
NPV	negative predictive value
N/V	nausea and/or vomiting
NVE	native valve endocarditis
OA	osteoarthritis
OCP	oral contraceptive pill
O/D	overdose
OG	osmolal gap
OGTT	oral glucose tolerance test
OI	opportunistic infection
OM	obtuse marginal coronary artery
p/w	present with
PA	pulmonary artery
PAD	peripheral arterial disease
PAV	percutaneous aortic valvuloplasty
pb	problem
PBC	primary biliary cirrhosis
PCI	percutaneous coronary intervention
PCWP	pulmonary capillary wedge pressure
PD	peritoneal dialysis
PDA	patent ductus arteriosus
PDA	posterior descending coronary artery
PE	pulmonary embolism
PEA	pulseless electrical activity
PEEP	positive end-expiratory pressure
PEFR	peak expiratory flow rate

PFO patent foramen ovale
PGA polyglandular autoimmune syndrome
PHT pulmonary hypertension
PID pelvic inflammatory disease
PIF prolactin inhibitory factor
PIP peak inspiratory pressure
proximal interphalangeal
PMHx past medical history
PMI point of maximal impulse
PMN polymorphonuclear leukocyte
PMV percutaneous mitral valvuloplasty
PMVT polymorphic ventricular tachycardia
PNA pneumonia
PND paroxysmal nocturnal dyspnea
PNH paroxysmal nocturnal hemoglobinuria
PPD purified protein derivative
PPH primary pulmonary hypertension
PPI proton pump inhibitors
P_{plat} plateau pressure
PPM permanent pacemaker
PPV positive predictive value
PR pulmonary regurgitation
PRBCs packed red blood cells
PRL prolactin
PRPP phosphoribosyl-1-pyrophosphate
PRWP poor R wave progression
PS pressure support
pulmonic stenosis
PSA prostate specific antigen
PSGN post streptococcal glomerulonephritis
PSHx past surgical history
PSV pressure support ventilation
Pt patient
PT prothrombin time
PTH parathyroid hormone
PTH-rP parathyroid hormone-related peptide
PTT partial thromboplastin time
PTX pneumothorax
PUD peptic ulcer disease
PV polycythemia vera
PVE prosthetic valve endocarditis
PVR pulmonary vascular resistance
qac before every meal
qhs every bedtime
Qw Q wave
RA refractory anemia
RA rheumatoid arthritis
RA right atrium
RAD right axis deviation
RAE right atrial enlargement
RAEB refractory anemia with excess blasts
RAEB-Tr refractory anemia with excess blasts in transformation
RAI radioactive iodine
RAIU radioactive iodine uptake
RARS refractory anemia with ringed sideroblasts
RAS renal artery stenosis
RBBB right bundle branch block
RBC red blood cell
RCA right coronary artery
RCMP restrictive cardiomyopathy
RCT randomized controlled trial
RDW red cell distribution width
RE reticuloendothelial
RF rheumatoid factor
RHD rheumatic heart disease
RI reticulocyte index
RIBA recombinant immunoblot assay
r/o rule out
RPGN rapidly progressive glomerulonephritis
RR respiratory rate
RUQ right upper quadrant
RUSB right upper sternal border
RV residual volume, right ventricle
RVAD RV assist device
Rx therapy
s/p status post
SAAG serum-ascites albumin gradient
SAARD slow-acting anti-rheumatic drug
SAH subarachnoid hemorrhage
SBE subacute bacterial endocarditis
SBP spontaneous bacterial peritonitis
systolic blood pressure
SCD sudden cardiac death
SCID severe combined immunodeficiency
sec second
sens. sensitivity
sev. severe
SIADH syndrome of inappropriate antidiuretic hormone
SIEP serum immunoelectrophoresis
SIMV synchronized intermittent mandatory ventilation
SLE systemic lupus erythematosus
SMA superior mesenteric artery
SMV superior mesenteric vein
spec. specificity
SPEP serum protein electrophoresis
SR sinus rhythm
s/s signs and symptoms
SSS sick sinus syndrome
ST sinus tachycardia
STE ST segment elevation
SV stroke volume
SVR systemic vascular resistance
SVT supraventricular tachycardia
sx symptom(s) or symptomatic
T_3RU T_3 resin uptake
TB tuberculosis
TBG thyroid binding globulin

TCA	tricyclic antidepressant
TCD	transcranial Doppler
TdP	torsades de pointes
TdT	terminal deoxynucleotidyl transferase
TEE	transesophageal echo
TFTs	thyroid function tests
TG	triglycerides
TIA	transient ischemic attack
TIBC	total iron binding capacity
TIPS	transjugular intrahepatic portosystemic shunt
TLC	total lung capacity
TP	total protein
TPO	thrombopoietin thyroid peroxidase
TR	tricuspid regurgitation
TRALI	transfusion-related acute lung injury
TRH	thyrotropin releasing hormone
TRUS	transrectal ultrasound
TS	tricuspid stenosis
TSH	thyroid stimulating hormone
TSI	thyroid-stimulating immunoglobulin
TTE	transthoracic echo
TTP	thrombotic thrombocytopenic purpura
TWI	T wave inversion
U/A	urinalysis
U/S	ultrasound
UA	uric acid
UAP	unstable angina pectoris
UC	ulcerative colitis
UCx	urine culture
UGIB	upper gastrointestinal bleed
UIP	usual interstitial pneumonitis
UPEP	urine protein electrophoresis
URI	upper respiratory tract infection
V/Q	ventilation-perfusion
VATS	video-assisted thoracoscopic surgery
VBI	vertebrobasilar insufficiency
VC	vital capacity
VLDL	very-low-density lipoproteins
VOD	veno-occlusive disease
VSD	ventricular septal defect
V_T	tidal volume
VT	ventricular tachycardia
vWD	von Willebrand's disease
vWF	von Willebrand's factor
w/	with
w/o	without
w/u	workup
WCT	wide-complex tachycardia
wk	week
WM	Waldenström's macroglobulinemia
WPW	Wolff-Parkinson-White syndrome

A

B

C

I

J

K

L

M

S

T

U

V

W

X

Z